CONTENTS

CONTRIBUTORS

David P. Adkison, M.D., MC, USNR
Head, Department of Orthopedic Surgery, National Naval Medical Center, Bethesda, Maryland

Julian S. Arroyo, M.D.
Formerly Resident, Department of Orthopaedics, University of Nebraska College of Medicine, Omaha, Nebraska

Brian E. Brigman, M.D.
Resident, Department of Orthopaedic Surgery, University of Nebraska Medical Center, Omaha, Nebraska

Marcia E. Bromley, B.S.
Medical Student, University of Nebraska College of Medicine, Omaha, Nebraska

David E. Brown, M.D.
Clinical Assistant Professor of Orthopaedic Surgery, University of Nebraska College of Medicine; Sports Medicine Center, Omaha, Nebraska

Peter K. Buchert, M.D.
Clinical Associate Professor, Department of Orthopaedic Surgery, University of Missouri–Columbia Medical School, Columbia, Missouri

James T. Canedy, M.D.
Orthopaedic Surgeon, Nebraska Health System, Omaha, Nebraska

Deepak V. Chavda, M.D.
Practicing Orthopaedic Surgeon, M-Star Orthopaedics, North Richland Hills, Texas

Kim J. Chillag, M.D.
Associate Clinical Professor, Department of Orthopaedics, University of South Carolina School of Medicine; The Moore Orthopaedic Clinic, P.A., Columbia, South Carolina

Ian D. Crabb, M.D.
Orthopaedic Surgeon, Sports Medicine Center, Omaha, Nebraska

Jeffrey P. Davick, M.D.
Des Moines Orthopaedic Surgeons, P.C., West Des Moines, Iowa

Gregory G. Degnan, M.D.
Assistant Professor of Orthopaedic Surgery, University of Virginia, Charlottesville, Virginia; Uniformed Services University of Health Sciences, Bethesda, Maryland

Stephen E. Doran, M.D.
Assistant Clinical Professor, Section of Neurosurgery, University of Nebraska Medical Center, Omaha, Nebraska

Paul W. Esposito, M.D., FAAP
Associate Professor, Department of Orthopaedic Surgery and Rehabilitation, and Department of Pediatrics, University of Nebraska Medical Center, Omaha, Nebraska; Assistant Professor of Surgery, Uniformed Services University of Health Sciences, Bethesda, Maryland

Edward V. Fehringer, M.D.
Resident, Department of Orthopaedic Surgery, Omaha, Nebraska

Timothy C. Fitzgibbons, M.D.
Assistant Clinical Professor of Orthopaedic Surgery, Creighton University School of Medicine, Omaha; Clinical Instructor, Department of Orthopaedics, University of Nebraska College of Medicine, Omaha, Nebraska

Keith R. Gabriel, M.D.
Associate Professor, Department of Orthopaedic Surgery, Saint Louis University School of Medicine, Saint Louis; Director, Pediatric Orthopaedics, Cardinal Glennon Children's Hospital, Saint Louis, Missouri

Glen M. Ginsburg, M.D.
Assistant Professor of Orthopaedic Surgery, Clinical Director, Munroe–Mayer Motion Analysis Laboratory, Department of Orthopaedic Surgery and Rehabilitation, University of Nebraska Medical Center, Omaha, Nebraska

Donald D. Graham, Jr., M.D.
Pulmonologist, Private Practice, Shelby, South Carolina

Thomas M. Heiser, M.D.
Clinical Assistant Professor, Department of Orthopaedics, University of Nebraska College of Medicine, Omaha, Nebraska

Michele Helzer-Julin, PA-C, M.S.
Physician Assistant and Exercise Physiologist, Sports Medicine Center, Omaha, Nebraska

Daniel P. Hoeffel, M.D.
Chief Resident, Department of Orthopaedics and Rehabilitation, University of Nebraska Medical Center, Omaha, Nebraska

Kirk S. Hutton, M.D.
Orthopaedic Surgeon, Sports Medicine Center, Omaha; Assistant Clinical Professor of Sports Medicine, Department of Orthopaedic Surgery and Rehabilitation, University of Nebraska Medical Center, Omaha, Nebraska

Walter W. Huurman, M.D.
Professor of Orthopedic Surgery, Department of Orthopedics and Rehabilitation, University of Nebraska Medical Center, Omaha, Nebraska

Atul B. Joshi, M.D.
Baylor College of Medicine, Houston, Texas

Christeen S. Kaga, M.D.
Franklin Orthopedic Specialists, P.A., Franklin, North Carolina

Todd A. Kile, M.D.
Assistant Professor of Orthopaedics, Mayo Medical School, Scottsdale; Chair, Division of Foot and Ankle Surgery, Mayo Clinic, Scottsdale, Arizona

David M. Lichtman, M.D.
Chairman and Director, Department of Orthopaedic Surgery, John Peter Smith Hospital, Fort Worth, Texas

Adolph V. Lombardi, Jr., M.D., FACS
Clinical Assistant Professor of Orthopaedic Surgery, The Ohio State University Hospitals, Columbus; Clinical Assistant Professor of Biomedical Engineering, The Ohio State University College of Medicine and Public Health, Columbus, Ohio

Craig R. Mahoney, M.D.
Resident, Department of Orthopaedics and Rehabilitation, University of Nebraska Medical Center, Omaha, Nebraska

Edward R. McDevitt, M.D., CAPT, MC, USN
Assistant Clinical Professor of Surgery, Department of Surgery, Uniformed Services University of the Health Sciences, Bethesda, Maryland

Scott T. McMullen, M.D.
Adjunct Assistant Professor Clinician, Department of Orthopedic Surgery, University of Nebraska Medical Center, Omaha, Nebraska

Stephanie A. Miske, M.D.
Department of Radiology, Clarkson Hospital, Omaha, Nebraska

John A. Miyano, M.D.
Assistant Professor, Department of Orthopaedics and Rehabilitation, University of Nebraska Medical Center, Omaha, Nebraska

Elizabeth A. Moran, M.D., MC, USNR
Resident, Department of Orthopaedic Surgery, National Naval Medical Center, Bethesda, Maryland

Matthew A. Mormino, M.D.
Assistant Professor, Department of Orthopaedic Surgery, University of Nebraska, Omaha, Nebraska

James R. Neff, M.D.
Professor and Chairman, Department of Orthopaedic Surgery, University of Nebraska Medical Center, Omaha, Nebraska

Kevin L. Nelson, M.D.
Chairman, Department of Radiology, and Director, Computed Tomography and Magnetic Resonance Imaging, Clarkson Hospital, Omaha, Nebraska

Randall D. Neumann, M.D.
Orthopaedic Surgeon, Sports Medicine Center, Omaha, Nebraska

Peter Norman Ove, M.D.
Anne Arundel Medical Center, Annapolis, Maryland

William R. Palmer, M.D.
Clinical Assistant Professor of Medicine, Department of Internal Medicine, University of Nebraska College of Medicine, Omaha, Nebraska

David A. Peterson, M.D.
Orthopaedic Clinic of Salina, Salina, Kansas

Stephen R. Pledger, M.D.
Staff Physician, Orthopaedic and Sports Medicine Consultants, Inc., Springfield, Ohio

J. Jeffrey Poggi, M.D., MAJ, USAF, MC
Assistant Chief, Department of Orthopaedics, Southern New England Orthopedics and Sports Medicine, Attleboro, Massachusetts

Vern J. Prochaska, M.D.
University of Nevada, Las Vegas, Nevada

Samar K. Ray, M.D., FRCS
Clinical Assistant Professor of Orthopaedic Surgery, University of Nebraska College of Medicine, Omaha, Nebraska

Jeffrey A. Rodgers, M.D.
Des Moines Orthopaedic Surgeons, P.C., West Des Moines, Iowa

Pamela S. Rolling, PA–C, A.T.C.
Formerly Sports Medicine Center, Omaha, Nebraska

Scott G. Rose, M.D.
General Surgeon, Methodist Hospital, Omaha, Nebraska

Michael J. Schmidt, M.D.
Orthopaedic Clinic and Sports Medicine, Topeka, Kansas

John A. Schneider, M.D.
Resident, Department of Orthopaedic Surgery, University of Nebraska Medical Center, Omaha, Nebraska

Jeffrey A. Senall, M.D.
Fellow, Foot and Ankle Surgery, Department of Orthopaedics, Mayo Clinic Scottsdale, Scottsdale, Arizona

Jeffrey J. Tiedeman, M.D.
Clinical Instructor, Department of Orthopaedic Surgery, University of Nebraska Medical Center, Omaha, Nebraska

Bradley K. Vaughn, M.D., FACS
Raleigh Orthopaedic Clinic, Raleigh, North Carolina

Donald J. Walla, M.D.
Lincoln Orthopaedic and Sports Medicine Clinic, Lincoln, Nebraska

W. Michael Walsh, M.D.
Orthopaedic Surgeon, Sports Medicine Center; Clinical Associate Professor, Department of Orthopaedic Surgery, University of Nebraska Medical Center, Omaha, Nebraska

Scott P. Wattenhofer, M.D., FACS
Assistant Professor, Department of Surgery, University of Nebraska College of Medicine, Omaha, Nebraska

Steven J. Wees, M.D.
Clinical Associate Professor of Medicine, Department of Internal Medicine, University of Nebraska Medical Center, Omaha, Nebraska

Joseph Yao, M.D.
Advanced Orthopaedics of Blytheville, Blytheville, Arkansas

DEDICATION

We dedicate this edition to our wives and families: Nancy, Casey, Claire, and Colleen Brown, and Diane, Ben, and Jon Neumann. We thank them for allowing us to take even more time away from them.

We also acknowledge the untiring efforts of our publisher Linda Belfus and our editor Aisha O'Connor. Their encouragement was instrumental in the completion of this edition.

Lastly, we thank our executive secretaries, Marilyn Novak and Keri Younker, for all their time in coordinating the work of all of the authors and editors.

PREFACE TO THE FIRST EDITION

This book continues the tradition of The Secrets Series® by presenting an overview of orthopedics in question and answer format. Comprehensive coverage is more properly the domain of the major textbooks in the field. *Orthopedic Secrets* is intended to be a handy reference that covers the common conditions encountered in orthopedic practice and that simplifies a vast amount of information without being overly simplistic.

A wide range of topics is addressed. An initial section on general considerations is followed by a section on congenital and developmental disorders. Subsequent sections cover the shoulder, the elbow and forearm, the hand and wrist, the spine, the hip and pelvis, the knee, the lower leg, and the foot and ankle.

The socratic foundation of The Secrets Series® is that the best way to teach is to question, and the goal of the authors is to ask the "right question" and to provide the best answer based on the current information available. Sometimes, there will be no right or wrong answer, or the answer will be controversial. In these areas, it is hoped that the points discussed will stimulate the reader to develop an ongoing appreciation of and interest in changing approaches in orthopedic care.

It is hoped that this book will carry on the successful Secrets tradition of providing for students and practitioners a resource that is instructive, thought-provoking, and enjoyable.

David E. Brown, M.D.
Randall D. Neumann, M.D.

PREFACE TO THE SECOND EDITION

In the tradition of The Secrets Series®, the second edition of *Orthopedic Secrets* is not a comprehensive textbook; rather, it is intended for students, residents, and practitioners who desire a concise reference about the most common conditions in orthopedic practice.

We have divided the text into ten sections: the first section covers general topics, such as the arthritides and diagnostic modalities; the second section discusses the diagnosis and treatment of congenital and developmental disorders; and the remaining eight sections are each devoted to a specific anatomic region.

Each chapter in the second edition has been updated and includes recent references. The chapters on bone tumors, shoulder instability, spinal trauma, spondylolisthesis, and scoliosis have been extensively revised. Several of the chapters detailing fractures also have been updated.

We have intentionally kept the section on pediatric orthopedics as concise as possible—an excellent *Pediatric Orthopaedic Secrets* text is already available. In addition, *Sports Medicine Secrets, 2nd edition* addresses many sports-related orthopedic injuries and conditions.

We hope that you find the question and answer format to be both useful and thought-provoking. Some of the questions may elicit a range of possible answers, because in medicine there may not always be a single "right" answer.

David E. Brown, M.D.
Randall D. Neumann, M.D.

I. *General*

1. OSTEOARTHRITIS

Randall D. Neumann, M.D.

1. What is osteoarthritis?

Osteoarthritis is a noninflammatory disorder of movable joints characterized by deterioration of articular cartilage and formation of new bone at the joint surfaces and margins. This disorder is also known as degenerative joint disease.

2. Describe the pathologic findings in osteoarthritis.

Early degeneration or disruption of the articular cartilage surface, which can be described as flaking or fibrillation, occurs most commonly on the weight-bearing surfaces of the joint. This early finding gradually proceeds to complete loss of articular cartilage and eburnation of the bone, which becomes highly polished and has a sclerotic surface, suggesting ivory. Cyst areas may occur in the subarticular bone, usually on the weight-bearing surface, and are thought to be related to microfractures that degenerate. New bone formation is usually found at the base of the articular cartilage and surrounding the cyst, creating an area of sclerosis.

3. What factors are important in the etiology of degenerative joint disease?

- Obesity
- Genetics and heredity
- Occupation (e.g., interphalangeal joint degeneration in the fingers of cotton mill workers)
- Multiple endocrine disorders, such as diabetes mellitus and acromegaly
- Multiple metabolic disorders, including Paget's disease, gout, and calcium pyrophosphate deposition (CPPD) disease

4. Discuss the epidemiologic features of osteoarthritis.

By age 40 years, 90% of all persons have some degenerative changes in the weight-bearing joints, even though clinical symptoms are generally absent. Roentgenographic manifestations of the disease commonly occur in the third decade. When minimal disease is excluded, the prevalence of osteoarthritis is approximately 20%. In one study 85% of patients aged 55–64 years had some degree of osteoarthritis in one or more joints. Men and women are equally affected by osteoarthritis. Under age 45 years the prevalence was greater among men, whereas prevalence was greater in women after age 55 years. Some studies show that patients with obesity have an increased frequency of osteoarthritis in the weight-bearing joints.

5. What are osteophytes? Why do they form?

Osteophytes, one of the main characteristics of osteoarthritis, are outgrowths, usually marginal, of ossified cartilage. Because of the vascularization in the subchondral bone, proliferation of adjacent cartilage and enchondral ossification occur. Outgrowths extend from the free articular space along the path of least resistance.

6. Describe the pathologic abnormalities of osteoarthritis in correlation with the radiographic abnormalities.

- Cartilage erosion—loss of joint space
- Increased cellularity and bone deposition of subchondral bone—bone eburnation

- Synovial fluid intrusion into bone—subchondral cysts
- Revascularization of the remaining cartilage and capsular traction—osteophytes
- Synovial membrane stimulation—osteophytes
- Compression of weakened bone—bony collapse
- Fragmentation of osteochondral surface—loose bodies
- Destruction and distortion of capsular ligaments—deformity and malalignment

7. Describe the symptoms in patients with osteoarthritis.

The cardinal symptom of osteoarthritis is pain, which first occurs only with joint use and motion but later is relieved only by rest. The pain is usually aching in character and poorly localized. In the severe stages of the disease, pain may awaken the patient from sleep because of loss of protective muscular joint splinting that during the waking hours limits painful motion. Pain may occur with minimal motion and even at rest. Muscle spasms around the joint, often described as sharp, may add to the pain. Most affected patients take nonsteroidal antiinflammatory drugs (NSAIDs) or pain pills for relief of the symptoms.

Stiffness on awakening in the morning and after periods of inactivity during the day is common. As the joint is "limbered up," patients feel better. If the patient sits down for any length of time, pain may develop after commencement of activity. The patient must "loosen" the joint. If loose bodies or meniscal tears are present, patients may complain of giving way or locking episodes. Typically there is some limitation of motion, often involving loss of extension and flexion. In the hip, patients usually maintain 90° of flexion but lose most abduction as well as internal and external rotation. In the knee, most patients develop a flexion contracture, usually mild. Loss of dorsiflexion in the ankle may occur, along with flexion contractures in the proximal and distal interphalangeal joints. Patients may describe crepitation, which generally occurs with any range of motion of the joint. The crepitation may be associated with pain and generally signifies the bone-on-bone quality of degenerative arthritis.

8. What are the clinical signs of patients with osteoarthritis?

Most patients have localized tenderness, generally along the area of the most significant degenerative changes. Patients may have palpable osteophytes. Crepitation may occur with attempts at range of motion. Generally range of motion is diminished compared with the normal extremity. Boggy synovitis, if present, is not as severe as with rheumatoid arthritis. Usually effusion is minimal. Increased effusion is common after slight twisting or giving way episodes.

9. What laboratory abnormalities are seen in primary osteoarthritis?

Erythrocyte sedimentation rate, complete blood count, rheumatoid factor, serum calcium, alkaline phosphates, and electrophoresis are usually within normal limits. Patients may have laboratory abnormalities in secondary osteoarthritis, such as the high levels of uric acid in gout or the high levels of alkaline phosphates in Paget's disease.

10. Describe the synovial fluid analysis in a patient with osteoarthritis.

Synovial fluid in osteoarthritis is generally noninflammatory. The increase in white blood cells is minimal. Viscosity is good. Uric acid or CPPD crystals are not found. Glucose is generally normal. No bacteria are seen on Gram stain.

11. What other radiographic abnormalities are seen with osteoarthritis?

Scanning with ^{99m}technetium shows increased uptake around osteoarthritic joints. Magnetic resonance imaging reveals areas of degenerative changes, subchondral cysts, and osteophyte formation. Such abnormalities are also commonly seen with computed tomography.

12. What is the differential diagnosis of osteoarthritis?

Differential diagnosis includes osteoarthritis, rheumatoid arthritis, gouty arthritis, calcium pyrophosphate arthropathy, osteonecrosis, and a neuropathic joint related to endocrine disease.

13. List the major complications of degenerative joint disease.

1. With loss of joint space, angulation in the affected extremity may occur. With complete collapse on the inner or outer side of one of the joints, such as the knee, deformity occurs.
2. Subluxation, as seen in the carpometacarpal joint of the thumb.
3. Ankylosis or complete bony fusion of a joint, such as the great toe metatarsophalangeal joint.
4. Interarticular loose bodies or joint mice related to subchondral fractures.

14. Name the most common disease processes in which secondary osteoarthritis may develop.

Acute trauma	Hyperparathyroidism
Chronic trauma	Overuse of interarticular corticosteroid therapy
Alcaptonuria	Neurologic diseases, including diabetes
Wilson's disease	Syringomyelia
Hemochromatosis	Frostbite
Acromegaly	Hemophilia

15. What is a Heberden's node?

Heberden's nodes are the detectable bony enlargements about the distal interphalangeal joints of the hands.

16. What is Bouchard's node?

Bouchard's nodes are bony enlargements in the proximal interphalangeal joints.

17. What is a mucinous cyst?

Mucinous cysts arise from the joint capsule in the distal or proximal interphalangeal joints. They generally contain degenerative myxomatous fibrous tissue from the degenerative arthritis.

18. Describe osteoarthritis of the first carpometacarpal joint of the thumb.

Osteoarthritis of the trapezoimetacarpal articulation is commonly seen in women. Patients have significant pain at the base of the thumb with loss of grip strength and range of motion. This syndrome typically occurs in women > 50 years of age.

19. List causes of degenerative arthritis in the wrist joint.

1. Kienböck's disease (osteonecrosis of the lunate)
2. Trauma
3. Nonunion of the scaphoid
4. Gout
5. CCPD disease
6. Carpal instability from ligamentous disruption of the scapholunate ligament

20. Which area of the shoulder has the highest incidence of degenerative arthritis?

The acromioclavicular joint has the highest incidence of degenerative arthritis.

21. What is a bunion?

A bunion is a combination of degenerative joint disease at the first metatarsal phalangeal joint and angulation or valgus at the same joint. Symptoms include progression of swelling and pain, difficulty with shoe wear and walking, and inflammation of the bursa of the medial aspect of the joint.

22. Describe the arthritis that occurs in the spine.

Formation is located both anteriorly and posteriorly adjacent to the intervertebral disk. Narrowing of the intervertebral disk is common with actual fusion of the adjacent vertebrae. Subluxation of one vertebral body on another may occur, especially in the lumbar spine. The facet joints with osteophyte formation may cause narrowing of the foraminal space, which may cause nerve root irritation.

23. Discuss the findings of osteoarthritis in the hip.
Osteoarthritis in the hip causes joint space narrowing, which is best seen on an anteroposterior view of the pelvis. Osteophytes occur inferiorly and superiorly on the acetabulum. Osteophytes may be found on the superior and inferior surface of the femoral head. Loose bodies are commonly seen. Sclerosis of the underlying bone with adjacent cystic areas may be seen in the head, neck, and acetabular area of the joint.

24. Describe the clinical and radiographic findings of osteoarthritis in the knee.
Any of the three compartments of the knee—medial, lateral, or patellofemoral—may be involved. Complete collapse of the lateral joint space causes the patient to be "knock-kneed" or in a valgus position. Complete joint space collapse in the medial compartment causes the patient to be bow-legged or in a varus position. Osteophytes may occur medially and laterally or along the patellofemoral joint. Often loose bodies are identified in the intercondylar notch region and in the posterior portions of the medial and lateral joint spaces. Subchondral cysts and sclerosis are common in the affected joint.

25. What is erosive osteoarthritis?
Erosive osteoarthritis involves primarily the distal and proximal interphalangeal joints. The disease may be hereditary. Severe inflammatory episodes lead to joint deformities and sometimes to ankylosis. Cysts may be painful and tender. Postmenopausal women are most frequently affected. Radiographs reveal severe bony erosions and subchondral bony sclerosis. Severe joint destruction is noted.

26. What is DISH?
DISH is the acronym for **d**iffuse **i**diopathic **s**keletal **h**yperostosis, a type of osteoarthritis with a significant amount of osteophyte formation. The spine shows calcification on the anterior longitudinal ligament and the peripheral disk margins. Calcification along the length of the ligaments has been described as following ossification along the vertebral bodies. The disk space height is generally preserved; calcification may be seen in the sacrotuberous, iliolumbar, and patellar ligaments. The main complaint is spinal stiffness, with surprisingly little pain. Patients generally have heel pain related to calcaneal spurs. Marginal osteophytes may be seen in all of the peripheral joints.

27. What new and experimental treatments for osteoarthritis and cartilage defects are available?
- **Soft tissue grafts.** Periosteal or perichondral grafts are sewn over defects (e.g., a small piece of rib perichondrium is transplanted into a metacarpophalangeal joint).
- **Chondrocyte transplantation.** Articular cartilage is harvested from the knee via arthroscopy. The chondrocytes are cultured and then placed in the defect. A periosteal flap is then sutured over the defect with the cells present. Medial femoral condyle defects are being treated this way.
- **Mosaic grafts.** A mosaic graft is an autograft. Osteochondral plugs are taken from the peripheral area of the anteromedial or anterolateral femoral condyle. Corresponding holes are drilled to match the size and depth of the plugs in the chondral defect, which are then inserted into the defect. Differing plug sizes create a "mosaic" look.
- **Artificial matrix.** Caron fiber, collagen, bone matrix, and polylactic acid are used to try to achieve a matrix upon which cartilage can grow.
- **Fresh osteochondral grafts**

BIBLIOGRAPHY

1. Buckwalter JA, Mankin HJ: Articular cartilage: Degeneration and osteoarthritis, repair, regeneration, and transplantation. J Am Acad Orthop Surg Instructional Course Lectures 47:487–504, 1998.
2. Hough AJ, McCarty DJ, Koopman WJ (eds): Pathology of osteoarthritis. In Arthritis and Allied Conditions: A Textbook of Rheumatology, 12th ed. Philadelphia, Lea & Febiger, 1993, pp 1699–1723.
3. Resnick D: Diagnosis of Bone and Joint Disorders, 3rd ed. Philadelphia, W.B. Saunders, 1995.

2. CRYSTALLINE ARTHROPATHIES

Steven J. Wees, M.D.

1. What are the major clinical crystalline arthropathies?
- Monosodium urate arthropathy
- Calcium pyrophosphate deposition (CPPD) disease

2. Is there more than one clinical manifestation of gouty arthropathy?
Yes. Gouty arthropathy may manifest clinically as acute inflammatory arthritis or chronic, erosive tophaceous arthritis.

3. What are the clinical features of calcium pyrophosphate dihydrate deposition (CPPD) disease?
- Acute pseudogout
- Several subsets of chronic arthritis (see table).

Subsets of Chronic CPPD

Pseudorheumatoid arthritis
Pseudoosteoarthritis
Pseudoneuropathic arthropathy

4. Describe the common clinical features of acute gouty arthritis and acute pseudogout.
The onset is usually abrupt. Involved joints rapidly become painful, swollen, warm, and tender. Patients are frequently awakened from sleep with gouty attacks. The joint may become so inflamed that the patient will not allow even a sheet to touch it. At times the overlying skin may resemble a bacterial cellulitis. Systemic signs of fever, leukocytosis, and elevated sedimentation rate often are present. Mild attacks may resolve spontaneously without treatment over several hours or 1–2 days. More severe untreated attacks may not subside for 7–10 days or, in the case of pseudogout, for as long as 2–4 weeks. Attacks may be provoked by surgery, trauma, and current illness.

5. What are the most commonly involved joints in acute gout?
In the majority of patients the first attack is monarticular. The first metatarsophalangeal joint is the most common site of involvement. Other frequent sites of initial involvement are the ankles, knees, wrists, fingers, and elbows. Distal and lower extremity joints tend to be involved most often.

6. What are the most commonly involved joints in acute pseudogout?
Larger joints are preferentially affected. Nearly 50% of attacks involve the knees. Other areas commonly involved are elbows, wrists, ankles, and, in contrast to gout, shoulders and hips.

7. What is the significance of hyperuricemia?
Large numbers of the general population have hyperuricemia, yet 19 out of 20 hyperuricemic patients remain asymptomatic throughout life. Hyperuricemia is often associated with other general medical conditions, such as hypertension, obesity, heavy alcohol use, atherosclerosis, ischemic heart disease, and impaired glucose tolerance.

8. List the major considerations in the differential diagnosis of acute gouty arthritis, chronic tophaceous gout, and acute pseudogout.
Acute gouty arthritis
Infectious arthritis, rheumatoid arthritis, acute pseudogout, and acute seronegative inflammatory arthritis (i.e., psoriatic arthritis)

Chronic tophaceous gout
Nodular rheumatoid arthritis and osteoarthritis
Acute pseudogout
Acute gouty arthritis and infectious arthritis

9. Explain the roles of laboratory and radiographic studies in the differential diagnosis of crystalline arthropathies.
Beyond joint aspiration and synovial analysis, all other laboratory studies are superfluous. The most critical diagnostic studies of synovial fluid are (1) cell count and differential; (2) crystal analysis under polarized microscopy; and (3) Gram stain and routine culture and sensitivity. In many patients who present with acute crystalline-induced arthritis, routine radiographs are normal. A helpful clue for the diagnosis of acute pseudogout is the finding of chondrocalcinosis on plain films.

10. What are the definitive diagnostic procedure and the definitive laboratory test for acute gout or acute pseudogout?
The definitive diagnostic procedure is joint aspiration; the definitive laboratory test is analysis of synovial fluid under polarized microscopy for the appropriate crystal (monosodium urate in acute gouty arthritis and calcium pyrophosphate in acute pseudogout).

11. Does the synovial fluid cell count distinguish acute gouty arthritis from acute bacterial arthritis?
No. Although synovial fluid white cell counts >50,000 cells/mm suggest bacterial infection, they occasionally are seen in crystal-induced arthritis and rheumatoid arthritis. Examination of fluid under polarized light and routine culture are most essential.

12. What is the treatment of choice in acute crystalline-induced arthritis?
The initial treatment is 75–100 mg orally of indomethacin, followed by 50 mg every 6 hours. As the attack subsides, the drug may be gradually tapered off. An equally effective alternative is to aspirate dry the involved joint and to inject a corticosteroid, such as triamcinolone.

CONTROVERSIES

13. What is the relationship of fever to crystal-induced arthritis?
Fever is frequent in acute gout and acute pseudogout, a fact that is frequently unrecognized. Temperatures may be $\geq 39°$ C. Leukocytosis also is common. Usually joint infection is suspected in the febrile patient, and crystal-induced arthritis is often forgotten as a diagnostic possibility. The fact that approximately 40% of patients with acute polyarticular gout are normouricemic during an attack compounds the problem. In patients hospitalized for serious medical problems, crystal-induced arthritis is often overlooked as a cause of fever, and antibiotics are prescribed for presumed infection. Defervescence occurs when antiinflammatory agents are introduced.

14. Describe the intravenous and oral role of colchicine.
Currently the use of colchicine has few indications. When given orally, colchicine typically induces significant gastrointestinal intolerance before joint symptoms subside. Intravenous colchicine may be strikingly effective but carries the risk of significant hematologic toxicity, particularly in elderly patients with underlying renal or hepatic disease and limited bone marrow reserve.

15. What is the appropriate management of hyperuricemia?
The physician often is faced with the question of whether or not to treat asymptomatic hyperuricemia. Because many years of silent deposition of urate are necessary before the first attack of gouty arthritis, it seems reasonable not to treat hyperuricemia solely to prevent its development.

Controversy also exists about when to begin antihyperuricemic therapy in the patient with gout arthritis. The first issue to resolve is whether the patient is in fact having attacks of acute gout. Hence the patient must be seen during an acute episode and have his or her synovial fluid carefully examined for the presence of intracellular, strongly negatively birefringent crystals (sodium urate). The absence of urate crystals in an attack of acute synovitis makes gout an unlikely cause of acute arthritis. An elevated serum urate level in a patient with acute inflammatory arthritis is not diagnostic of gout; examination of synovial fluid is mandatory.

After the clinician is sure that the patient has suffered acute gout but is now asymptomatic, the decision to begin antihyperuricemic treatment may be made. The large number of patients who have only infrequent gouty attacks even in the absence of therapy probably do not require antihyperuricemic treatment. Patients suffering recurrent acute attacks of gout may find that small daily doses of colchicine (0.5 mg 2 times/day) provide adequate prophylaxis against further attacks. Other patients have found that using indomethacin (25–50 mg 3–4 times/day) at the first sign of an acute attack will abort a full-blown incident. Nevertheless, some patients suffer recurrent gouty attacks despite adequate prophylaxis with colchicine or indomethacin. Such patients are good candidates for long-term treatment with allopurinol. Patients with tophaceous deposits also require long-term treatment with allopurinol. It is important not to administer allopurinol during the acute phase of gouty arthritis, because it typically prolongs the acute attack; wait at least 2 weeks before initiating such treatment.

BIBLIOGRAPHY

1. Dieppe PA, Bacon PA, Bamji AN, Watt I (eds): Atlas of Clinical Rheumatology. New York, Gower, 1986.
2. Kelley WN, Harris ED Jr, Ruddy S, Sledge CB (eds): Textbook of Rheumatology, 5th ed. Philadelphia, W.B. Saunders, 1997.
3. Krey PR, Lazaro DM (eds): Analysis of Synovial Fluid. Summit, NJ, Ciba-Geigy Corporation, 1992.
4. Maddison PJ, Isenberg DA (eds): Oxford Textbook of Rheumatology, 2nd ed. New York, Oxford University Press, 1998.
5. McCarty DJ, Koopman WJ (eds): Arthritis and Allied Conditions. Philadelphia, Lea & Febiger, 1993.
6. Pinals RS: Polyarthritis and fever. N Engl J Med 330:769–774, 1994.
7. Wees SJ: Practical Points in Rheumatology. New York, Medical Examination Publishing, 1983.

3. INFLAMMATORY ARTHROPATHIES

William R. Palmer, M.D.

1. What are the seronegative spondyloarthropathies?

The seronegative spondyloarthropathies are a group of rheumatic diseases that share common clinical, genetic, and radiologic features. Examples include ankylosing spondylitis, psoriatic arthritis (Reiter's syndrome), juvenile ankylosing spondylitis, and arthropathies that complicate inflammatory bowel diseases (regional enteritis and ulcerative colitis).

2. Name the common features of the seronegative spondyloarthropathies.

1. Predilection for inflammatory lesions of axial skeleton in many (sacroiliitis and spondylitis)
2. Oligoarticular peripheral joint arthritis
3. Enthesitis—inflammation at bony insertion of tendons, ligaments, and articular capsules
4. Frequent extraarticular inflammation of eye (uveitis), heart (aortitis), skin, and mucous membranes
5. Tendency to afflict young adults (mostly men)
6. Strong association with HLA-B27
7. Negative rheumatoid factor

3. What are characteristic features of low-back pain in patients with ankylosing spondylitis (AS)?

Onset before age 40
Insidious onset
Daily symptoms for more than 3 months

Prolonged morning stiffness
Improvement of symptoms
 with exercise

4. What steps should be taken to diagnose ankylosing spondylitis?
- Compatible history
- Compatible physical exam
- Radiologic demonstration of sacroiliitis—absolutely essential

5. How is sacroiliitis best demonstrated radiographically?
An anteroposterior radiograph of the pelvis usually suffices to demonstrate the bilateral sacroiliitis of AS. Occasionally a computed tomographic (CT) scan of the pelvis and sacroiliac (SI) joints is necessary in early adult disease or juvenile AS.

6. What is the most common extraskeletal manifestation of AS?
Acute uveitis (anterior iridocyclitis), usually unilateral, occurs in 30% of patients.

7. What treatment modalities are commonly used in the management of AS?
- Nonsteroidal antiinflammatory drugs (NSAIDs); indomethacin widely used
- Patient education
- Physical therapy—as important as medical therapy (range-of-motion exercises, back extension, done at home)

8. What is osteitis condensans ilii (OCI)?
OCI is a disorder primarily of young multiparous women, who often are asymptomatic. It is usually discovered radiographically and frequently confused with sacroiliitis. OCI is characterized by a triangular area of dense sclerotic bone limited to iliac bones of the pelvis adjacent to the lower half of normal SI joints.

9. Is disability common in AS?
Fewer than 20% of patients have significant work disability. Those who do frequently have deterioration of the hips and spinal fusion (bamboo spine).

10. Name the clinical features of psoriatic arthritis.
- Psoriasis
- Asymmetric peripheral arthritis with frequent involvement of distal interphalangeal (DIP) joints
- Negative rheumatoid factor
- Sausage digits (dactylitis)
- Spondylitis and sacroiliitis (in a minority of patients)

11. List the five clinical patterns of psoriatic arthritis.

15%	Classic psoriatic arthritis confined to DIP joints of hands and feet
5%	Arthritis mutilans
15%	Symmetric polyarthritis similar to rheumatoid arthritis
60%	Asymmetric, oligoarticular involvement of small joints, dactylitis
5%	Spondylitis/sacroiliitis with or without arthritis

12. Are nail changes common in psoriatic arthritis?
Yes. Changes include pitting, onycholysis, and transverse ridging. In patients with few psoriatic skin lesions the nail changes may be the most prominent clue to the presence of psoriasis.

13. How many patients with psoriasis develop psoriatic arthritis?
Approximately 5%.

14. Is it advisable to treat psoriasis as part of the comprehensive therapy for psoriatic arthritis?

Yes. The consensus is that the more active and severe the psoriasis, the more severe the psoriatic arthritis.

15. What systemic pharmacologic agents are used in the treatment of psoriatic arthritis?
- Nonsteroidal drugs
- Disease modifiers—hydroxychloroquine, gold, methotrexate, sulfasalazine
- Corticosteroids—low-dose systemic prednisone; intraarticular corticosteroids (e.g., triamcinolone hexacetonide)

16. What are the unique radiographic findings of psoriatic arthritis?
- Lack of paraarticular osteopenia
- "Pencil-in-cup" deformity of DIP or proximal interphalangeal (PIP) joints (pathognomonic)

17. Is the prognosis of psoriatic arthritis similar to that of rheumatoid arthritis?

The prognosis of psoriatic arthritis is actually much better. Five percent or fewer of patients have significant disability; mortality is minimal.

18. What is the most common extraintestinal manifestations of inflammatory bowel disease (Crohn's disease, ulcerative colitis)?

Up to 20% of patients have arthritis in one of two patterns:

1. Peripheral arthritis—oligoarticular involvement of the lower limbs; remitting (parallels activity of bowel disease) and nondeforming

2. Sacroiliitis/spondylitis—identical to that of AS

19. Define reactive arthritis.

Reactive arthritis is joint inflammation initiated by an infection in which the causative agent cannot be isolated from the joint. Reactive arthritis is included in the family of spondyloarthropathies because of a similar pattern of involvement, occurrence of enthesopathy and sacroiliitis, and high association with HLA-B27.

20. Where do the infections that precipitate reactive arthritis usually occur?

Gastrointestinal (GI) tract
Urogenital tract (especially in young men)

21. Describe the symptom complex of classic reactive arthritis (Reiter's syndrome).
- Infection (GI or genital)—may be barely symptomatic
- Urethritis or cervicitis
- Conjunctivitis ⎫ Develop 1–4 weeks
- Mucocutaneous lesions ⎬ after infection
- Arthritis/spondylitis/enthesitis ⎭

22. What is incomplete Reiter's syndrome?

Incomplete Reiter's syndrome is defined as typical reactive arthritis of the musculoskeletal system without other manifestations (e.g., skin, eyes); it occurs in 40% of all patients with reactive arthritis.

23. List the musculoskeletal manifestations of reactive arthritis.

1. Asymmetric oligoarthritis of lower extremities
2. Sausage digits (dactylitis)
3. Enthesitis—Achilles' heel ("lover's heel")
4. Spondylitis/sacroiliitis in 20% (asymmetric)

24. What are the common mucocutaneous features of reactive arthritis?
1. Keratoderma blenorrhagicum—palms, soles, penis
2. Circinate balanitis—penis
3. Oral ulcerations—tongue, palate
4. Nail changes—no pits; onycholysis and yellow color

25. What is Lofgren's syndrome?
Lofgren's syndrome is a benign, self-limited, acute arthropathy that occurs in patients with sarcoidosis. Classic manifestations include (1) hilar lymphadenopathy, (2) erythema nodosum, and (3) symmetric migratory, additive polyarthritis with a predilection for the ankles (erythema), knees, wrists, hands. The syndrome usually resolves within 2–3 months and requires supportive (NSAID) therapy.

26. Name the common viral disorders that may be accompanied by arthritis.

Hepatitis B	Mumps
Parvovirus B19 (fifth disease)	Chickenpox
Rubella	Human immunodeficiency virus (HIV)

27. Define Lyme disease.
Lyme disease is a tick-borne inflammatory disorder caused by the spirochete *Borrelia burgdorferi*. Disease onset frequently is heralded by a characteristic skin lesion (erythema chronicum migrans) at the site of the tick bite. Most untreated patients subsequently develop disseminated infection that results in a variable and occasionally chronic inflammatory process affecting joints, nervous system, heart, or skin.

CONTROVERSIES

28. Are the seronegative spondyloarthropathies related to rheumatoid arthritis?
No. Although once classified as part of the spectrum of rheumatoid arthritis ("rheumatoid variants"), the seronegative spondyloarthropathies now stand apart on the basis of clinical, genetic, and epidemiologic investigations. This distinction is necessary because of differing articular and nonarticular complications, responses to therapy, and prognosis.

Major Differences between Rheumatoid Arthritis and the Spondyloarthropathies

	RHEUMATOID ARTHRITIS	SPONDYLOARTHROPATHIES
Peripheral arthritis	Symmetric Polyarticular	Asymmetric Pauciarticular
Sacroiliitis	No	Yes
Spondylitis	No	Yes
Enthesopathy	No	Yes
Rheumatoid factor	Present (85%)	Absent
Subcutaneous nodules	Yes	Absent
Associated with HLA-B27	No	Yes

Comparison of Ankylosing Spondylitis and Related Disorders

CHARACTERISTIC	ANKYLOSING SPONDYLITIS	REACTIVE ARTHRITIS (REITER'S SYNDROME)	PSORIATIC ARTHROPATHY	ENTEROPATHIC ARTHROPATHY
Usual age at onset	Young adult age < 40 yr	Young to middle-aged adult	Young to middle-aged adult	Young to middle-aged adult
Sex ratio	Three times more common in males	Predominantly males	Equally distributed	Equally distributed

Table continued on following page.

Comparison of Ankylosing Spondylitis and Related Disorders (Continued)

CHARACTERISTIC	ANKYLOSING SPONDYLITIS	REACTIVE ARTHRITIS (REITER'S SYNDROME)	PSORIATIC ARTHROPATHY	ENTEROPATHIC ARTHROPATHY
Sacroiliitis or spondylitis	Virtually 100%	< 50%	~ 20%	< 20%
Symmetry of sacroiliitis	Symmetric	Asymmetric	Asymmetric	Symmetric
Peripheral joint	~ 25%	~ 90%	~ 95%	15–20%
HLA-B27 (in Caucasians)	~ 90%	~ 75%	< 50%	~ 50%
Eye involvement	25–30% (iritis)	~ 50% (conjunctivitis)	~ 20% (conjunctivitis)	≤ 15% (iritis)
Skin or nail involvement	None	< 40%	Virtually 100%	Uncommon

29. Is HLA-B27 a useful test in the diagnosis of AS and other spondyloarthropathies?

Even though HLA-B27 is found in a large percentage of patients with AS and other spondyloarthropathies (see table below), this relatively expensive test is rarely necessary to make an accurate diagnosis. A careful history and physical exam, frequently supplemented by appropriate radiographs (sacroiliitis), are the best and most accurate tools for diagnosis. The HLA-B27 test should be ordered primarily in the following situations:

1. Classic history and physical exam for AS but radiographic findings do not permit the diagnosis;
2. Suspected juvenile AS; and
3. Suspected atypical reactive arthritis.

Frequency of HLA-B27

Normal	2–13%
Ankylosing spondylitis	90%
Reactive (Reiter's) arthritis	75%
Psoriatic arthritis	
Sacroiliitis	50%
Without sacroiliitis	Normal
Enteropathic arthritis	
Peripheral arthritis	Normal
Sacroiliitis	50%

30. Can psoriatic arthritis precede the clinical appearance of psoriasis?

Yes. Psoriatic arthritis precedes the clinical appearance of psoriasis in 10–15% of adult patients. In 15–20% of patients, psoriasis and arthritis occur simultaneously. In the remainder, psoriasis precedes the arthritis.

31. Is there a difference in the outcome of joint replacement surgery in the seronegative spondyloarthropathies?

Many physicians may still believe that the outcome of total joint replacement in patients with AS or psoriatic arthritis is poor. Anecdotal reports have raised the possibility of reankylosis and mechanical failure of total hip replacements. A more optimistic report concluded that 75% of total hip replacements were graded as excellent or good. In another retrospective study, 86% of 87 patients who underwent 150 total hip replacement procedures considered the outcome to be good or very good. Such statistics compare favorably with total hip replacement for other conditions.

Patients with psoriatic arthritis undergoing joint surgery have been thought to be at risk of wound infections from the heavy bacterial contamination of psoriatic plaques. Because the

peripheral joints in psoriatic arthritis tend to ankylose, reankylosis and mechanical failure of a replaced joint have been speculated but rarely reported. The problem of infection may be controlled by careful antiseptic skin preparation and perioperative antibiotic therapy against the
common psoriasis contaminants (staphylococci and streptococci). On rare occasions psoriasis
may occur in the incision site, but is not a major problem.

The indications for joint replacement surgery are the same for psoriatic arthritis, AS, and
other spondyloarthropathies. Steps to prevent early postoperative loss of motion and appropriate
perioperative antibiotic therapy are appropriate.

32. Can reactive arthritis (Reiter's syndrome) be chronic and disabling?

In years past medical students were taught that reactive arthritis was a self-limited disorder
that usually resolved without sequelae. We now know that the course and progression of reactive
arthritis are more varied and unpredictable. The majority of patients have an initial episode of
arthritis lasting 3–12 months. Many then experience recurrent attacks, frequently after disease-
free intervals. Between 20 and 50% of patients have a chronic course of persistent disease activity with the potential for a destructive arthropathy and/or progressive spondylitic change. Several
studies have shown that < 15% of patients experience severe disability, which usually is due to
severe arthropathy of lower extremities or aggressive spondylitis. The overall prognosis is better
than for most other arthropathies. Death is rare.

BIBLIOGRAPHY

1. Arnett FC: Seronegative spondyloarthropathies. Bull Rheum Dis 37(1):1987.
2. Beyer CA, Hanssen AD, et al: Primary total knee arthroplasty in patients with psoriasis. J Bone Joint Surg 73B:258–259, 1991.
3. Calin A, Elswood J: The outcome of 138 total hip replacements and 12 revisions as AS: High success rate after a mean followup of 7.5 years. J Rheumatol 16:955–958, 1989.
4. Calin A, Kaye B, et al: The prevalence and nature of back pain in an industrial complex. Spine 5:201–205, 1980.
5. Kelley WN, Harris ED Jr, Ruddy S, Sledge CB (eds): Textbook of Rheumatology, 5th ed. Philadelphia, W.B. Saunders, 1997.
6. Klippel JH, Dieppe PA (eds): Rheumatology, 2nd ed. St. Louis, Mosby, 1998.
7. McCarty DJ, Koopman WJ (eds): Arthritis and Allied Conditions, 12th ed. Philadelphia, Lea & Febiger, 1993.
8. Maddison PJ, Isenberg DA, Woo P, Glass D (eds): Oxford Textbook of Rheumatology. New York, Oxford University Press, 1993.
9. Stern SH, Insall TM, et al: Total knee arthroplasty in patients with psoriasis. Clin Orthop 248:108–111, 1989.

4. RHEUMATOID ARTHRITIS

Steven J. Wees, M.D.

1. Give a brief clinical definition of rheumatoid arthritis (RA).

Rheumatoid arthritis is a symmetric inflammatory arthritis, involving small and large joints,
of at least 6 weeks' duration.

2. List the seven diagnostic criteria for RA.

1. Morning stiffness
2. Arthritis of at least 3 areas lasting > 6 weeks
3. Arthritis of hand joints lasting > 6 weeks
4. Symmetric arthritis lasting > 6 weeks
5. Rheumatoid arthritis
6. Serum rheumatoid factor
7. Radiographic changes

Establishing a diagnosis of RA requires adherence to the 1987 revised criteria from the
American College of Rheumatology. At least four criteria must be fulfilled to diagnose RA.

3. What is the most common pattern of onset?

Most patients have an insidious, slow onset over weeks to months, often accompanied by complaints of fatigue, malaise, anorexia and weight loss, arthralgias, myalgias, and morning stiffness. A smaller number of people have an acute or subacute onset.

4. Name the main sites of joint involvement.

Wrists	Ankles and metatarso-	Shoulders
Metacarpophalangeal and proximal	phalangeal joints	Hips
interphalangeal finger joints	Knees	Elbows

5. What are the most common extraarticular manifestations of RA?

Nodules, dry eyes, dry mouth, and carpal tunnel syndrome.

6. What are the four major pharmacologic treatment groups used in the management of RA?

Narcotic analgesics	Corticosteroids
Nonsteroidal antiinflammatory	Disease-modifying agents
drugs (NSAIDs)	

7. Describe the role of corticosteroids in the management of RA.

Most patients with RA demonstrate significant improvement with conservative use of corticosteroids. Men are given up to 7.5 mg of prednisone and women up to 5 mg each morning. This regimen can be tolerated on a long-term basis with minimal adverse effect. Selective intraarticular installation of corticosteroids is also highly effective. Triamcinolone hexacetonide has the longest-lasting effect.

8. Name the most commonly used disease-modifying drugs.

Plaquenil, methotrexate, and parenteral gold.

9. What is the indication for initiation of disease-modifying treatment?

Patients with uncontrolled synovitis, despite optimal use of low-dose corticosteroids and NSAIDs, need additional medical treatment. The detection of bony erosions on plain films of the hands and feet in a patient with active rheumatoid synovitis also is an important indication for beginning such treatment.

CONTROVERSIES

10. Does a positive rheumatoid factor (RF) test result definitively diagnose RA?

Contrary to widespread belief among physicians, RF is not specific for RA. RF is found in a small percentage of seemingly normal people, and with increasing age a greater percentage of normal people test positive for RF. Positive tests are found in a large number of acute and chronic inflammatory diseases (see table below). In most nonrheumatic diseases and with increasing age, titers of RF are lower than in RA ($< 1:320$). Furthermore, approximately 20% of patients with bona fide RA have negative RF tests and are categorized as having seronegative RA.

Occurrence of Rheumatoid Factor in Selected Conditions

Rheumatic diseases	Acute viral infections	Miscellaneous
Adult rheumatoid arthritis	Infectious mononucleosis	Elderly but otherwise
Sjögren's syndrome	Infectious hepatitis	healthy individuals
Systemic lupus erythematosus	Influenza	Sarcoidosis
Scleroderma	Rubella	Chronic active hepatitis
Mixed connective tissue	**Chronic inflammatory diseases**	Chronic persistent hepatitis
disease	Tuberculosis	Hyperglobulinemic
Polymyositis	Syphilis	purpura
Juvenile rheumatoid	Infective endocarditis	After transfusions
arthritis	**Neoplasms**	After renal transplantation

11. Can RA be diagnosed without objective physical evidence of joint inflammation?

No. One may suspect the diagnosis, but a patient with joint pain but no objectively demonstrable synovitis cannot be said to have RA, regardless of the positivity of the serum RF test. Many patients are erroneously diagnosed with RA solely on the basis of joint pain and a positive serum RF test, often as low titer. In essence, RA is diagnosed at the bedside. Laboratory and radiologic tests are ancillary.

12. Does a positive serum antinuclear antibody test result exclude a diagnosis of RA?

No. A large number of antinuclear antibodies are present in patients with RA.

13. Discuss the current role of synovectomy.

Over the past two decades the use of synovectomy has diminished substantially. Although the procedure is still effective in relieving pain, no retardation of radiologic progression is achieved. More intensive pharmacologic management, including earlier institution of disease-modifying agents, is the preferred approach. The major indication for synovectomy at present is extensor tenosynovectomy for prophylaxis of extensor tendon rupture.

BIBLIOGRAPHY

1. Dieppe PA, Bacon PA, Bamji AN, Watt I (eds): Atlas of Clinical Rheumatology. New York, Gower, 1986.
2. Kelley WN, Harris ED Jr, Ruddy S, Sledge CB (eds): Textbook of Rheumatology, 5th ed. Philadelphia, W.B. Saunders, 1997.
3. Maddison PJ, Isenberg DA (eds): Oxford Textbook of Rheumatology, 2nd ed. New York, Oxford University Press, 1998.
4. McCarty DJ, Koopman WJ (eds): Arthritis and Allied Conditions. Philadelphia, Lea & Febiger, 1993.
5. Wees SJ: Practical Points in Rheumatology. New York, Medical Examination Publishing, 1983.

5. SEPTIC ARTHRITIS

Randall D. Neumann, M.D.

1. What is septic arthritis?

Septic arthritis is a bacterial infection of the synovium and joint space that causes an intense inflammatory reaction with migration of polymorphonuclear leukocytes and subsequent release of proteolytic enzymes. Bacterial infection remains one of the most rapidly destructive and potentially lethal forms of arthritis; one-third of affected patients suffer residual loss of function in the involved joint.

2. Describe the process of articular damage in septic arthritis.

Hematogenous infection results from bacterial seeding of the synovium. When the bacteria in the synovium begin to multiply, products from the bacteria stimulate the migration of polymorphonuclear leukocytes into the joint. The leukocytes release proteolytic enzymes, which cause acute damage to the articular cartilage.

3. List the major predisposing conditions for septic arthritis.

Underlying chronic joint disease	Immunosuppressive drug treatment
Trauma	Malignancy
Joint involvement in rheumatoid arthritis	Parenteral drug abuse
Diabetes mellitus	Recent joint infection
Steroid administration	Injection or aspiration
Renal failure	Vascular insufficiency

4. What are the common sites affected with septic arthritis?

In reviews of bacterial arthritis, 443 joints were identified; 85% of cases were monarticular.

Knee	53%	Shoulder	11%	Wrist	9%
Hip	20%	Elbow	17%	Ankle	8%

5. What are the most common sites of bacterial septic arthritis in pediatric patients?

The knee is affected 39% of the time and the hip 32% of the time, with a broad mixture in all other joints.

6. Name the common bacteria found in nongonoccocal joint infection.

Staphylococcus aureus, *Streptococcus* sp., gram-negative rods, and *Pneumococcus* sp.

7. What bacteria are found most often in children under 2 years of age with septic arthritis?

Haemophilus influenzae.

8. Discuss the microbiology of nongonococcal bacterial arthritis.

In the past, *Staphylococcus aureus* has been involved in approximately 50% of joint infections. *Staphylococcus epidermidis* accounts for 6–10% of infections. Streptococci account for 20% and pneumococci for 10%; numerous other bacteria, including *Pseudomonas aeruginosa* and *Haemophilus influenzae*, an anaerobic bacteria, also may be involved. Polymicrobial infection occurs in approximately 5–7% of patients.

9. Discuss the microbiology of septic arthritis in children.

The most striking difference between adults and children is the high incidence of cases caused by *Haemophilus influenzae* in children < 5 years of age. *Haemophilus influenzae* is the single most common pathogen in children 2 years of age or younger. Infection in the hip in older children is caused more frequently by *Staphylococcus aureus* than by *Haemophilus influenzae*.

10. Describe septic arthritis from an animal bite.

Animal bites are most frequently inflicted by dogs, cats, and rodents. *Pasturella multocida* is commonly associated with cat bites. *Staphylococcus aureus* and *Streptococcus* sp. also are quite common. Treatment for *P. multocida* infection should include penicillin G and appropriate coverage for other microorganisms. Drainage is commonly necessary.

11. Give an example of direct implantation of infection.

Examples include surgery, such as open reduction with internal fixation of a fracture, or an endoprosthesis for joint replacement.

12. Describe the clinical findings found in patients with septic arthritis.

Patients present with pain that often is extreme. The pain is described as constant and may wake the patient out of a sound sleep. The patient has loss of motion and severe pain with any attempt to move the affected joint. Children and adults may walk with a limp. Joint fluid with effusion may be mild to severe. Fever is present in only 50% of patients. Septic arthritis is generally monarticular; polyarticular disease may be found in chronically ill and elderly patients.

13. What percentage of patients with septic arthritis have monarticular disease? What percentage have polyarticular disease?

Ninety percent of patients have monarticular septic arthritis; 10% have polyarticular septic arthritis.

14. Describe patients who present with polyarticular septic arthritis.

Patients with polyarticular disease are usually elderly and chronically ill. They present with multiple sites of infection and have multiple predisposing conditions, including rheumatoid arthritis, prosthetic joints, diabetes, corticosteroid usage, immunosuppressive drug usage, renal failure,

and parenteral drug abuse. The mortality rate is approximately 25%. The microbes involved include *Staphylococcus aureus*, *Streptococcus* sp., *Pneumococcus* sp., and *Haemophilus influenzae*.

15. What common diseases are considered in the differential diagnosis of septic arthritis?

Trauma	Rheumatoid arthritis
Osteoarthritis	Crystalline arthropathies

16. What is the most accurate tool for the diagnosis of septic arthritis?
The most accurate diagnostic tool is joint aspiration with joint fluid analysis.

**17. Which diagnostic tests should be included in the analysis of the synovial fluid in pa-
tients with septic arthritis?**

Gram stain	Glucose level
Culture and sensitivity	Crystals
White blood cell count	

18. Describe the analysis of synovial fluid in an aspirate from a patient with septic arthritis.
The white blood cell count is 50,000–100,000 mm^3, with 80% being polymorphonuclear
leukocytes. The glucose level is low. A positive Gram stain is found in approximately 60% of patients; of these, 60% involve gram-positive cocci. Tests for crystals of uric acid and calcium pyrophosphate are negative.

19. What abnormalities are seen in laboratory tests in patients with septic arthritis?
Approximately 60% of patients with bacterial infections have an elevated WBC count. The
erythrocyte sedimentation rate (ESR) is elevated above 20 mm/hr in approximately 95% of patients. The ESR is a sensitive test for septic arthritis, but it lacks specificity for the cause of the
acute synovitis; rheumatoid arthritis, Reiter's syndrome, and crystalline-induced arthritis also
may be associated with an elevated ESR. Most joint infections develop as a result of bacteremia;
blood cultures are positive in 35–50% of cases.

20. What radiographic tests are helpful in the evaluation of septic arthritis?
Plain radiographs show soft-tissue swelling, joint effusions, and possible preexisting joint
disease. Baseline radiographs may be used for later comparison. Often juxtaarticular osteoporosis is identified on subsequent films, along with juxtaarticular osteomyelitis. Computed tomography is helpful in evaluation of an infectious process in the sacroiliac joints. Scanning with
[99m]technetium polyphosphate has been sensitive in detecting infections in the peripheral joints
before radiographic changes develop. Such scans may not be helpful in differentiating rheumatoid arthritis from septic arthritis.

21. What is the treatment for septic arthritis?
Patients must be appropriately diagnosed by Gram stain and culture. Appropriate antibiotics
are given intravenously. Surgical drainage is necessary.

22. What is the optimal method for drainage of an infected joint?
The optimal method of drainage is open to debate. Most surgical textbooks and clinicians
believe that open surgical drainage is the treatment of choice. Needle aspiration has been used to
drain infected joints, especially in the pediatric population. A series of patients treated with
arthroscopic decompression had a highly favorable outcome with arthroscopic surgery of the
knee. Septic arthritis of the hip in children requires surgical drainage. Complications such as subluxation of the hip and avascular necrosis are common.

23. What is the duration of treatment with intravenous antibiotics?
Duration of treatment remains controversial, but most authors believe that a 2–4 week
course of parenteral antibiotics is necessary for eradication of bacteria in the joint space. Some

authors believe that children may be treated for 7–10 days intravenously followed with high oral dosages.

24. Which antibiotics should be used in the treatment of patients with septic arthritis?
The antibiotic is chosen by the infectious disease consultant. Multiple factors come into play when treating patients with septic arthritis, including the patient's age and condition, location and extent of the infection, microbiology of the infection, and potential side effects.

25. What are the common complications of antibiotic therapy in orthopedic patients?
Hypersensitivity reaction is the most common complication of the penicillin and cephalosporin agents. Ototoxicity and renal toxicity remain the major complications associated with aminoglycosides. Pseudomembranous colitis may be associated with short- and long-term administration of cephalosporins. Affected patients may develop significant diarrhea and should be checked by culture for *Clostridium difficile*. Vancomycin may cause nephrotoxicity.

26. Is physical therapy appropriate in the treatment of septic arthritis?
During the acute phase of bacterial joint infection, motion of the infected joint is exquisitely painful. Therefore, decompression of the joint and external splinting should provide early relief. The optimal time for initiating exercises with passive range of motion is usually within the first week of treatment, followed by active motion as soon as the patient feels comfortable.

27. What is the prognosis in bacterial septic arthritis?
Patients who are not diagnosed and remain untreated for more than 1 week appear to do poorly. Other factors associated with a poor outcome are infections with gram-negative rods, positive blood culture results, polyarticular infection, existence of other serious illness, prior arthritis, and old age. After treatment has begun, the persistence of high levels of synovial fluid, high WBC count, or positive synovial fluid cultures points to a poor outcome.

28. What is the treatment for septic arthritis in a joint that has previously been replaced with total knee or hip arthroplasty?
The patient should be questioned about the chronicity of the infection. Infections of < 3 weeks' duration are considered acute, those > 3 weeks' duration are considered chronic. Patients should be treated with immediate aspiration of the joint. If the Gram stain reveals a positive cocci, such as *Staphylococcus aureus* or *Staphylococcus epidermidis*, the joint should be debrided. Controversy exists as to whether debridement with antibiotics is the best treatment in the acute phase. Some authors believe that acute infections should be treated as chronic infections, which require debridement of the joint with removal of prosthesis, cement, and infected synovium. A cement spacer with antibiotics may be used for 6 weeks. Reimplantation after sterile aspiration and 6 weeks of IV antibiotics may be appropriate. Patients infected with a gram-negative rod have a poor prognosis for retaining the joint and for subsequent reimplantation. Such patients may have a chronic indolent infection and require surgical fusion of the knee or a Girdlestone procedure of the hip.

29. What unusual locations of septic arthritis are found in parenteral drug abusers?
Sacroiliac joint
Sternal articulations
Pubic symphysis

30. Which bacteria are commonly found in septic arthritis in patients with parenteral drug abuse?
Staphylococcus aureus
Pseudomonas aeruginosa
Serratia marcescens

31. What microbe is commonly found in septic arthritis in patients with sickle-cell disease?
Salmonella has a much higher rate of occurrence in patients with sickle-cell disease.

32. Describe the infection that occurs when children or adults step on a nail.
Patients who step on a nail usually have septic arthritis of the metatarsophalangeal (MTP) joint. *Pseudomonas aeruginosa* is commonly found in cultures taken from sneakers and has a high incidence in bacterial septic arthritis of the MTP joint caused by a nail injury.

33. What are the clinical characteristics of patients with septic bursitis?
Septic bursitis causes painful swelling in the bursa overlying the olecranon process or the patella. Joint effusion is normally absent, and the range of motion is normal. Pain may be caused with full flexion of the joint but is due to stretching of the overlying soft tissues. Fever is found only in 30–40% of patients. Local skin abrasions, lacerations, or draining sinuses are frequently noted. Cellulitis surrounds the bursa. In adults, infection of olecranon bursa is 4 times more common than septic prepatellar bursitis. In children, however, the ratio of septic prepatellar bursitis to olecranon bursitis is close to 8:1.

34. Which bursa are most commonly affected by septic bursitis?
The prepatellar bursa and the olecranon bursa are the most common sites.

35. What is the pathogenesis of septic bursitis?
Septic bursitis usually results from transcutaneous inoculation of pathogens, whereas septic arthritis typically results from hematogenous spread. The most common organism in septic prepatellar bursitis is *Staphylococcus aureus*. The second most common organism is *Streptococcus* sp.

36. Describe the treatment for septic bursitis.
Both parenteral and oral routes of antibiotic administration have been used successfully for the treatment of septic bursitis. Antibiotic levels can be maintained in bursal fluid by both routes, sometimes at levels higher than simultaneous serum levels. Patients with overwhelming bursal infection, which is manifested by extensive local skin infection, marked peribursal cellulitis, or signs of systemic illness, should be hospitalized and given parenteral antibiotic therapy. Proper drainage of the infected bursa is essential for successful therapy. Most cases respond to percutaneous needle aspiration, a procedure that may be performed daily or every other day, depending on the severity of the infection. Open surgical drainage should be done when the infection does not respond to standard treatment. The duration of antibiotic treatment for septic bursitis should be adjusted for each individual; the average duration of antibiotic therapy, however, is approximately 10 days, which is the length of time necessary to sterilize bursal fluid.

BIBLIOGRAPHY

1. Abrams RA, Botte MJ: Hand infections: Treatment recommendations for specific types. J Am Acad Orthop Surg 4:219–230, 1996.
2. Lane JG, Falahe MH, Wojtys EM: Pyarthrosis of the knee: Treatment considerations. Clin Orthop 252:198–204, 1990.
3. Leslie BM, Harris JM III, Driscoll D: Septic arthritis of the shoulder in adults. J Bone Joint Surg 71A:1515–1522, 1989.
4. Ruthberg AD, Ho G: Nongonococcal bacterial arthritis. In D'Ambrosia R, Marier R (eds): Orthopedic Infections. Thorofare, NJ, Slack, 1989.
5. Schoifet SD, Morrey BF: Treatment of infection after total knee arthroplasty by debridement with retention of components. J Bone Joint Surg 72A:1383–1390, 1990.
6. Shaw BA, Kasser JR: Acute septic arthritis in infancy and childhood. Clin Orthop 257:212–225, 1990.

6. OSTEOMYELITIS

Randall D. Neumann, M.D.

1. What is osteomyelitis?
Acute bacterial osteomyelitis is a musculoskeletal infection specifically related to bone infection.

2. Describe the clinical classifications for hematogenous osteomyelitis.
1. **Acute hematogenous osteomyelitis** is characterized by systemic illness, absence of bony radiologic changes at presentation, duration of less than 10 days, and, in most cases, no history of a previous episode.
2. **Subacute hematogenous osteomyelitis** is characterized by lack of systemic illness, established bony radiographic changes at presentation, duration of more than 10 days, and no history of a previous episode.
3. **Chronic hematogenous osteomyelitis** is characterized by presence or absence of systemic illness, depending on presentation; bony radiologic changes (common); and a history of previous episodes of infection.

3. Describe the pathogenesis involved with acute hematogenous osteomyelitis.
Hematogenous osteomyelitis in adults begins as an acute infection within the medullary canal. Edema and breakdown of products increase local compromise and herald the necrosis of fat, hematopoietic tissue, and trabecular bone. Increased osteoclastic activity, induced by hyperemia, enlarges cortical haversian and Volkmann's canals. Macrophages, white blood cells, and fibroblasts gain access to the site. The pathogens and/or inflammatory byproducts pass through these channels into the soft tissues to produce induration and periosteal abscesses. The virulence of the organism, condition of the host, and status of the local milieu determine the end result.

4. Describe the pathogenesis in chronic hematogenous osteomyelitis.
The original cortex is replaced by thickened, reactive involucrum and sequestra within the bone. The sequestered, lamellar fragments reflect the seemingly endless struggle to contend with a persistent osteomyelitis. Spontaneous drainage may occur from the medullary canal through the soft tissues and out the skin. A breakdown of the soft-tissue envelope either begins or perpetuates the exposure of normal bone to a constant bacterial inoculum. Cortical penetration may lead to medullary extension and abscess formation.

5. Describe the natural history of osteomyelitis in its untreated form.
Typical acute hematogenous osteomyelitis involves the metaphysis of the long bone in a child. A septic focus begins with the lodging of bacteria or septic emboli in the metaphyseal vessels. This infection may be contained as a small local abscess, or it may extend along the metaphyseal aspect of the growth plate. Extension may occur to the local haversian canals, into the subperiosteal space, and subsequently into the soft tissues. Patchy bone reabsorption and periostitis become apparent in 10–14 days. Periosteal abscesses may become quite large, stripping the periosteum completely from the shaft of the bone and resulting in occlusion of nutrient vessels and death of the cortical shell. The periosteum subsequently lays down new bone in a shell around the shaft.

6. What are the clinical findings in acute metaphyseal osteomyelitis?
Patients nearly always describe severe, localized bone pain and can readily identify the affected area. Dramatic local tenderness is present, along with soft-tissue inflammation.

Approximately 75–80% of patients have fever. Loss of function around the major joint atypically occurs within 12–48 hours after the onset of infection. Painful and tense joint effusion may indicate septic arthritis, but osteomyelitis also may cause a sympathetic effusion.

7. What preexisting conditions may negatively affect the host's response to infection?

Malnutrition	Immune deficiency	Extremes of age
Renal failure	Chronic hypoxia	Steroid therapy
Liver failure	Malignancy	Tobacco use
Alcohol abuse	Diabetes mellitus	

8. What local factors may negatively affect host response to infection and treatment?

Chronic lymphedema	Major vessel compromise	Extensive scarring
Venous stasis	Arteritis	Radiation fibrosis

9. What diagnostic tests are useful in acute osteomyelitis?

White blood cell count and sedimentation rate are usually elevated. The bone is aspirated for a Gram stain and culture and sensitivity. Bacteria are isolated from local aspiration in up to 70% of cases. The objective is to obtain infected material from the subperiosteal or the soft-tissue abscess.

10. Which lab test is commonly used to screen for osteomyelitis?

Erythrocyte sedimentation rate (ESR), a nonspecific test for an inflammatory process, is commonly used. A normal ESR should be < 20 mm/hr. Other conditions with elevated ESR include rheumatoid arthritis, neoplasia, collagen vascular disease, other infections, or recent surgery. As treatment proceeds, the ESR should slowly return to normal.

11. What are the most common pathogens isolated from acute osteomyelitis?

In descending order, the most common pathogens are *Staphylococcus aureus, Streptococcus* sp., gram-negative bacilli, and *Staphylococcus epidermidis.*

12. Describe an imaging approach for the diagnosis of osteomyelitis.

In the presence of clinical suspicion, a plain radiograph of the affected extremity is taken. If the radiograph is positive for osteomyelitis, treatment is begun. If the radiograph is negative for osteomyelitis, a bone scan is done. If the bone scan is negative, a search for other causes is begun. If the bone scan is positive with a normal radiograph, treatment is begun for osteomyelitis. If the radiograph is abnormal (e.g., as a result of fracture or previous surgery), a radionuclide scan with indium-labeled white blood cells is performed. If the scan is negative, a search is begun for other causes. If the scan is positive, the patient is treated for osteomyelitis.

13. What are the radiographic findings in acute osteomyelitis?

The main radiographic findings are punched-out or irregular lucencies in the cancellous bone without marginal reactions. Erosive lesions involving the cortex with reactive changes are also identified in diffuse disease. The diaphysis shows a reactive periosteal response, and sequestration may occur. Demineralization of the surrounding bone may be detected with osteoporosis. Soft-tissue edema is present in 35–50% of patients. Trabecular alterations signify rapid bone turnover.

14. If plain radiographs reveal abnormalities, what is the clinical stage of infection?

Abnormalities on plain radiographs indicate a subacute infection, because radiographic evidence appears after approximately 10 days.

15. What is the standard imaging method for establishing the diagnosis of osteomyelitis?

Several types of radionuclide scans are available for the diagnosis of osteomyelitis, including technetium-99m or gallium-67 and indium-111–labeled leukocytes. The uptake of technetium phosphorate is related primarily to osteoblastic activity. Because technetium is rapidly cleared from the blood and absorbed into the bone, maximal uptake occurs within 1 hour of injection. The usual procedure in evaluating areas of suspected osteomyelitis is to perform the so-called three-phase bone scan. The first phase includes a flow study at the time of injection. The second stage is the equilibrium, or intermediate, stage, in which increased uptake of tracer aids in the differentiation of superficial nonosseous and joint infections from osteomyelitis. A delayed phase, generally performed 2–4 hours after injection of the radioisotope, shows active osteoblastic activity and is positive in various disease states, including osteomyelitis, tumor, degenerative joint disease, trauma, and postsurgical changes. A focus of osteomyelitis presents as an area of increased tracer uptake on the delayed image. On occasion, a "cold" area may result from decreased delivery of tracer due to edematous occlusion of flow and intramedullary vessels. Indium-labeled leukocytes have been suggested for differentiating between osteomyelitis and reactive involucrum without the necessity for delayed imaging. The test requires drawing approximately 50 cc of venous blood. The leukocytes are separated from the other blood elements and labeled with indium-111. The indium-labeled leukocytes are then reinjected into the patient, and scans are performed 18–24 hours later. The scan is interpreted as positive if a focal accumulation of activity exceeds adjacent normal bone activity.

16. Describe the computed tomography (CT) findings in osteomyelitis.

The CT diagnosis of acute osteomyelitis is based on the detection of interosseous gas, decreased density of infected bone in association with soft-tissue masses, and destructive lesions of bone.

17. Describe magnetic resonance imaging (MRI) findings in acute osteomyelitis.

MRI imaging is superior to the CT scan in displaying soft tissues and bone marrow. Thus MRI may be a sensitive tool for detecting the marrow edema associated with early osteomyelitis, although later bony changes, such as periosteal reaction or sequestrum formation, may remain unapparent.

18. What is a sequestrum?

A sequestrum is death of the cortical shell from occlusion of the nutrient vessels caused by intense infection.

19. What is the involucrum?

The involucrum is the new bone laid down by the periosteum around the shell of the old shaft that has necrosed because of infection.

20. Describe the biologic classification of adult osteomyelitis.

The classification for adult osteomyelitis was developed by Cierny and Mader in 1981. Type I is medullary osteomyelitis; lesions include hematogenously infected fractures and nonunions. Type I is also seen in patients with intramedullary rods. Type II is superficial osteomyelitis, usually limited to the surface of the bone exposed by inadequate soft-tissue envelope. Type III is a localized infection involving stable, well-demarcated lesions characterized by full-thickness cortical sequestration and cavitation. Usually debridement does not lead to segmental instability. Infected nonunions and refractory pintrack infections are common type III lesions. Type IV is diffuse osteomyelitis, involving circumferential lesions. Type IV osteomyelitis includes infected nonunions and septic joints, which generally are considered mechanically unstable, either at presentation or after appropriate treatment.

21. Describe the physiologic classification in the Cierny-Mader system.

The class A host has a normal response to infection and surgery. Class B includes patients who are compromised with local, systemic, or combined deficiencies in wound healing. Class C is a result of treatment or development of a condition potentially more compromising than the presenting infection.

22. What is the surgical treatment for stage I medullary osteomyelitis?

Treatment consists of drainage and curettage of the dead space with simple closure of tissue and administration of related antibiotics.

23. What is the treatment for stage II osteomyelitis?

Stage II osteomyelitis is limited to the surface of the bone that is exposed by an inadequate soft-tissue envelope. Treatment includes drainage and curettage of the dead space but also involves a complex closure, such as free-flap treatment.

24. What is the treatment for stage III osteomyelitis?

Treatment which focuses on the usually infected unions and refractory pintrack infections commonly seen in type III lesions, includes complex drainage and curettage of dead space with removal of bone and general complex closure. Patients do not require stabilization, because there is no segmental instability.

25. What is the treatment for stage IV osteomyelitis?

Treatment includes complex drainage and curettage of dead space for debridement of bone with complex closure and complex stabilization.

26. Describe the common soft-tissue coverage for orthopedic infections.

1. **Conventional rotation flaps** have very limited place for skin coverage in the extremity.

2. **Rotation muscle flaps.** The gastrocnemius flap is by far the most useful and has the least morbidity at the donor site. The muscle with available skin is taken, along with the blood supply branching from the popliteal artery. This flap is most useful for defects of the tibial plateau or in the knee.

3. **Free tissue transfer.** The most versatile technique of skin coverage is the free tissue transfer, which includes the scapular, radial arm, groin, and dorsal pedis flaps. Skin and muscle pedicles are transferred with a branch of local artery, and microscopic anastomosis of the transferred vessel to a local vessel results in free blood flow to the musculocutaneous flap.

4. **Osteocutaneous flaps.** The most commonly used is the free fibular graft; vascularity is based on the peroneal blood supply. The graft may be taken with or without skin.

5. **Free muscle flaps.** The most popular free muscle flaps are the latissimus, gracilis, and rectus abdominis. Vascularity is based on local blood supply and allows coverage of large areas. Skin is then grafted over the muscle.

27. What are the principal isolates in hematogenous osteomyelitis in patients with sickle-cell disease?

The predominant organism is *Salmonella* species. Other common organisms include *Staphylococcus aureus, Streptococcus pneumoniae*, and *Haemophilus influenzae*.

28. What are the principal isolates in hematogenous osteomyelitis in patients with drug addiction?

The predominant organism is *Staphylococcus aureus. Pseudomonas aeruginosa* also occurs, as do gram-negative bacilli.

29. What are the common principal isolates in hematogenous osteomyelitis in patients on hemodialysis?

The predominant organism is *Staphylococcus aureus.* Other common organisms include *Staphylococcus epidermidis* and *Mycobacterium tuberculosis*.

BIBLIOGRAPHY

1. Bateman JL, Pevzner MM: Spinal osteomyelitis: A review of 10 years' experience. Orthopedics 18:561–565, 1995.

 2. Cierny G III, Mader JT: Adult chronic osteomyelitis: An overview. In D'Ambrosia RD, Marier RL (eds): Orthopedic Infections. Thorofare, NJ, Slack, 1991, pp 33–47.
 3. Carragee EJ, Kim D: The clinical use of erythrocyte sedimentation rate in pyogenic vertebral osteomyelitis. Spine 22:2089–2093, 1997.
 4. Green NE, Edwards K: Bone and joint infections in children. Orthop Clin North Am 18:555, 1987.
 5. Gustilo RB (ed): Orthopedic Infections: Diagnosis and Treatment. Philadelphia, W.B. Saunders, 1989.
 6. Mader JT, Pennick J: The chemical staging of adult osteomyelitis. Contemp Orthop 10:17–37, 1985.
 7. Reilly KE, Linz JC, Stem PJ: Osteomyelitis of the tubular bones of the hand. J Hand Surg Am 22:644–649, 1997.
 8. Schurman DJ, Fitzgerald RH, Nelson CL, Patzakis MJ: Symposium: Antibiotics in bone and joint infections. Contemp Orthop 15:47, 1987.
 9. Spangehl MJ, Younger A, Masri BA, Duncan CP: Diagnosis of infection following total hip arthroplasty. AAOS Instructional Course Lecture 47:285–295, 1998.
10. Warner WC: Osteomyelitis. In Canale ST (ed): Campbell's Operative Orthopedics, 9th ed. St. Louis, Mosby, 1998, pp 578–800.

7. OPEN FRACTURES

David A. Peterson, M.D.

1. How are open fractures classified?

The Gustilo classification system is commonly used for evaluating open fractures and deciding on the most appropriate treatment:

Type I   ≤ 1 cm wound
Type II > 1 cm wound with moderate soft-tissue damage
Type III Extensive soft-tissue damage and crushing due to high-velocity trauma. Type III is further subdivided into three subtypes:
   A   **A**dequate coverage
   B   **B**one exposed with periosteal stripping
   C   **C**irculation disrupted; arterial repair required

2. What is the initial treatment for patients with open fractures?

Many open fractures are associated with motor vehicle accidents, gunshot wounds, falls, and other major trauma. Consequently, the first objective of treatment is to ensure that the ABCs—airway, breathing, and circulation—are stable. An examination that includes neurologic status, head, spine, abdomen, and pelvis is completed before starting treatment of the open fracture.

3. What is the initial objective in the treatment of open fractures?

The initial objective is to remove all contamination from the wound and fracture site. Aerobic and anaerobic cultures are taken before starting antibiotics. "Dilution is the solution to the pollution" describes the role of irrigation in open fractures. Liters of normal saline (usually with antibiotics or Betadine) may be used to clean fractures of long bones. All foreign material must be removed, including the wadding from gunshot wounds and pieces of clothing driven inward by the force of injury.

4. Which tissues are removed during debridement of an open fracture?

The four major principles of debridement are described in a poem by James Learmonth:
   On the edges of the skin take a piece very thin (1);
   The tenser the fascia, the more you should slash'er (2);
   Of muscles much more, 'til you see fresh gore (3);
   And the bundles contract at least the impact;
   Hardly any of bone, only bits quite alone (4).

Nonviable tissues (i.e., dead muscle, fascia, and small pieces of bone not attached to soft tissue) that provide a focus for infection are removed. Skin should be preserved; only the contaminated edge is removed.

5. In the open fracture, how can you differentiate viable from nonviable muscle tissue?

The four Cs—color, contractility, consistency, and capacity to bleed—help the surgeon to decide which muscles to debride. Pale muscle that does not (1) bleed when cut or (2) contract when touched should be excised.

6. What is the difference in treatment of open fractures between low-velocity and high-velocity gunshot wounds?

High-velocity wounds (e.g., from a rifle) result in more disruption and destruction of soft tissue due to the high energy involved. Multiple debridements may be required to ensure that no nonviable tissue is left behind as a focus of infection. Low-velocity wounds may require only local irrigation, debridement of the entry and exit wounds, and supportive antibiotic treatment.

7. Which antibiotics are used on open fractures with severe contamination, as in a barnyard injury?

Most open fractures of the long bones require a cephalosporin and an aminoglycoside. If clostridial infection is present due to soil or barnyard contamination, intravenous penicillin G is added. Cultures of the wound should be taken before starting antibiotics.

8. What is the best time to close the wounds of type III open fractures?

The ideal time frame is 5–7 days. Closure may be accomplished if no necrotic tissue or contamination is present. Local muscle flaps or vascularized free-tissue transfers may be required for larger soft-tissue defects. The flaps may provide the additional benefit of improved circulation to the area, which assists healing of the fracture site and protects against infection with increased O_2 tension.

9. What type of fixation is used to stabilize open fractures?

This is complex and controversial. The surgeon needs to stabilize the fracture site to protect viable soft tissue, but the metal provides a potential source of infection, because bacteria are isolated from the immune system and circulation. In general, external fixation is used when multiple irrigation and debridements are required (e.g., type III) and subsequent soft-tissue transfers may be necessary. Internal fixation with plates and screws may be used in type I open fractures and articular fractures that require anatomic reduction. Primary and delayed intramedullary fixation have been used in types I and II open fractures of the long bones.

10. In a type IIIC fracture, which is completed first—arterial repair or fracture fixation?

Fracture stability, usually with external fixation, is achieved before arterial repair. Occasionally a temporary arterial shunt may be used before skeletal repair, but attempts at achieving fracture fixation after arterial repair may disrupt the vascular reconstruction with the repetitive motion of reduction and correction of alignment.

CONTROVERSIES

11. Which is the better treatment for type IIIC open fractures of the tibia: amputation or salvage?

Amputation is the better treatment, although it still has disadvantages. The obvious disadvantage is loss of limb and dependence on a prosthesis. Participation in strenuous sports or employment in a job requiring heavy labor or fine foot movements may be impossible. Advantages include shorter hospitalization, fewer operations, and a quick return to work.

Salvage of the leg may require many procedures and more operating time for vascular repair, fracture fixation, soft-tissue transfers, removal of infected bone, nerve repair and reconstruction, and removal of fixation. Amputation may still be required if infection, nonunion, or a painful limb results from attempted salvage. The four Ds—divorce, destitution, depression, and disability—may be the final result of attempted salvage.

12. What factors assist the surgeon in deciding whether to amputate or salvage a type IIIC open fracture of the tibia?

Warm ischemia time over 6 hours and disruption of the posterior tibial nerve are considered to be absolute indications for amputation by Lange. In addition, the Mangled Extremity Severity Score (MESS) may help determine whether amputation or salvage should be performed. A score of at least 7 points indicates that amputation should be strongly considered over salvage.

The Mangled Extremity Severity Score

TYPE	CHARACTERISTICS	INJURIES	POINTS	SCORE
Skeletal and soft-tissue group				
1	Low energy	Stab wounds, simple closed fractures, small-caliber gunshot wounds	1	_____
2	Medium energy	Open or multiple-level fractures, dislocations, moderate crush injuries	2	_____
3	High energy	Shotgun blast (close range), high-velocity gunshot wound	3	_____
4	Massive crush	Logging, railroad, oil-rig accidents	4	_____
			Subtotal	_____
Shock group				
1	Normotensive	Blood pressure stable in field and OR	0	_____
2	Transient hypotension	Blood pressure unstable in field, but responsive to intravenous fluids	1	_____
3	Prolonged hypotension	Systolic blood pressure < 90 mmHg in field hypotension responsive to intravenous fluids only in OR	2	_____
4	Advanced	Pulseless, cool, paralyzed, and numb	3	_____
			Subtotal	_____
Ischemia group (points double if ischemia > 6 hrs)				
1	None	Pulsatile leg without signs of ischemia	0	_____
2	Mild	Diminished pulses only	1	_____
3	Moderate	No pulse by Doppler, sluggish capillary refill, paresthesias, diminished motor activity	2	_____
4	Advanced	Pulseless, cool, paralyzed, numb	3	_____
			Subtotal	_____
Age group				
1	< 30 yrs		0	_____
2	30–50 yrs		1	_____
3	> 50 yrs		2	_____
			Subtotal	_____
Total mangled extremity severity score			Total	_____

From Helfet DL, Howey T, Sanders R, Johansen K: Limb salvage versus amputation: Preliminary results of the mangled extremity severity score. Clin Orthop 256:80–86, 1990, with permission.

BIBLIOGRAPHY

1. Bartlett C, Weiner L, Young E: Treatment of type II and type III open tibia fractures in children. J Orthop Trauma 2:357–362, 1997.
2. Chapman MW: Open fractures. In Rockwood CA, Green DP, Bucholz RW (eds): Rockwood and Green's Fractures in Adults, 3rd ed. Philadelphia, J.B. Lippincott, 1991, pp 223–333.
3. Christian CA: General principles of fracture treatment. In Canale ST (ed): Campbell's Operative Orthopaedics, 9th ed. St. Louis, Mosby, 1998, pp 1993–2041.
4. Connolly JF: Management of open fractures. In Connolly JF (ed): DePalma's The Management of Fractures and Dislocations, vol. 1, 3rd ed. Philadelphia, W.B. Saunders, 1981, pp 125–135.
5. Gustilo RB, Anderson JT: Prevention of infection in the treatment of one thousand and twenty-five open fractures of long bones: Retrospective and prospective analyses. J Bone Joint Surg 58A:453–458, 1976.
6. Gustilo RB, Mendoza RM, Williams DN: Problems in the management of type III (severe) open fractures: A new classification of type III open fractures. J Trauma 24:742–746, 1984.
7. Hansen ST Jr: Editorial. The type-IIIC tibial fracture: Salvage or amputation. J Bone Joint Surg 69A:799–800, 1987.
8. Hansen ST Jr: Overview of the severely traumatized lower limb: Reconstruction versus amputation. Clin Orthop 243:17–19, 1989.
9. Helfet DL, Howey T, Sanders R, Johansen K: Limb salvage versus amputation: Preliminary results of the mangled extremity severity score. Clin Orthop 256:80–86, 1990.
10. Henley M, Chapman J, Agel J, et al: Treatment of type II, IIIA, and IIIB open fractures of the tibial shaft: A prospective comparison of unreamed interlocking intramedullary nails and half-pin external fixators. J Orthop Trauma 12:1–7, 1998.
11. Lange RH: Limb reconstruction versus amputation decision making in massive lower extremity trauma. Clin Orthop 243:92–99, 1989.
12. Sanders R, Swiontkowski M, Nunley J, Spiegel P: The management of fractures with soft tissue disruptions. J Bone Joint Surg 75A:778–789, 1993.

8. COMPARTMENT SYNDROME

J. Jeffrey Poggi, M.D.

1. Define compartment syndrome.

Compartment syndrome is a condition in which elevated pressure in an enclosed space can damage irreversibly the contents of the space.

2. What are the major causes of compartment syndrome?

The causes of compartment syndrome are divided into two categories: those that decrease or constrict the compartment and those that increase the contents of the space. Closure of fascial defects or application of compressive dressings, a tight cast, or military antishock trousers (MAST) may limit the compartment's ability to expand to accommodate an increased volume. Compartment volumes may be increased by hemorrhage after a fracture, surgery, or blunt injury, or by postischemic swelling resulting from arterial injury or restoration of blood flow after arterial injury.

3. How does compartment syndrome occur?

Increased compartmental tissue pressures obstruct venous return initially, resulting in vascular congestion and further increase in intracompartmental pressure. Capillary beds become occluded, and blood is shunted away from occluded areas, resulting in muscle and nerve ischemia. Capillary basement membranes become leaky, allowing transudation of fluid into the surrounding tissues and thus compounding the problem. If the condition is uncorrected, arterial flow to the affected compartment becomes so impaired that the muscle and nerve tissues within the compartment die.

ACUTE COMPARTMENT SYNDROME

4. What are the four Ps?

The four Ps of compartment syndrome are pain, paresthesias, paralysis, and pulselessness. Although they are commonly cited for the diagnosis of compartment syndrome, if one waits for all four signs to appear, it will be too late to initiate treatment.

5. In the alert, responsive patient, what are the signs of impending acute compartment syndrome?

The patient complains of pain out of proportion to the injury. On physical examination, the most reliable sign is pain with passive motion or stretch of the involved muscle(s), especially in association with paresthesias in the distribution of the sensory nerve traversing the involved compartment. Usually, the involved portion of the upper or lower extremity is tensely swollen to palpation, and the overlying skin is shiny and smooth.

6. How specific are the signs of pulselessness and paralysis?

Unless arterial injury has occurred, peripheral pulses and capillary refill of the digits remain normal in most cases of acute compartment syndrome. If treatment is delayed until muscle paralysis is noted clinically, full function rarely returns.

7. Where is acute compartment syndrome most often seen?

Acute compartment syndrome occurs most commonly in the forearm and leg. Other locations include the hand and foot. In rare instances, the upper arm or thigh also may develop compartment syndrome.

8. When should compartment pressures be measured?

Measurements should be obtained in any unresponsive or unreliable patient who has sustained a fracture or other injury to the leg or forearm, especially if the compartment feels tense. In the alert patient, the clinical findings for compartment syndrome often are inconclusive. Pressure readings in such cases help to determine which patients require fasciotomy. As a general rule, if one merely considers compartment pressure measurements, they should be obtained.

9. How are compartment pressures measured?

Needle manometer, wick or slit catheter, and Stic catheter techniques have been described to measure intracompartmental pressures. Specific instructions on the use of such techniques may be found in this chapter's bibliography.

10. What is the threshold for intracompartmental pressures?

The threshold for intracompartmental pressures is debatable. Some advocate fasciotomy for all patients who demonstrate a resting pressure > 30 mmHg, whereas others suggest waiting until the pressure is > 45 mmHg. Still others believe that it is more important to relate the intracompartmental pressure to the patient's systolic, diastolic, or mean arterial pressures; i.e., intracompartmental pressure raised to within 20 mmHg of the patient's diastolic pressure indicates the need for fasciotomy. In general, whenever compartment pressures are > 30 mmHg, the patient should be followed closely. Fasciotomy should be performed whenever pressures are > 40 mmHg or fall within 20 mmHg of the diastolic pressure and are associated with clinical findings suggestive of impending compartment syndrome.

11. What is the proper initial management of a responsive patient demonstrating the signs of early impending compartment syndrome?

All constrictive dressings should be removed or split down to the skin. Any circumferential cast should be bivalved, with the underlying cast padding split down to the skin. The limb should not be elevated but placed at the level of the heart to promote arterial inflow.

12. Describe the definitive treatment for acute compartment syndrome.

The definitive treatment is fasciotomy, the open release of the restrictive fascial compartment dividers. In performing this procedure, the skin and fascia are left open; skin is grafted at a later date.

13. How many compartments are in the forearm? What approach is used for decompression of the forearm?

The forearm is divided into three compartments: superficial volar, deep volar (flexor digitorum profundus), and dorsal. Decompression is performed with either a one-incision or two-incision technique. The one-incision technique uses an ulnar incision to access all three compartments, whereas in the two-incision method the volar compartments are decompressed via Henry's volar approach and a separate dorsal incision is used to decompress the dorsal compartment.

14. What is the result of an unrecognized acute compartment syndrome of the forearm?

If left untreated, compartment syndrome of the forearm in a child or adult results in muscle necrosis with permanent contracture of the wrist flexors to the hand. This entity is termed *Volkmann's contracture* in honor of the man who recognized its etiology. In severe cases, contracture of the extensor muscles to the wrist and hand also may occur.

15. How many compartments are in the leg?

The leg is divided into four compartments: anterior, lateral, and deep and superficial posterior. Some researchers suggested that the posterior tibialis muscle is contained within a fifth compartment. A recent cadaveric study, however, shows that a fifth compartment does not exist.

16. What approach is used to decompress the leg?

Most commonly, a two-incision technique is used. The anterior and lateral compartments are opened through an anterolateral incision centered over the fascia dividing the two compartments, whereas the two posterior compartments are accessed through a posteromedial incision. A perifibular fasciotomy in which all four compartments are accessed through a single lateral incision also has been described. Larger incisions (16 cm) have been shown to decompress the compartments more completely than shorter incisions (8 cm).

17. How is acute compartment syndrome of the foot decompressed?

Compartment syndrome of the foot is difficult to diagnose clinically. A high index of suspicion is necessary in conjunction with a palpably tense foot and pain out of proportion to the injury. Nine different compartments in the foot are now recognized. They are best decompressed through two dorsal incisions and a medial longitudinal incision.

18. Can compartment syndrome occur in the thigh?

For many years it was believed that compartment syndrome occurs only rarely, if at all, in the thigh. Recently, however, the disorder has been reported more frequently, especially in patients sustaining blunt injury to the thigh with prolonged compression by body weight (with or without femoral fracture) and in patients with vascular injury. Compartment syndrome may occur in any of the three thigh compartments (quadriceps, hamstring, adductor), but the quadriceps compartment is involved most often.

19. When should a fasciotomy be done prophylactically?

Postischemic compartment syndromes occur commonly in patients who have sustained ischemic insult to an extremity, either from an arterial injury or a thrombus or after bypass procedures. Prophylactic fasciotomy of the forearm or leg should be performed at the time of reperfusion if arterial ischemia has been present for ≥ 4–6 hours. Prophylactic fasciotomy also should be considered seriously whenever an open tibia fracture is debrided or a tibial osteotomy is performed.

CHRONIC COMPARTMENT SYNDROME

20. What is chronic compartment syndrome?
Chronic exertional compartment syndrome occurs most often in the anterior compartment of the leg in athletes and is manifest by pretibial pain induced by exercise.

21. How is the diagnosis made?
The diagnosis of chronic compartment syndrome is confirmed by elevated intracompartment pressures at rest (>15 mmHg) or during exercise (>30 mmHg) and by prolonged elevated pressures after completing the exercise (>20 mmHg for ≥5 minutes).

22. What clinical finding is often associated with chronic compartment syndrome?
Frequently, a soft-tissue mass is present over the anterolateral portion of the lower third of the leg. This mass results from the herniation of fat or muscle tissue through the fascial defect often found in the lower third of the leg.

23. What structure passes through the fascial defect found in the anterolateral third of the lower leg?
One or both branches of the superficial peroneal nerve traverse the fascial defect in the anterolateral third of the leg and must be protected during fascial release.

24. Describe the management of chronic compartment syndrome.
Initial treatment consists of altering or decreasing the patient's level of activity. If this solution fails or if the patient finds it unacceptable, decompression of the involved compartment(s) is performed, as outlined above, through a limited incision.

25. What is the differential diagnosis of chronic compartment syndrome?
The differential diagnosis of exercise-induced pretibial pain relieved by rest includes tibial stress fracture and periostitis ("shin splints") in addition to chronic compartment syndrome.

BIBLIOGRAPHY

1. Browner BD, Jupiter JB, Levine AM, Trafton PG: Skeletal Trauma, 2nd ed. Philadelphia, W.B. Saunders, 1997.
2. Chapman MW: Operative Orthopaedics, 2nd ed. Philadelphia, J.B. Lippincott, 1993.
3. Canale ST (ed): Campbell's Operative Orthopaedics, 9th ed. St. Louis, Mosby, 1998.
4. Hansen ST Jr, Swiontkowski MF (eds): Orthopaedic Trauma Protocols. New York, Raven Press, 1993.
5. Kasser JR: Orthopaedic Knowledge Updates. Rosemont, IL, American Academy of Orthopedic Surgeons, 1996.

9. DEEP VENOUS THROMBOSIS

Scott P. Wattenhofer, M.D., FACS, and Pamela S. Rolling, PA–C, A.T.C.

1. Describe the classic triad for the pathogenesis of venous thrombosis as described by Virchow.
1. **Venous stasis:** prevents clearance of activated coagulation factors, retards inflow of clotting inhibitors, promotes endothelial cell hypoxia and injury, and increases blood viscosity.
2. **Vascular damage:** intact endothelial cells inhibit platelet adherence and initiation of blood clotting; injury to the endothelial layer of the vessel wall exposes the underlying tissue that initiates platelet adherence and initiation of the clotting cascade.

3. **Hypercoagulability:** alteration of the normal clotting mechanism that predisposes to thrombus formation (e.g., congenital or acquired hypercoagulable states, hypercoagulability associated with malignancies, and hypercoagulability associated with oral contraceptives).

2. What risk factors are associated with an increased risk of development of deep venous thrombosis (DVT)?
- Previous episode of DVT or pulmonary embolism (most important risk factor)
- Pregnancy (fivefold increase)
- Age > 40 years
- Surgery in the pelvis or lower extremities
- Prolonged immobility
- Congestive heart failure
- Obesity
- Malignancy
- Oral contraceptives (reduce antithrombin III levels)
- Venous valvular reflux and varicose veins
- Hypercoagulable states

3. Where do most DVTs originate?
The calf veins.

4. What is the natural history of calf vein thromboses?
Seventy-eight percent spontaneously lyse with little or no sequelae; 22% propagate into the popliteal and femoral veins, where they have a greater potential for embolization and chronic venous stasis.

5. What is the frequency of DVT after surgery?
- Major abdominal surgery: 30–40%
- Prostatectomy: 38%
- Elective orthopedic operation: 52%
- Emergency orthopedic operation: 70%
- Peripheral vascular procedure: 7%
- Cardiothoracic operation: 3%
- Medical intensive care (nonsurgical): 70%

6. What is the incidence of DVT after total hip arthroplasty and total knee arthroplasty in patients unprotected by anticoagulation therapy?
The incidence of DVT after total hip replacement is 40–70%. Thromboembolic disease is the most common serious complication after total hip arthroplasty. It is the most common cause of death within 3 months after surgery and accounts for > 50% of the postoperative mortality after total hip arthroplasty.

The incidence of DVT after total knee arthroplasty was originally thought to be 1–10% on the basis of clinical diagnosis. Studies using radioactive fibrinogen, however, have reported DVT at rates of 50–70%, indicating that DVT is more common than clinical diagnosis suggests and that prophylactic treatment is warranted.

7. When do most postoperative DVTs occur?
Fifty percent occur within the first 24 hours; 85% occur within the first 4 days.

8. What are the signs and symptoms of DVT?
The clinical findings of DVT can vary from obvious to elusive. The classic signs and symptoms are unilateral pain and swelling (pain is due to venous engorgement and inflammation associated with the thrombus; swelling is caused by venous outflow obstruction). Other signs and symptoms may include warmth, erythema, engorged superficial veins, and low-grade fever.

9. What is Homan's sign?

Homan's sign is a clinical test for evaluation of DVT. With a positive Homan's sign, calf pain is produced with dorsiflexion of the ankle. The absence of Homan's sign does **not** rule out DVT, and a positive sign is not diagnostic of DVT.

10. Describe the clinical picture of phlegmasia alba dolens (milk leg).

Phlegmasia alba dolens is characterized by a swollen, white painful leg secondary to extensive acute DVT of the iliac and femoral veins. Initially it was described in the 18th century in postpartum patients. Physicians attributed the condition to suppression of lactation and accumulation of milk in the blood vessels of the leg, hence the term *milk leg*.

11. Describe the more serious condition phlegmasia cerulea dolens.

This condition presents with a swollen, blue painful leg secondary to extensive acute DVT of the iliac and femoral veins. The popliteal, tibial, and superficial veins may be thrombosed as well. This serious condition has a high risk of limb loss and death. Extensive venous outflow obstruction interferes with arterial inflow and results in leg ischemia.

12. How is DVT diagnosed?

Diagnosis of DVT begins with a high **clinical suspicion**. The greater the number of risk factors, the higher the suspicion for DVT. Because the diagnosis of DVT cannot reliably be made on physical examination, diagnostic study is required.

Radioactive-labeled fibrinogen, Doppler ultrasound, and impedance plethysmography are not currently routinely available for diagnosis of DVT, but they may be used in select circumstances. The two studies currently used to diagnose DVT are contrast venography and venous duplex scan.

Contrast venography remains the gold standard for diagnosis of DVT; however, it has largely been replaced by the venous duplex scan. The venogram is useful when duplex scanning capability is not available or when the duplex scan is not diagnostic or is equivocal. Venography is invasive, uncomfortable for the patient, expensive, potentially may induce adverse reaction to contrast material, and has a small risk of initiating venous thrombosis.

Venous duplex scans have replaced contrast venography because they are noninvasive, cause little or no patient discomfort, and are low-risk and less expensive than venography. The reliability of the duplex scan is dependent on a number of factors, including the quality of the equipment used, the experience, skill, and training of the technologist performing the study, as well as the skill of the physician interpreting the study. When properly performed, the duplex scan can accurately diagnose DVT in the femoral, popliteal, and tibial veins. Due to technical difficulties, accurate diagnosis of iliac vein thrombosis is limited.

13. What is the most serious complication of DVT?

Pulmonary embolism is the most serious complication. The annual incidence of fatal and nonfatal pulmonary embolism is >500,000. Approximately 95% of pulmonary emboli arise from the lower extremity. The risk of embolism is higher with thrombi located above the knee versus below the knee.

14. What are the long-term complications of DVT?

The most common long-term complication of DVT is chronic venous insufficiency. Patients with chronic lower extremity edema eventually develop stasis pigmentation, stasis dermatitis, and stasis ulceration after 10–20 years.

15. What prophylactic measures are recommended to prevent DVT?

• Early ambulation
• Extremity elevation
• Range-of-motion exercises (calf muscles act as a pump to empty the calf veins)
• Graduated elastic stockings (only decrease DVT by 5–10%)

- Intermittent pneumatic compression stockings (highly effective after knee surgery but less effective after hip surgery)
- Anticoagulation

16. Outline the medical treatment for DVT.

1. Obtain baseline coagulation studies
2. Bed rest and lower extremity elevation to reduce swelling and discomfort
3. Begin heparinization:
   - Average-sized adult: bolus of 5,000–10,000 U followed by IV infusion at 1,000 U/hr **or** loading dose of 100–150 U/kg IV with a maintenance dose of 10–15 U/kg/hr.
   - Check activated partial thromboplastin time (aPTT) every 6 hours initially and adjust heparin infusion to maintain aPTT at 1.5–2.5 times normal.
   - Administer until therapeutic level of warfarin achieved.
4. Administer warfarin (Coumadin):
   - Daily prothrombin time (PT) and daily maintenance dose of 2.5–10 mg to achieve PT 1.5–2.0 times normal or internationally normalized ratio (INR) of 2–3.
   - Continue Coumadin for 3–6 months.
5. Monitor for bleeding complications

17. Which patients require DVT prophylaxis?

The greater the number of risk factors that a patient has, the more they benefit from DVT prophylaxis. Patients < 40 years of age undergoing uncomplicated abdominal or thoracic operations do **not** require DVT prophylaxis.

18. What methods are available for DVT prophylaxis?

Mechanical
- Graduated compression stockings worn before and after surgery. Knee-high stockings are as effective as the thigh-high variety; each decreases the risk of DVT by only 5–10%.
- Intermittent pneumatic compression devices are as effective as low-dose heparin; they are highly effective after knee surgery but less effective after hip surgery.

Anticoagulants
- Low-dose heparin (2 hr SQ before surgery and 8–12 hr after surgery) decreases the risk of DVT by 15–20% with no increased risk of major bleeding episodes, but the risk of wound hematomas increases. Anticoagulants work well for general surgery patients but lower the risk of DVT by only 15% in orthopedic patients.
- Low–molecular-weight heparin has a different mechanism of action than regular heparin, equivalent antithrombotic effect, and less bleeding potential. It is superior to low-dose heparin for orthopedic patients.
- Warfarin (low fixed dose 2 mg/day or adjust PT to achieve mildly prolonged PT) reduces the risk of DVT after elective hip procedures, but has a slow onset and a slow reversal.

BIBLIOGRAPHY

1. Canale ST (ed): Campbell's Operative Orthopedics, 9th ed. St. Louis, Mosby, 1998.
2. Ferree BA, Stern PJ, Jolson RS, et al: Deep venous thrombosis after spinal surgery. Spine 18:515–319, 1993.
3. Greenfield LJ: Venous and lymphatic disease. In Schwartz SI (ed): Principles of Surgery, 6th ed. New York, McGraw-Hill, 1994, pp 989–1003.
4. Kassir JP (ed): Current Therapy in Internal Medicine, 3rd ed. Philadelphia, B.C. Decker, 1991.
6. McNally MA, Kernohan WG, Croal SA, Mollan RAB: Deep venous thrombosis in orthopedic patients. Clin Orthop 295:275–280, 1993.
7. Raju S: Pathophysiology of venous thrombosis. In Ernst CB, Stanley JC (eds): Current Therapy in Vascular Surgery, 3rd ed. St. Louis, Mosby, 1995, pp 874–879.
8. Kumar V, Cotran RS, Robbins SL (eds): Basic Pathology, 6th ed. Philadelphia, W.B. Saunders, 1997.
8. Sumner DS: Diagnosis of deep venous thrombosis. In Rutherford RB (ed): Vascular Surgery, 4th ed. Philadelphia, W.B. Saunders, 1995, pp 1698–1743.

9. Swayze OS, Nasser S, Roberson JR: Deep venous thrombosis in total hip arthroplasty. Orthop Clin North Am 23:359–364, 1992.
10. Vitti MJ, Barnes RW: Nonoperative treatment of acute thrombophlebitis and femoral venous thrombosis. In Ernst CB, Stanley JC (eds): Current Therapy in Vascular Surgery, 3rd ed. St. Louis, Mosby, 1995, pp 888–893.
11. Wilde AH, Colwell CW, Paiement G, et al: Symposium: Advances in the prevention of venous thromboembolic disease in orthopedics: The introduction of LWMH. Contemp Orthop 27:551–577, 1993.

10. PULMONARY PROBLEMS

Donald D. Graham, Jr., M.D.

1. What are the most common pulmonary problems in orthopedic medicine?
- Fat emboli
- Acute respiratory distress syndrome (ARDS)
- Pulmonary embolus
- Atelectasis
- Postoperative pneumonia

2. What are fat emboli?
Fat emboli characterize a syndrome due to the entry of neutral fat into the vascular system. The syndrome usually develops 24–48 hours after the inciting event. The most common inciting event is traumatic fracture of long bones; the incidence increases with the number of fractures. Orthopedic procedures and trauma to other fat-laden tissues, such as a fatty liver, occasionally are followed by the same syndrome.

3. What are the most common signs and symptoms of fat emboli syndrome?
Mental aberrations are common and may progress to delirium and coma. Patients also may develop high fever, marked dyspnea, and a petechial rash, usually over the thorax and upper extremities. Examination of the lungs may reveal fine rales, and the typical chest radiograph shows a diffuse alveolar filling pattern throughout both lung fields. Analysis of arterial blood gases may reveal hypoxemia and hypocapnia; a decrease in the hematocrit count and thrombocytopenia also may be present.

4. What is the treatment for fat emboli?
Current treatment of fat emboli is primarily supportive. Various therapies have been suggested, including ethanol infusion, heparin, and corticosteroids, but to date none has been proved to be effective. Most patients survive with meticulous supportive therapy.

5. Define ARDS.
The American Thoracic Society defines ARDS as a clinical syndrome with the four following findings in a patient with acute respiratory failure:

1. Severe hypoxemia, refractory to supplemental oxygen therapy. The partial pressure of oxygen (PO_2) is less than 75 in patients receiving > 50% oxygen.

2. Diffuse pulmonary infiltrates, which generally are fluffy and involve both lungs.

3. The absence of increased pulmonary capillary hydrostatic pressure (which suggests a cardiogenic cause). The pulmonary wedge pressure is generally < 18.

4. The absence of other clinical explanations for the above findings. Physiologically the lungs demonstrate diffuse alveolar damage (DAD). The lungs generally become stiff with reduced lung-thoracic compliance.

6. With what clinical conditions does ARDS commonly develop?

In orthopedic medicine, the most common underlying clinical conditions are trauma, multiple fractures, lung contusion, and fat emboli. Other underlying conditions include sepsis, prolonged hypotension, gastric aspiration, drug overdose, and massive blood transfusion.

7. Describe the management of a patient with ARDS.

The best approach to patients with ARDS is to treat the underlying condition. If necessary, a pulmonary artery catheter may be used for measurement of the pulmonary capillary wedge pressure to rule out a cardiogenic cause. No pharmacologic agent has been demonstrated to alter the course of ARDS. Many patients develop respiratory distress that necessitates mechanical ventilation. No specific form of mechanical ventilation has been proved to be superior in the treatment of ARDS. The most important concern is meticulous attention to the prevention of complications.

8. What is the mortality rate of ARDS?

The mortality rate of ARDS is 50–60%. Death within the first week generally is due to the underlying condition. At later dates, common causes of death include sepsis and infection. Most survivors return to near-normal activity.

9. What predisposing factors increase the risk for deep venous thrombosis (DVT) and pulmonary emboli (PE)?

- Prolonged anesthesia and postoperative convalescence
- Injury or surgery to the pelvis and lower extremities
- Right ventricular failure
- Long periods of travel, immobility, and bed rest
- Obesity
- Cancer
- Previous history of DVT
- Coagulation disorders

10. What orthopedic procedure places the patient at high risk for DVT and possible PE?

Hip surgery or replacement.

11. What signs and symptoms suggest PE?

The clinical presentation of PE is quite variable. PE should be considered in patients who develop unexplained dyspnea, pleuritic chest pain, hypoxia, tachypnea, tachycardia, or signs of cor pulmonale. Patients may present with a low arterial oxygen tension, but a normal value does not rule out PE.

12. How is PE diagnosed?

Because the clinical presentation of PE is variable, further testing is needed to establish a diagnosis. Because the chest radiograph in PE is most often normal, the first diagnostic test is usually a ventilation/perfusion (VQ) scan. The recent PIOPED study clarified the usefulness of a VQ scan in diagnosing PE. In patients with high clinical suspicion and a high-probability scan, the accuracy rate was 96%. Unfortunately, only 41% of the patients with PE had high-probability scans. For the definitive diagnosis of PE, a pulmonary angiogram should be done. If noninvasive leg studies reveal DVT, anticoagulation therapy should be initiated without angiography to document a PE.

13. What is the treatment for PE?

With the diagnosis of PE, heparin therapy is indicated. Anticoagulation, however, does not speed the resolution of the thrombus; it only prevents formation of new thrombi. Heparin is usually begun with an initial bolus followed by intravenous infusion with monitoring of partial thromboplastin time (PTT). Platelet counts also should be checked to identify heparin-induced thrombocytopenia. In patients with massive PE (proved by angiography) and hemodynamic instability, thrombolytic therapy should be considered. In patients in whom anticoagulation is contraindicated or who have recurrent embolism despite adequate anticoagulation, vena cava interruption with filter placement is indicated. The mortality rate among patients with treated PEs is about 10%.

14. List the common risk factors for postoperative atelectasis.
- Upper abdominal surgery
- Thoracotomy
- Smoking
- Chronic obstructive pulmonary disease (COPD)
- Restrictive pulmonary disease
- Obesity
- Age greater than 70 years
- Postoperative immobility

15. What methods may be used to improve postoperative pulmonary function?
Methods to improve postoperative pulmonary function include incentive spirometry, deep breathing, intermittent positive pressure breathing, and continuous positive airway pressure. Persistent, clinically significant atelectasis requires therapy.

16. How serious a problem is postoperative pneumonia in orthopedic medicine?
Nosocomial pneumonia occurs most frequently in surgical patients and has a mortality rate that approaches 50%.

17. What are the most prevalent organisms in postoperative pneumonia?
The most prevalent organisms include gram-negative organisms such as *Pseudomonas aeruginosa, Klebsiella pneumoniae*, and *Escherichia coli*. Gram-positive organisms such as staphylococci also may be seen. Postoperative pneumonia also may develop from the subclinical aspiration of oropharyngeal secretions.

BIBLIOGRAPHY

1. American College of Physicians: Pulmonary Medicine. Medical Knowledge Self-Assessment Program. Philadelphia, American College of Physicians, 1994.
2. Canale ST (ed): Campbell's Operative Orthopaedics, 9th ed. St. Louis, Mosby, 1998.
3. Coosling H, Pelligrini V: Fat embolism syndrome. Clin Orthop 165:68–92, 1982.
4. George RB, Light RW, Matthay MA, Matthay RA: Chest Medicine. Baltimore, Williams & Wilkins, 1990.
5. Moser KM: Diagnosing pulmonary embolism. J Respir Dis 13(7), 1992.
6. Moylan J, Evenson MA: The diagnosis and therapy of fat embolism. Ann Rev Med 28:85–94, 1977.
7. O'Donohue WJ Jr: Postoperative pulmonary complications. Postgrad Med 91(3), 1992.
8. The PIOPED Investigators: Value of the ventilation/perfusion scan in acute pulmonary embolism. JAMA 263(20), 1990.

11. SURGICAL NUTRITION

Scott G. Rose, M.D.

1. How is a patient evaluated for nutritional intervention?
Evaluation for nutritional intervention depends on a combination of factors derived from the physical examination, prehospital nutritional deficiencies, expected clinical course, anthropometric measurements, and biochemical tests. The subjective global assessment (SGA) is made at the bedside without the input of sophisticated metabolic, biochemical, or anthropometric measurements. It is based on clinical appearance, history of weight loss preceding the illness, extent of metabolic demands during the illness, and the patient's ability to maintain an adequate oral intake during the hospitalization. Some authors suggest that the SGA alone can adequately identify 60–80% of patients in need of nutritional intervention. The SGA should be undertaken during the admission of any patient to the hospital, and plans for further nutritional testing or nutritional intervention should be entertained early in the hospitalization. Other studies show that if the physician waits until a severe complication develops to begin nutritional support, morbidity and mortality are markedly increased. Early intervention in appropriate patients has been shown to decrease morbidity and mortality. The restoration of normal metabolic activities, the development of an anabolic state, and the return to a normal immune functioning system have been found to be beneficial in patients with nutritional deficiencies.

2. What are the components of a nutritional assessment?

Components of an adequate nutritional assessment generally include a detailed history of a patient's weight changes before hospitalization. The clinical course and expected surgical intervention also are noted. The patient's current weight is evaluated and compared with expected ideal body weight. Although no specific weight loss in an adult is considered critical, the amount of weight lost over a period of time is an important factor in deciding on early intervention. Anthropometric measurements, based on standards recommended by the World Health Organization, include measurement of triceps skinfold and mid-arm circumference. Additional laboratory tests often included are albumin, prealbumin, transferrin, and retinol-binding protein. A decreased lymphocyte count has been found to be an early marker of a catabolic state.

Immune skin testing has been recommended for evaluation of reactivity to delayed cutaneous antigens, but in a study of over 3,000 patients at Methodist Hospital, Omaha, Nebraska, it was not found to be a critical determinant. The tests are so sensitive that >90% of the studied population showed evidence of anergy or relative anergy. Because negative results were so common in the identified population, the test is no longer recommended routinely.

Determination of urine urea nitrogen (UUN) to measure excretion of nitrogen in urine is also recommended. Although the test does not reflect all nitrogen degradation that is excreted, it tends to reflect accurately total urinary nitrogen. Increased losses of UUN are seen in a hypermetabolic state and in patients with closed head injuries and spinal injuries. Sometimes the dramatic increase in UUN in this setting is the normal result of denervation of muscle mass and should not be used as a target for delivery of protein. In most circumstances, however, nitrogen delivery to the patient should be equal to or in excess of nitrogen lost through the urine. Each day the average adult patient loses an additional 4 gm of nitrogen that is not measured in the UUN. This additional loss should be calculated in nitrogen balance studies. In patients on aggressive nutritional support, this author recommends weekly determinations of UUN to adjust nutritional support.

3. What is indirect calorimetry?

Indirect calorimetry is a measurement of caloric demands over a period of time. It is done through the hospital's pulmonary laboratory. The patient's O_2 consumption and production of CO_2 are measured over a period through a closed system. When these data are fed into a computer, caloric demand over a 24-hour period can be accurately estimated. Substrate utilization also can be detailed from the same data. A respiratory quotient (RQ) is useful in adjusting total calories during nutritional support. An RQ >1.0 indicates overfeeding of the patient, which not only has metabolic consequences but also is expensive. The author recommends an RQ between 0.7 and 0.9 to keep the patient in a positive caloric balance. The RQ is evaluated each week, along with the UUN, for better adjustment of nutritional balance support products. The RQ is a ration of CO_2 production divided by O_2 consumption, and does not take into account activity during the day. Most hospitalized patients, however, are physically inactive and do not require increased nutritional requirements. It was originally thought that caloric demand would exceed 3,500 cal/day in a severely traumatized patient. Experience with RQs, however, has shown that the demand rarely exceeds 1,500–2,000 cal/day. As a standard guideline, the delivery of 2,000–2,500 cal/day parenterally, enterally, or orally is usually sufficient for the hospitalized patient, even in the setting of trauma. This author currently uses a peripheral parenteral solution delivering 1,520 kcal/day for the majority of surgical/trauma patients.

4. Which fuels are used as preferred fuel sources during increased metabolic demands?

The three fuels commonly available for utilization under any circumstances include glucose, fat, and protein. During periods of starvation glucose and glycogen stores are initially the preferred fuel. Because both are generally exhausted in the first day or two, ketosis becomes a prominent fuel source. Ketones are broken down into free fatty acids and glycerol, which are then metabolized as the preferred fuel source in the absence of glucose. Ketosis is followed by a slow but chronic breakdown of visceral and somatic protein stores. Nutritional intervention should help to reduce the amount of ketosis, to eliminate protein degradation, and to supply adequate glucose and fat calories for daily metabolic activity.

5. What routes are available for administration of calories?

In evaluation of a patient, all routes of administration of calories should be considered, including oral delivery and consumption of adequate calories. Sometimes the addition of between-meal snacks and nutritional supplements is sufficient to meet caloric requirements. If oral feedings are not adequate, enteral feedings can be administered through a nasogastric tube, nasoduodenal tube, percutaneous endoscopic gastrostomy tube, laparoscopically placed gastrostomy tube, or surgically placed jejunostomy tube. In general, routes of administration that deliver nutrients directly into the stomach can deliver larger quantities in a bolus fashion. Nutrients delivered directly into the small intestine need to be administered by continuous infusion, because no reservoir function is present. If the GI tract must be bypassed, intravenous options include peripheral total parenteral nutrition and central total parenteral nutrition. Both can deliver adequate parenteral products.

6. When should nutritional support be considered in a patient who is not allowed or not able to eat?

In a healthy adult under maximal stress, parenteral or enteral support can be safely initiated 3–5 days after admission without causing undue risk. Patients with multiple trauma often have a hyperglycemic/hypermetabolic response immediately after injury. Early intervention during a period of rapid volume resuscitation is not indicated. In general, once fluid requirements have stabilized, parenteral or enteral support may be initiated. Some evidence, however, suggests that early enteral nutritional support in burn patients not only decreases morbidity and mortality during hospitalization but also attenuates the acute metabolic response to the burn. The patient should be evaluated for the need for invasive enteral or parenteral nutrition on a daily basis during rounds.

7. What is the most common metabolic abnormality associated with central total parenteral nutrition?

Hyperglycemia remains the main metabolic problem associated with total parenteral nutrition. Most formulas deliver a solution with a 25% concentration of dextrose (comparable to a blood sugar of 25,000 mg/dl). Thus glucose intolerance may develop in some individuals. Close monitoring of serum glucose during the initiation of parenteral nutrition is essential for a successful outcome. Glucosuria and hyperglycemia should be treated by decreasing the glucose concentration of the delivered fluid or by adding insulin to combat the exogenous hyperglycemia. Insulin may be delivered subcutaneously or intravenously by a pump or mixed directly with the parenteral nutritional solution. Blood sugar should generally be < 200 mg/dl. If severe glucose intolerance develops and the glucose content is reduced, the lipid protein portion of nonnitrogen calories may be increased. In a patient who develops hyperglycemia but otherwise has been stable on glucose infusion, evaluation for subclinical sepsis should be considered. Often sepsis is first recognized by newly developed glucose intolerance. If hyperglycemia is not treated, hyperosmolarity may result, leading to dehydration, coma, and death.

8. Describe the appropriate enteral formula.

Although enteral products are currently under intensive investigation, presently they are evaluated in two major categories:

1. **Elemental diets** include basic nutrients—amino acids, carbohydrates, and fats—delivered in forms that require little sophisticated change during digestion. Elemental diets are generally recommended for patients who have a short amount of GI tract available for absorption, who have poorly functioning GI mucosa, or who are intolerant of other formulas. These are the most expensive diets.

2. **Nonelemental diets** include combinations of proteins, polypeptides, and dipeptides, along with more complex fats and carbohydrates. Most use complete formulas that include the micronutrients, vitamins, minerals, and free water required for normal metabolic activities.

Selection of an enteral formula may be a hit-or-miss proposition. Some patients may tolerate one formula but not another for no identifiable reason. Intolerance of all enteral formulas may be due to poor gastric emptying, which often results from injury, ileus, or drugs. Malabsorption may be secondary to atrophic jejunal villi with inability to digest nutrients appropriately. Intolerance due to diarrhea may be secondary to bacterial overgrowth from use of broad-spectrum antibiotics or histamine blockers that alkalinize the gastric contents. Such problems may require adjustment in the enteral formula.

9. What is the appropriate ratio of nonnitrogen calories for each gram of nitrogen delivered in parenteral and enteral formulas?

Most parenteral formulas have a ratio of 150–300 nonnitrogen cal/gm of nitrogen, usually in the form of carbohydrates and lipids. Under normal metabolic activities, this ratio supplies enough nonnitrogen fuels so that nitrogen products can be used for metabolic activities. Because the early posttraumatic period is associated with glucose intolerance, formulas with a ratio of < 100 nonnitrogen cal/gm of nitrogen may be appropriate. A similar ratio for enteral formulas has been recommended. If the caloric density of enteral formulas is increased, the solution often becomes hyperosmotic and intolerance develops. In general, enteral formulas with > 1 cal/ml carry a higher risk of intolerance. Most parenteral formulas at full strength deliver 1 cal/ml.

10. What causes metabolic bone disease associated with total parenteral nutrition? How is it treated?

Metabolic bone disease is a poorly understood complication of long-term home parenteral nutrition. It is clinically manifested by development of compression fractures, usually of the thoracic and lumbar spine, at some point after the first year of home parenteral therapy. Many theories have been suggested to explain this process, but none has proved consistently true. At one point, aluminum toxicity was implicated because of aluminum salts. After elimination of such salts, however, the incidence does not appear to change. Perhaps a micro- or macronutrient excess or deficiency develops as a result of long-term parenteral nutrition. Levels of trace elements, including copper, zinc, chromium, magnesium, manganese, calcium, and selenium, should be monitored in all patients on long-term home parenteral nutrition. Correcting metabolic serum deficiencies is the only known treatment other than supportive care. Over time metabolic bone disease seems to become less active, and patients complain less of new fractures as the years pass.

11. What specialty was instrumental in the development of parenteral nutrition?

Laboratory experiments and the clinical use of parenteral nutrition were begun in the late 1960s by a group of general surgeons at the University of Pennsylvania. Their initial experiments were in beagle puppies. They found that puppies from the same litter could grow and develop at a normal rate whether they received parenteral nutrition or standard puppy formula. The first human patient to be maintained successfully on the new parenteral nutrition formula was a newborn infant.

12. What are the potential pulmonary complications of hypermetabolic state?

The end-products of metabolism of carbohydrates are CO_2 and H_2O. The patient who receives excessive glucose may develop an excess of CO_2 that needs to be eliminated through the pulmonary system. Patients with severe pulmonary problems may not be able to excrete the CO_2 and thus may become hyperbaric due to its retention. Because of this potential problem, it is best to decrease the glucose concentration for patients with severe respiratory compromise.

BIBLIOGRAPHY

1. Fischer JE (ed): Nutrition and Metabolism in the Surgical Patient, 2nd. ed. Philadelphia, Lippincott-Raven, 1996.
2. Silk DBA: Nutritional Support in Hospital Practice. Oxford, Blackwell, 1983.
3. Wright R, Heymsfield S (eds): Nutritional Assessment. Boston, Blackwell, 1984.

12. DIAGNOSTIC RADIOLOGY

Stephanie A. Miske, M.D.

1. What are the usual radiographic views for evaluating shoulder problems?

The anteroposterior view is the most common; it may be taken in a neutral position or in internal and external rotation. A transthoracic lateral view or axillary view assesses positioning of the humeral head in the glenoid.

2. Which is more common—anterior or posterior dislocations of the shoulder?

Anterior dislocations are much more common, occurring in approximately 95% of cases, whereas posterior dislocations occur in 5%.

3. What radiographic examination best differentiates anterior and posterior dislocations?

Anterior and posterior dislocations are best differentiated by an axillary view of the shoulder. The x-ray beam is directed from an inferior position through the axilla to a superior plate.

Axillary view of the shoulder. *Left,* This view demonstrates any anteroposterior dislocation. In this radiograph, the humeral head is normally seeded in the glenoid. A small avulsion fracture of the glenohumeral ligament is identified at the superior aspect of the glenoid. *Right,* Supraspinatus outlet view demonstrates the morphology of the acromion.

4. What is a Hill-Sachs lesion?

A Hill-Sachs lesion is a defect of the posterolateral aspect of the humeral head. It occurs with anterior dislocation of the shoulder when the posterior superior surface of the humeral head impinges on the anteroinferior portion of the glenoid. The Hill-Sachs deformity is easily visualized by anteroposterior view of the shoulder with the arm in full internal rotation.

5. What is a Bankart lesion?

A Bankart lesion is an avulsion of the anterior capsular structures with a fragment of bone. This lesion is the hallmark of radiographic findings for recurrent dislocations of the shoulder. It is best seen on an axillary view of the shoulder.

6. What is the radiographic appearance of an acromioclavicular dislocation?

An acromioclavicular dislocation is a disruption of the coracoclavicular and acromioclavicular ligaments. The space between the clavicle and the coracoid is widened. Dissociation of the acromioclavicular joint is complete, and the clavicle is displaced superiorly in comparison with the acromion. The best view to visualize an acromioclavicular dislocation is attained with the patient holding 10–15 pounds of weight in each arm. Anteroposterior radiographs are then taken simultaneously of the affected and nonaffected acromioclavicular joint.

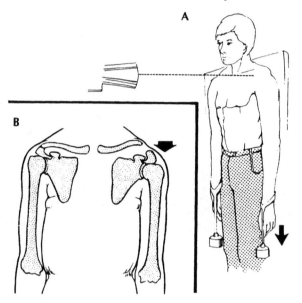

Technique of obtaining stress views of the acromioclavicular joint. *A,* Anteroposterior radiographs are made of both acromioclavicular joints with 10–15 pounds of weight hanging from the wrists. *B,* The distance between the superior aspect of the coracoid and the undersurface of the clavicle is measured to determine whether or not the coracoclavicular ligaments have been disrupted. One large horizontal 14 × 17-inch cassette can be used in small patients to visualize both shoulders on the same film. In large patients it is better to use two horizontal smaller cassettes and to take two separate radiographs for the measurements. (From Rockwood CA Jr, Green DP, Bucholz RW (eds): Rockwood and Green's Fractures in Adults, 3rd ed. Philadelphia, J.B. Lippincott, 1991, p 1201, with permission.)

7. What radiographic view is used to evaluate impingement syndrome?

The supraspinatus outlet view is used to evaluate impingement syndrome. In this view the patient is positioned for the scapular lateral radiograph, and the tube is angled inferiorly at approximately 10°. This view shows the morphology of the acromion for the treatment of impingement syndrome.

8. What are the most common views for evaluating elbow symptoms?

Anteroposterior and lateral radiographs are most commonly used. Fractures are common around the radial head with trauma. Loose bodies may be identified in the olecranon fossa or anteriorly in the anterior joint. Osteochondritis dissecans may be seen as irregularities along the capitellum.

9. Is it normal to visualize the anterior fat pad on lateral radiographs of the flexed elbow?

The normal anterior fat pad appears as a lucid stripe paralleling the anterior margin of the supracondylar region. If the anterior fat pad has assumed a "sail-shaped" configuration, the elbow capsule is distended. This finding signifies recent trauma, most likely a hemarthrosis.

10. Is it normal to visualize a posterior fat pad on lateral radiographs of a flexed elbow?
The posterior fat pad is not visible on routine lateral views of the flexed elbow. Visualization of the posterior fat pad indicates capsular distension, most likely due to hemarthrosis and often caused by a nondisplaced radial head fracture.

11. What radiographic examination is invaluable for evaluating patients with rheumatologic diseases?
An anteroposterior radiograph of the hand shows many joints of the wrist and phalanges. Rheumatoid arthritis has a predilection for an entire wrist and metacarpophalangeal joint. Osteoarthritis generally affects the interphalangeal joints and the first carpometacarpal joint. Erosive osteoarthritis is characterized by interphalangeal joint destruction with subluxation and severe erosions. Radiographs of patients with calcium pyrophosphate dihydrate deposition disease (CPDD) may show small subchondral cysts and interarticular soft-tissue calcification, most notably over the radial styloid and triangular fibrocartilage. Erosions in gout may show a characteristic overhanging margin.

12. What radiographic studies should be taken for evaluation of hip disease?
An anteroposterior view of the pelvis, not just the affected hip, should be taken. This view gives clues to the diagnosis of other disease processes by visualizing the pelvic bones, lower portion of the spine, sacroiliac joint, and pubic symphysis. Joint changes may give clues to diagnoses such as ankylosing spondylitis and rheumatoid arthritis. Bone destruction commonly occurs in the pelvis of patients with metastatic disease or multiple myeloma. Fractures generally occur in the ring of the pelvis and can be seen in the contralateral iliac crest and pubic and ischial rami.

13. What are the standard radiographs for evaluation of knee pathology?
The standard radiographs are anteroposterior and lateral views of the knee, which show the metaphyseal bone of the femur and fibula joint surfaces and the surrounding soft tissue. A tunnel view shows the intercondylar notch and may visualize loose bodies not seen on the anteroposterior radiographs. It is also the best view to see osteochondritis dissecans of the medial or lateral femoral condyles. A sunrise Hughston view shows subluxation or dislocations of the patella from the trochlear groove.

Tunnel view. The tunnel view radially shows osteochondritis dissecans on the medial femoral condyle.

14. What is a Segond fracture?
A Segond fracture is an avulsion fracture of the capsular ligament on the lateral side of the tibia, best seen on the anteroposterior view of the knee (see figure, top of next page, left). It is highly suggestive of an anterior cruciate ligament tear because the two are commonly associated.

Segond fracture.   Talar dome fracture *(arrow)*.

15. Which radiographs are used in evaluation of the ankle injuries?

Anteroposterior and lateral radiographs are used in conjunction with a mortise view, an oblique view with approximately 20–30° of internal rotation that attempts to show the ankle mortise. The medial and lateral malleolus are on the same plane in the mortise view, which can be used to evaluate the congruity of the talus as it sits adjacent to the medial and lateral malleolus and the tibial plafond.

16. What talar abnormalities are seen on ankle radiographs?

Fractures of the talar neck or talar dome may be seen on ankle radiographs (see figure above, right). Dome fractures are usually related to inversion or eversion injuries and occur on the superolateral or superomedial portion of the talar dome. The radiographic appearance suggests a small, separated fracture. Dome fractures are sometimes best visualized on an anteroposterior film in full plantar flexion.

17. What radiographic abnormality is seen in patients with peroneal tendon dislocations?

Peroneal tendon dislocations involve avulsion of the osteocartilaginous attachment of the peroneal tendon sheath to the fibula. The result is a small avulsion fracture that is best seen on the posterolateral corner of the distal fibula. This fracture is the hallmark of the radiographic appearance of peroneal tendon subluxation.

Peroneal tendon subluxation avulsion.

Stress view of the ankle *(left)*. Stress views of the ankle show the opening on the lateral side of the joint from an inversion stress injury.

Jones fracture *(right)*. This typical stress fracture occurs in the diaphyseal portion of the fifth metatarsal.

18. Describe the radiographic features of an inversion injury of the ankle.

With inversion injuries of the foot and ankle, avulsive forces affect the lateral structures and compressive forces affect the medial structures (see figure, above left). Lateral injuries may consist of a sprain or avulsion of the lateral ligamentous complex, neither of which is apparent on radiographs. If, however, a fracture is involved, it is usually a transverse fracture in which the ligaments have been avulsed with bone. Fractures appear on the anteroposterior and oblique views. Medial injuries with inversion sprains may show an oblique fracture of the medial malleolus. In general, oblique fractures are usually due to compressive forces and transverse fractures to avulsion forces.

19. Describe the radiographic appearance of an eversion injury of the ankle.

With eversion injuries of the foot, avulsive forces act on the medial structures and compressive forces on the lateral. Depending on the rotation involved, a sprain or avulsion of the medial deltoid ligament may occur; neither is apparent on radiographs. However, if a fracture is involved, it is usually a transverse fracture of the medial malleolus below the ankle mortise. Lateral injuries consist of an oblique or spiral fracture of the lateral malleolus with rupture of the syndesmosis. The tibiofibular ligament may rupture with or without a fracture of the fibula.

20. What is a Jones fracture?

A Jones fracture is a transverse fracture of the proximal fifth metatarsal shaft (see figure, above right). The fracture is located approximately 1.5–2 cm distal to the tip of the metatarsal and usually is a stress fracture. It is differentiated from a styloid fracture, which occurs in the metaphysis, on an oblique view of the foot (see figure, top of next page). The normal apophysis may not be entirely fused in children and may give the appearance of a fracture (see figure, top of next page).

Fifth metatarsal fractures.

Jones fracture   Styloid fracture   Normal apophysis

21. What types of stress fractures are seen?

Stress fractures generally can be divided into two categories: fatigue fractures and insufficiency fractures. Fatigue fractures are due to repetitive prolonged stress on normal bone. Insufficiency fractures result from normal stresses on abnormal bone, such as that in osteomalacia or osteoporosis.

22. Name the common sites for fatigue fractures.

Tibial shaft	Metatarsals	Patella
Midfibula	Calcaneus	Pars interarticularis
Pubic ramus		

23. Name the major predisposing conditions for insufficiency fractures.

Osteomalacia	Radiation	Osteoporosis
Paget's disease	Fibrous dysplasia	Hyperparathyroidism

24. What is the radiographic appearance of a stress fracture?

Stress fractures generally are seen as transverse fractures in the shaft of the bone. Stress fractures of the metatarsals may be seen as a slight, thin, radiolucent line, whereas in larger bones, such as the tibia or the femur, they are better visualized. Some fractures show no lines, but only signs of healing, such as new bone formation. Often callus formation is abundant in metatarsal fractures but minimal in fractures of the tibia and femur.

Stress fracture of the third metatarsal. This anteroposterior radiograph of the foot shows the third metatarsal stress fracture. Note the transverse radiolucent line with the formation of new cortical bone.

25. What is avascular necrosis?

Avascular necrosis, also known as osteonecrosis, is bone death caused by vascular insult. The vessels may be damaged directly by trauma or occluded by emboli or elevated marrow pressure. The most common sites include the hips, shoulders, medial femoral condyle, and talus.

Avascular necrosis of the right hip. This anteroposterior radiograph shows loss of joint space and collapse and sclerosis of the superior segment of the femoral heal.

26. What are the common causes of avascular necrosis?

Steroids	Sickle-cell disease	Emboli
Alcohol abuse	Lupus erythematosus	Caisson disease
Congenital problems such as Gaucher's disease	Radiation therapy	Pancreatitis

27. Which radiographic features suggest a slow-growing or benign process?

- Preservation of cortical margin
- Well-demarcated boundary of the lesion
- Sclerotic margin
- Solid, uninterrupted periosteal reaction
- Little or no soft-tissue mass, except in acute osteomyelitis

Osteochondroma of femur. Osteochondroma is a slow-growing, benign process. A good cortical margin is present. The boundary of the lesion is well defined. No host reaction is present.

28. What are the radiographic findings in patients with osteonecrosis?

In the early stages radiographs may be nondiagnostic; bone scans may be the only positive test. In the later stages, radiographic changes include (1) bone cysts with sclerotic changes in the bone; (2) subchondral collapse, with or without flattening of the articular surface; (3) narrowing of joint spaces; and (4) other degenerative signs. Degenerative changes may be minimal but generally progress to include joint space narrowing, osteophytes, subchondral cysts, and subchondral sclerosis.

29. List the common radiographic features of a malignant bone lesion.

- Cortical erosion and destruction
- Irregular periosteal reaction, including sunburst, onion peeling, and Codman's triangle
- Indistinct boundaries of the lesion, which seems to permeate into the adjacent soft tissue and bone
- Absence of sclerotic margin
- Associated soft-tissue mass

Renal cell carcinoma metastasis to the hip. Complete destruction of the inferior portion of the femoral head is seen on the hip. A stress fracture is noted in the superior cortex of the femoral neck. Note the indistinct margins, along with the moth-eaten appearance and significant destruction of bone.

Giant cell tumor of bone. Malignant giant cell tumor of bone is characterized by bone destruction with breach of the medial cortex of the tibia and a soft-tissue mass.

30. What is Codman's triangle?

Codman's triangle is a radiographic pattern, usually in patients with infection or tumor. When infection or tumor elevates the periosteum of the bone, a gap occurs between the periosteum and bone. Where the gap is elevated, bone is formed, creating a triangular shape on radiographs. Codman's triangle, which denotes soft-tissue extension of the tumor or infectious process, was first described in 1914 by Rubbert. Although long considered to be a manifestation of malignancy, Codman's triangle may result from any disorder that lifts the periosteum, whether benign or malignant.

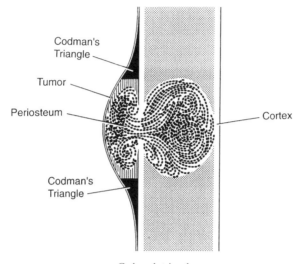

Codman's triangle.

31. What is a pathologic fracture?

A pathologic fracture occurs when the bone has been weakened by infection, neoplasm, or metabolic bone disease. Common causes include benign tumors, osteomyelitis, and tuberculosis.

Pathologic fracture of bone. This pathologic fracture is due to multiple myeloma of the radius.

32. What are radiologic features of acute osteomyelitis?

The earliest sign may be blurring or obliteration of soft-tissue fat planes. Soft-tissue changes are followed by intramedullary destruction, usually in a permeative pattern. Subsequent findings are cortical destruction, endosteal scalloping, and periosteal reaction. Radiographic changes lag behind onset of infection by 10–14 days.

33. What is the study of choice in diagnosis of suspected acute osteomyelitis?
Initial radiographic findings may be nonspecific. A 3-phase bone scan is useful in diagnosing early acute osteomyelitis. Increased activity on perfusion, blood pool, and delayed images in the areas of bony involvement are compatible with a diagnosis of osteomyelitis.

34. What is a Charcot joint?
Charcot joint, also called neuropathic joint, occurs in patients who have neurologic neuropathy secondary to diabetes mellitus, paraplegia, syphilis, leprosy, and various other peripheral neuropathies. Patients generally have lost sensations of pain and proprioception, but motion is maintained. Subtle fractures occur, along with significant degenerative changes. Radiographic features include joint destruction, significant amounts of bony debris from fractures and loose bodies, and disorganization of the joint with subluxation and dislocation.

35. What is the initial film to obtain in evaluating a patient for cervical spine trauma?
The first film to obtain is a cross-table lateral view. All seven cervical vertebrae and the upper thoracic vertebrae need to be visualized. The cervicothoracic junction is a common site of traumatic injury.

36. If the cross-table lateral view is normal, is further imaging needed?

Type I   Epiphyseal plate separation—the fracture line is in the cartilage and is not visible radiographically.

Type II   A fragment from the metaphysis is associated with the epiphyseal plate fracture; this is the most common injury.

Type III The fracture runs through the epiphysis and growth plate.

Type IV   A vertically oriented fracture extends through the epiphysis and growth plate into the metaphysis; growth arrest and joint deformities are possible complications.

Type V   Crushing injury to the epiphyseal plate; a frequent complication is shortening or angulation of the bone due to premature closure of the epiphyseal plate.

BIBLIOGRAPHY

1. Keats TE: Emergency Radiology. Chicago, Year Book, 1989.
2. Mettler FA, Guiberteau MJ: Essentials of Nuclear Medicine Imaging. Philadelphia, W.B. Saunders, 1991.
3. Resnick D, Niwayama G: Diagnosis of Bone and Joint Disorders. Philadelphia, W.B. Saunders, 1988.
4. Rockwood CA, Green DP, Bucholz RW (eds): Rockwood and Green's Fractures in ADults, 3rd ed. Philadelphia, J.B. Lippincott, 1991.
5. Rockwood CA, Wilkins KE, King RE (eds): Fractures in Children, 3rd ed. Philadelphia, J.B. Lippincott, 1991.
6. Rogers LF: Radiology of Skeletal Trauma. New York, Churchill Livingstone, 1992.

13. NUCLEAR MEDICINE

Stephanie A. Miske, M.D.

1. What is nuclear medicine?
Nuclear medicine imaging studies physiology through administration of radiolabeled drugs. Selection of radiolabeled drugs extracted by specific organs allows observation of how the organs function through recorded images of activity distribution.

2. What is a bone scan?
A bone scan uses a physiologic marker to detect abnormalities of bone metabolism. The imaging agents used are radiolabeled phosphorus-based compounds. Depending on the clinical indication, imaging may include the whole body or be limited to a specific region.

3. What is a 3-phase bone scan?

A 3-phase bone scan consists of the following:

1. A radionuclide angiogram centered over the area of interest and performed during injection;
2. Blood pool images of the area of interest obtained after injection; and
3. Delayed images obtained 2–3 hours after injection.

4. What are the scintigraphic features of osteomyelitis?

A 3-phase bone scan is needed for evaluation of possible osteomyelitis. If osteomyelitis is present, the radionuclide angiogram reveals focally increased blood flow. Blood pool and delay images also show increased activity, which is more focal on the delayed scans.

5. What scintigraphic features distinguish osteomyelitis from cellulitis?

On a 3-phase bone scan cellulitis presents as increased activity on the perfusion (radionuclide angiogram) and blood pool images. Normal activity is demonstrated on delayed images. Osteomyelitis has abnormal activity in all three phases.

6. What additional nuclear medicine examinations may be performed if bone scan findings for osteomyelitis are equivocal?

Gallium-67 citrate and leukocytes labeled with indium 111 are useful in the diagnosis of inflammatory and infectious disease of soft tissue and bone. Labeled white blood cells have a lower sensitivity than gallium in detecting chronic osteomyelitis.

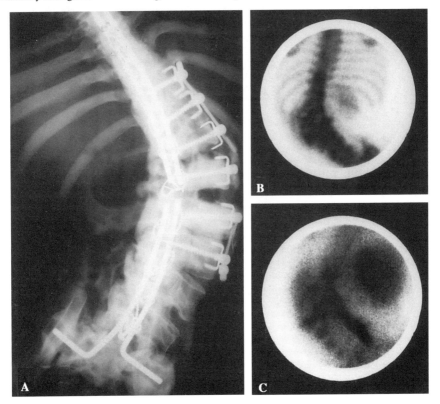

A, Patient with instrumentation of the thoracolumbar spine for scoliosis. Patient complains of fever and back pain. *B,* Bone scan delay images demonstrate multiple sites of abnormal increased activity. *C,* Gallium scan demonstrates abnormal increased activity corresponding to the left psoas muscle. Increased activity is noted in an upper lumbar vertebral body. Findings consistent with osteomyelitis and left psoas abscess.

7. Name three bones that are studied more effectively with nuclear medicine than with plain film in cases of trauma.

Nuclear medicine is more effective than plain film for studies of the three S's—sternum, scapula, and sacrum.

8. What does the H-shaped pattern of increased activity in the sacrum indicate?

Bilateral linear areas of increased activity in the sacral alae with transverse increased activity in the mid sacrum are characteristic of sacral insufficiency fractures. Osteoporosis is the most common underlying etiology.

Abnormal increased activity superior to the bladder corresponding to the sacrum. Findings are consistent with a sacral fracture, which may be an insufficiency type.

9. Which is the more sensitive in the detection of stress fractures—plain film or bone scan?

Bone scan is more sensitive in the detection of stress fractures. If the stress injury is acute, angiogram and blood pool images show increased uptake. In both acute and subacute stress fractures, delayed images show increased uptake. The activity is focal and corresponds to the area of pain.

Areas of abnormal increased activity in the right proximal tibia and left tibial shaft consistent with stress fractures in a runner.

10. Shin splints occur in the same location as tibial stress fractures—the distal third of the tibia in the posteromedial cortex. What are the scintigraphic features of shin splints?

The angiogram and blood pool images are normal. Delayed images show longitudinal linear uptake on the posteromedial tibial cortex. Involvement covers approximately one-third of the length of the bone.

11. What is osteitis pubis?

A common site of overuse inflammation is the symphysis pubis. The mechanism of injury is believed to be secondary to stress exerted on the joint by the adductor muscles when they adduct the pelvis against the foot in external rotation and abduction. The injury may be seen in runners, ballet dancers, and football, basketball, and soccer players.

12. What are the scintigraphic findings of osteitis pubis?

Bilateral increased activity at the pubic rami by the symphysis is demonstrated with osteitis pubis.

13. What is Legg-Calvé-Perthes disease?

Legg-Calvé-Perthes disease refers to primary avascular necrosis of the capital femoral epiphysis. It occurs most frequently between the ages of 5–7 years and is more common in boys. In early disease, radionuclide scanning is used to evaluate the vascular supply to the femoral head. Scintigraphic studies show a cold area in the proximal femoral epiphysis with early disease.

14. Name the other common sites of avascular necrosis.

Other common sites of avascular necrosis include the femoral head, lunate, scaphoid, body of the talus, and knee.

Left, Abnormal increased activity in left femoral head in 30-year-old male on steroids for lupus. Findings are consistent with avascular necrosis. *Right,* Plain film of left hip demonstrates early collapse of the articular surface.

15. Are the scintigraphic features always the same with osteonecrosis?

No. Scintigraphic findings vary with the stage of disease. In early disease, decreased uptake is seen. With reparative process and degenerative changes, increased activity is noted.

16. What is reflex sympathetic dystrophy syndrome (RSDS)?

Reflex sympathetic dystrophy is a syndrome characterized by pain, vasomotor instability, swelling, and dystrophic skin changes. Patients frequently report a history of trauma or injury. RSDS may follow a self-limited course or become chronic and irreversible. RSDS usually involves the upper extremity.

17. What are the scintigraphic features of RSDS?

Three-phase bone scan shows increased blood flow to the affected limb with increased activity on blood pool images. On delayed images, increased juxtaarticular activity is noted around all the joints.

18. What are the most frequent complications of hip replacement?

The most frequent complications of hip replacement are loosening of the prosthesis and infection. Other complications include dislocation, hematoma, and heterotopic bone formation. Loosening is the most common cause of pain.

19. What are the scintigraphic findings in loosening of a prosthesis?

On a bone scan, loosening of a prosthesis appears as an area of increased activity, usually at the distal aspect of the femoral component or around the shaft of the femur or acetabulum. The bone scan should be correlated with plain films. The bone scan is not reliable in the first 9–12 months after surgery.

20. Name the primary cancers that most frequently metastasize to bone.

Tumors most likely to spread to bone include breast cancer, lung cancer, prostate cancer, lymphoma, renal cell carcinoma, and thyroid cancer, both papillary and follicular. Bone scans are more sensitive than plain films in identification of metastatic disease. Whole bone images show multiple areas of abnormal increased activity.

Multiple areas of abnormal increased activity are demonstrated in a random distribution consistent with diffuse bony metastatic disease.

21. What is a superscan?

Diffuse increased uptake of activity is noted throughout the skeleton, along with a lack of renal activity and nearly complete absence of soft-tissue activity.

22. What are the causes of superscans?

Metastatic disease is the most common cause, usually from the prostate or breast. Additional etiologies include hyperparathyroidism, osteomalacia, Paget's disease, and fibrous dysplasia.

BIBLIOGRAPHY

1. Datz FL, Patch GG, Arias JM, Morton KA: Nuclear Medicine: A Teaching File. St. Louis, Mosby, 1992.
2. Fogelman I, Collier DB: An Atlas of Plenar and SPECT Bone Scans. St. Louis, Mosby, 1989.
3. Freeman LM (ed): Nuclear Medicine Annual 1997. Philadelphia, Lippincott-Raven, 1997.
4. Mettler FA, Guiberteau MJ: Essentials of Nuclear Medicine Imaging, 4th ed. Philadelphia, W.B. Saunders, 1998.

14. COMPUTED TOMOGRAPHY

Kevin L. Nelson, M.D.

1. When a complex pelvic fracture is identified on radiographs, what is the best imaging study for further evaluation and surgical planning?

Computed tomography (CT) of the pelvis provides a cross-sectional image to evaluate the degree of displacement of bone fragments as well as soft-tissue injuries, including hematomas.

2. A complex fracture of the hip is best visualized with what imaging modality?

CT provides the orthopedic surgeon with the greatest amount of information about the extent of fractures, displacement, and fracture fragments within the joint space. Three-dimensional CT images may also enhance the anatomic depiction of the fractures.

3. A suspected acute fracture of the sacrum that cannot be defined on plain films is probably best imaged with what modality?

CT is the preferred modality. Acute fractures may not be identified on nuclear medicine bone scans for several days.

Sacral stress fracture. Axial CT image reveals an acute fracture of the sacrum that could not be demonstrated on radiographs.

4. A fracture dislocation of the sternoclavicular joint is best defined with what imaging modality?

CT is more rapid and accurate in identifying fractures of the sternoclavicular joint than plain radiographs. Subtle fractures or dislocations are easily ascertained, and underlying mediastinal trauma also may be evaluated with CT.

5. Complex fractures of the foot such as the Lisfranc fractures are best evaluated by what imaging methods?

The preferred protocol is plain radiographs followed by CT reformatted in the coronal plane.

6. After radiographs, what additional studies are useful for evaluation of tarsal coalition?

CT is the most appropriate imaging study, particularly to define the bony coalition and to identify facets. CT indirectly images fibrous coalitions by demonstrating irregular or roughened cortical surfaces. Magnetic resonance imaging (MRI) is becoming increasingly useful in tarsal coalition because of its direct multiplanar imaging capabilities.

7. A suspected fracture of the triquetrum not identified on plain radiographs is best defined on what imaging study?

CT is generally more useful in displaying fracture morphology and cortical detail than MRI.

8. What is the best imaging study to obtain in a case of a suspected cartilaginous intraarticular loose body in a joint?

CT arthrography or MRI is the preferred study. MR arthrography is also useful; however, the Food and Drug Administration (FDA) has approved no MR contrast agent for intraarticular use.

9. What is the most sensitive imaging modality for evaluation of glenoid labral tears?

CT arthrography or MR arthrography are probably more sensitive in detecting glenoid labrum tears than routine MRI alone. Sensitivity for detection of glenoid labral tears by CT or MR arthrography is believed to be greater than 95%.

10. What is the imaging procedure of choice for identifying a suspected lumbar disc herniation?

This issue is controversial. There is little disagreement, however, that MRI is more sensitive in identifying early changes in degenerative disc disease and offers the added advantage of direct sagittal imaging. CT, however, is a highly sensitive test for identifying a suspected lumbar disc herniation (see figure, top of next page) and is generally less expensive than MRI. CT offers the added advantage of superior cortical bone detail (see figure, middle of next page). In some instances, the examinations are complementary, and both may be needed.

11. What is the appropriate imaging modality for evaluating the patient with recurrent low back pain after lumbar discectomy?

Contrast-enhanced MRI is more accurate than CT in differentiating recurrent nonenhancing lumbar disc herniation from enhancing postoperative epidural scar. Other etiologies of recurrent low back pain may include spinal stenosis, which is effectively evaluated with MRI, and arachnoiditis, which also is evaluated more effectively with MRI than with CT.

12. What is the most sensitive imaging examination for identifying a cervical disc herniation?

Although MRI is an excellent screening examination, postmyelogram thin-section CT is considered by many to be the most sensitive imaging study to identify subtle cervical disc herniations (see figure, bottom of next page).

13. What imaging modality is appropriate in the clinical setting of cervical spine trauma when plain radiographs are equivocal but suspicious for fracture?

Thin-section CT of the suspected area is the modality of choice.

Normal lumbar discs *(top, left)*. Axial CT scan at the level of the lumbar intervertebral discs shows the posterior margin of the intermediate density disc *(arrows)* is confined to the posterior margin of the vertebral body with no abnormal protrusion of the disc.

Lumbar disc herniation *(top, right)*. Axial CT scan at the level of the lumbar intervertebral disc reveals an abnormal protrusion of the disc *(arrow)*.

Central lumbar spinal canal stenosis *(right)*. Axial CT scan at the level of the lumbar intervertebral disc shows narrowing of the central spinal canal. There is hypertrophy of the ligamentum flavum *(arrows)* and low-density vacuum *(arrowhead)* in the nucleus pulposus of the degenerated disc. CT is very useful in evaluating suspected lumbar spinal stenosis due to eloquent definition of bony encroachment of the spinal canal.

Cervical disc herniation. Axial CT image at the level of the cervical intervertebral disc following myelography reveals a cervical disc herniation *(arrow)* compressing the high-density myelogram contrast agent that has been placed in the intradural space.

14. If a spinal cord contusion is suspected after cervical spine trauma, what is the appropriate imaging study?

MRI is the study of choice. Although CT provides high-resolution bone detail of the osseous elements, the intradural structures, including the cervical spinal cord, are best imaged with MRI.

15. What is the best imaging modality for identifying a pseudarthrosis in the patient who has undergone a bone fusion of the lumbar spine?

CT is the modality of choice. Plain radiographs in flexion and extension are also useful to define the degree of instability.

16. What are the two types of spondylolisthesis?

The two types are lytic and degenerative spondylolisthesis. **Lytic spondylolisthesis** is due to bilateral fractures or congenital defects in the pars intraarticularis (classically described as the "collar on the neck of the Scottie dog" on oblique plain radiographs of the lumbar spine). Lytic spondylolisthesis results in posterior displacement of the superior vertebral body with respect to the inferior vertebral body. **Degenerative spondylolisthesis** is due to degenerative erosion of the superior facet of the inferior vertebral body. Such erosion allows forward movement of the inferior facet of the superior vertebral body and results in spondylolisthesis. CT scanning can document the degree of displacement and the pars intraarticularis defects.

17. A suspected soft-tissue mass in the extremity is best evaluated first with what imaging modality?

With direct multiplanar imaging capabilities and excellent soft-tissue discrimination, MRI is the initial imaging modality of choice in evaluating soft-tissue masses in an extremity. CT usually is reserved for cases that require a clearer depiction of bony detail.

BIBLIOGRAPHY

1. Greenfield GB (ed): Radiology of Bone Diseases, 5th ed. Philadelphia, Lippincott-Raven, 1990.
2. Lee JKT, Sagel SS, Stanley RJ, Heiken JP (eds): Computed Body Tomography with MRI Correlation, 3rd ed. Philadelphia, Lippincott-Raven, 1997.
3. Magid D, Fishman EK, Gregerman MB (eds): Computed Tomography with Multiplanar Reconstructions: An Atlas of the Normal and Abnormal Hip. New York, Field & Wood, 1989.
4. Resnick D (ed): Diagnosis of Bone and Joint Disorders, 3rd ed. Philadelphia, W.B. Saunders, 1995.
5. Stiles RG, Otto MT: Imaging of the shoulder. Radiology 188:603–613, 1993.

15. MAGNETIC RESONANCE IMAGING

Kevin L. Nelson, M.D.

1. What pulse sequences are most commonly used in magnetic resonance imaging (MRI) of the musculoskeletal system?

Conventional spin-echo T1-weighted, proton density, and T2-weighted images are used most often. Gradient-echo and inversion recovery (STIR) images are also common.

2. What are the absolute contraindications to MRI?

Patients with an internal cardiac pacemaker, brain aneurysm clip, metallic foreign body in the eye, cochlear implant, and surgically implanted drug infusion pumps, neurostimulators, or bone growth stimulators cannot undergo MRI.

3. May a patient who has a metallic hip or knee prosthesis undergo an MRI examination?
Yes. Metallic distortion artifact may cause signal void on MR images of anatomic structures in the immediate region of the metal implant. If the patient has a hip or knee prosthesis in place, the contralateral hip or knee can be readily imaged with MRI. Orthopedic screws or wire usually do not cause significant distortion of the MR signal. For example, an anterior cruciate ligament reconstruction stabilized with metallic screws usually can be well visualized with MRI.

4. What is the accuracy rate of MRI in detecting meniscal tears of the knee?
The accuracy rate of MRI in detecting meniscal tears is greater than 90% in most series. With three-dimensional imaging the rate of concurrence between MRI and arthroscopy is 95%.

5. What is the normal MRI appearance of a meniscus?
The intact meniscus demonstrates homogeneous low signal intensity on all pulse sequences.

Normal medial meniscus. The normal meniscus demonstrates homogeneous low signal intensity on this sagittal proton-density-weighted image. The anterior *(short arrow)* and posterior *(long arrow)* horns are triangular in configuration and sharply marginated.

6. How many grades of abnormal signal intensity are used to classify an abnormal meniscus on MRI?
There are three grades of abnormal signal intensity. Grade 1, which correlates with globular foci of early mucinous degeneration, may be observed in normal volunteers and has no clinical significance. Grade 2 is a linear horizontal area of increased signal intensity that does not extend to an articular surface but may contact a capsular margin. Grade 1 and 2 menisci are arthroscopically normal. An abnormal signal intensity that extends to an articular surface is considered grade 3, which represents a torn meniscus and is visible at arthroscopy.

Torn posterior horn medial meniscus. The sagittal proton-density–weighted image reveals abnormal grade III high-signal intensity *(arrow)* in the posterior horn of the medial meniscus, which extends in an oblique fashion to the inferior or tibial articular surface of the meniscus. This tear was confirmed at arthroscopy.

7. What is a discoid meniscus of the knee? What are the complications of a discoid meniscus?

A discoid meniscus is a dysplastic meniscus that has a broad, disclike configuration. Lateral discoid menisci are more common than medial discoid menisci. Complications include tears and cysts.

8. What is the appearance of an anterior cruciate ligament (ACL) tear on MRI?

A complete tear results in nonvisualization of the normal low-signal–intensity ACL. If the tear is acute, the MRI usually shows an effusion in the joint space and an edematous pseudomass where the ACL is normally visualized. Most tears occur in the mid to proximal portion of the ACL. If the tear is chronic, the ACL is not visualized in its normal oblique course, and the distal portion of the remaining intact ACL may be seen lying inferiorly within the joint.

Normal anterior cruciate ligament *(left)*. The normal anterior cruciate ligament is identified as a low-signal band *(arrows)* on this sagittal proton-density–weighted image.

Torn anterior cruciate ligament *(right)*. As compared with the normal anterior cruciate ligament seen at left, the torn anterior cruciate ligament *(arrow)* is identified lying inferiorly in the knee joint space on the sagittal proton-density–weighted image. The normal posterior cruciate ligament *(open arrow)* is also visualized.

9. Certain bone contusions of the knee are commonly associated with a complete tear of the ACL. Where are these contusions located?

Bone contusions of the knee commonly associated with a complete tear of the ACL are located on the posterolateral tibial plateau and lateral femoral condyle, presumably because of impaction of the lateral femoral condyle into the posterior tibia during injury.

10. Chondromalacia patella is usually best defined on which MR pulse sequence and plane?

Axial T2-weighted or gradient-echo T2 images usually offer the best depiction of the changes of chondromalacia patella.

11. Which pathologic findings of a lateral patellar dislocation may be demonstrated with MRI?

- Torn medial retinaculum
- Osteochondral fracture of the patella
- Impaction bone bruise of the lateral femoral condyle
- Lateral subluxation of the patella
- Joint effusion and dysplastic patella without a medial facet
- Shallow or hypoplastic femoral groove

12. Where is osteochondritis dissecans of the knee classically located?

Osteochondritis dissecans of the knee is classically located in the non–weight-bearing lateral aspect of the medial femoral condyle. It is usually seen in men, and up to 50% of patients may have a history of trauma. Early osteochondritis dissecans is best visualized with MRI.

13. A complete rupture of the medial collateral ligament is often associated with what other injuries of the knee that can be visualized on MRI?

Complete tears of the medial collateral ligament may be associated with tears of the anterior cruciate ligament, medial meniscus, or medial and posterior capsule of the knee as well as impaction injuries of the lateral femoral condyle and lateral tibial plateau.

14. What is the best imaging modality for evaluation of a suspected popliteal fossa mass?

MRI accurately differentiates most popliteal fossa masses, including cysts, aneurysms, and soft-tissue masses.

15. What is the imaging procedure of choice for early detection of avascular necrosis (AVN) of the femoral head?

MRI is reported to be the most sensitive imaging modality for differentiating AVN from non-AVN of the femoral head with a specificity of 98% and a sensitivity of 97% (see figures, below). In addition to MRI, nuclear scintigraphy with technetium-99m–labeled phosphate compounds is the second most sensitive imaging modality. Radiographs become positive in later stages of AVN (see figure, top of next page). Early diagnosis is critical because all treatment procedures are more successful in the initial stages of AVN.

Normal hips *(top, left)*. On this coronal T1-weighted image, the normal femoral heads demonstrate high-signal intensity fat in the bone marrow space.

Early avascular necrosis femoral head *(top, right)*. Compared with figure at left, this patient shows early changes of avascular necrosis of the femoral head. Abnormal low-signal intensity *(arrowheads)* observed in the femoral head is indicative of early avascular necrosis.

Late changes of avascular necrosis humeral head *(right)*. More advanced changes of avascular necrosis are demonstrated in the humeral head of this patient. Multiple loose fragments *(arrows)*, which are surrounded by a rim of high-signal–intensity fluid *(curved arrows)*, are seen on the sagittal T2-weighted image.

16. What imaging study is appropriate when a nondisplaced femoral neck fracture is suspected clinically but radiographs are negative?

MRI is useful in identifying nondisplaced femoral neck fractures that cannot be detected on routine radiographs. Although bone scintigraphy is also useful, it is not as specific. MRI is able to depict the morphology of the nondisplaced fracture more accurately than bone scintigraphy.

17. What nerve is entrapped or compressed in the tarsal tunnel syndrome?

In the tarsal tunnel syndrome the posterior tibial nerve is entrapped or compressed. Etiologies of this compression neuropathy that can be effectively imaged with MRI include neuromas, ganglion cysts, lipomas, varicose veins, and tenosynovitis.

18. What is the most likely tendon to be torn in the patient presenting with a unilateral flat-foot deformity?

The tibialis posterior tendon is the most likely candidate. MRI is the best imaging modality to confirm a partial or complete tear of the tendon.

19. What is the most common site of rupture of the Achilles tendon?

The Achilles tendon is most susceptible to rupture 2–6 cm above the os calcis. Because rupture may be missed on clinical examination in up to 25% of patients, MRI is invaluable in confirming the diagnosis.

20. The rotator cuff comprises which muscles?

The SIT muscles (supraspinatus, infraspinatus, teres minor) and the subscapularis muscle.

21. Which tendon of the rotator cuff is most likely to tear first?

The tear usually begins along the anterolateral leading edge of the supraspinatus tendon at its insertion into the greater tuberosity of the humerus.

22. Describe the difference between a partial-thickness and full-thickness tear of the rotator cuff.

A full-thickness tear extends through the entire width of the tendon and appears as an area of high signal intensity, approximating fluid, on T2-weighted MR images (see figure, top of next page). A partial-thickness tear does not extend through the width of the tendon. It may involve either the inferior or articular surface or the superior or bursal surface of the tendon. Partial-thickness tears can—and probably often do—progress to full-thickness tears.

23. How are abnormal tendons of the rotator cuff classified on MRI?

There are three grades of abnormal rotator cuff tendons. Grade 1 tendinitis demonstrates normal morphology of the tendon with high signal intensity on T1-weighted images and normal low signal intensity on T2-weighted images. Grade 2 lesions are partial-thickness tears on either the articular or bursal surface of the tendon and are seen as high-signal–intensity lesions on T2-weighted images. Grade 3 lesions are full-thickness tears that show a high-signal–intensity gap in the tendon on T2-weighted images.

24. What important abnormal anatomic etiologies of impingement syndrome of the shoulder can be effectively imaged with MRI?
- Shape and slope of the acromion process
- Subacromial osteophytes
- Morphology of the acromioclavicular joint

25. Which pathologic bone and soft-tissue lesions of recurrent anterior dislocations of the shoulder can be demonstrated on MRI?

The bone lesions are a Hill-Sachs deformity of the humeral head and a fracture of the inferior glenoid. The soft-tissue lesions are tears of the anterior glenoid labrum and anterior capsule.

Normal supraspinatus muscle and supraspinatus tendon *(left)*. A normal supraspinatus muscle *(open arrows)* and low-signal–intensity supraspinatus tendon *(arrow)* are seen on this coronal T2-weighted image.

Full-thickness tear supraspinatus tendon *(right)*. A coronal T2-weighted image demonstrates a large full-thickness tear of the supraspinatus tendon. The torn supraspinatus tendon *(arrowhead)* is retracted from its normal insertion on the humeral head and is surrounded by high-signal–intensity fluid. The humeral head is also noted to be superiorly subluxed in the glenoid fossa *(arrows)*.

26. What is the site of insertion of the biceps tendon in the elbow? What is the appropriate imaging modality when a torn biceps tendon is suspected?

The biceps tendon inserts at the tuberosity of the radius. Partial- or full-thickness tears of the tendon are best imaged with MRI.

27. What is the most common appearance of avascular necrosis of the scaphoid on MRI?

The most common appearance of AVN of the scaphoid is low signal intensity on both T1- and T2-weighted images. Occasionally an increased signal on T2-weighted images may be noted because of marrow edema and local fluid accumulation.

28. What carpal bone is affected by Kienböck's disease?

Kienböck's disease is avascular necrosis of the lunate. MRI is the imaging modality of choice in diagnosing Kienböck's disease.

Kienböck's disease. Compared with the other normal high-signal–intensity carpal bones of the wrist on this coronal T1-weighted image, the lunate demonstrates low signal intensity *(arrow)* as a result of avascular necrosis.

29. What is the imaging procedure of choice to identify a suspected lesion of the brachial plexus?

The procedure of choice is MRI.

30. What is the first imaging modality to order in screening for pathology of the cervical or thoracic spine?

MRI provides the most information in a single imaging examination for pathology of the cervical and thoracic spine. Both the extradural structures, including the vertebra and intervertebral discs, and the intradural anatomy, including the spinal cord, are clearly depicted on MRI.

31. For evaluating congenital abnormalities of the pediatric spine, what is the first imaging study to order?

Plain radiographs always should be obtained first to evaluate bony anatomy for such abnormalities as spina bifida, butterfly vertebra, or other congenital bony abnormalities. MRI is commonly used next for evaluating the neural elements of the spine for abnormalities such as myelomeningocele, tethered cord, syrinx, diastematomyelia, and other congenital abnormalities of the neural elements.

32. What is the first imaging modality to order in evaluating spinal infections?

The first imaging modality to order for discitis, vertebral osteomyelitis, and epidural abscess is MRI.

33. What is the best imaging modality for evaluating bone marrow?

MRI directly images bone marrow and is highly sensitive in detecting early disease such as metastases, lymphoma, and myeloma. Nuclear bone scintigraphy is the best modality in screening for metastatic disease in the asymptomatic patient with a known malignancy.

34. Is MRI able to differentiate confidently between benign and malignant lesions of soft tissue and bone?

No. No specific characteristic of MR signal intensity determines whether the lesion is benign or malignant. If the mass is extensive and has poorly circumscribed margins involving soft tissue, bone, and the neurovascular bundle, it is more likely to be malignant.

Rhabdomyosarcoma. A large heterogeneous signal intensity mass *(arrows)* is demonstrated in the gluteal muscles.

BIBLIOGRAPHY

1. Berquist TH (ed): MRI of the Musculoskeletal System, 3rd ed. Philadelphia, Lippincott-Raven, 1996.
2. Deutsch AL, Mink JH, Kerr R (eds): MRI of the Foot and Ankle. New York, Raven Press, 1992.
3. Mink JH, Reicher MA, Crues JV III, Deutsch AL (eds): MRI of the Knee. New York, Raven Press, 1993.
4. Reicher MA, Kellerhouse LE (eds): MRI of the Wrist and Hand. New York, Raven Press, 1990.
5. Stoller DW (ed): Magnetic Resonance Imaging in Orthopaedics and Sports Medicine, 2nd ed. Philadelphia, Lippincott-Raven, 1997.
6. Uri DS: MR imaging of shoulder impingement and rotator cuff disease. Radiol Clin North Am 35:77, 1997.
7. Virolainen H, Visuri T, Kuusela T: Acute dislocation of the patella: MR findings. Radiology 189:243–246, 1993.
8. Zlatkin MB (ed): MRI of the Shoulder. New York, Raven Press, 1991.

16. MULTIPLE TRAUMA

Matthew A. Mormino, M.D.

1. How should a patient with multiple injuries be evaluated?

All trauma patients should be evaluated using standard ATLS protocols, which include the ABCDE of initial evaluation: **a**irway, **b**reathing, **c**irculation, **d**isability (neurologic evaluation), and **e**xposure (undress the patient). The primary survey is followed by a secondary survey to identify non–life-threatening injuries.

2. Which radiographs are required in the initial assessment of a trauma patient?

Initial films include an anteroposterior (AP) view of the chest, an AP of the pelvis, and a lateral view of the cervical spine.

3. What is the "golden hour" of trauma management?

Death from trauma has a trimodal distribution. The first peak is within the first seconds to minutes after injury. Very few such patients can be saved due to the severity of their injuries. The second peak is within the next few hours. The first hour of care following injury is characterized by the rapid assessment and repair of life-threatening injuries. Within this "golden hour" an organized trauma system can have the greatest impact on patient outcome. The third death peak occurs within several days or weeks of injury and is most often due to sepsis and multiorgan failure.

4. How should an unstable pelvic fracture be managed acutely in a patient with hemodynamic instability?

The unstable pelvis is most easily stabilized in the emergency room by binding the pelvis with a sheet. This method may temporarily reduce pelvic volume and promote tamponade until more definitive measures can be taken. The emergent application of an external fixator and angiographic arterial embolization are more definitive ways to address hemodynamic instability in a patient with a pelvic fracture.

5. What does MAST stand for?

Military antishock trousers (MAST) were developed to stabilize shock victims during transport. The idea was to put compression on the lower extremities to shunt blood to more vital organs. The use of MAST is controversial because of associated complications (e.g., compartment syndrome, skin slough).

6. What is the best way to control external hemorrhage?

External bleeding is best controlled by direct pressure. The use of tourniquets and clamping should be avoided.

7. What noninvasive methods are available to evaluate the vascular status of an extremity?

The vascular status of an injured extremity can be evaluated by palpation of pulses, Doppler examination of pulses, and the ankle brachial index (ABI). The ABI is the ratio of the arterial occlusive pressure of the arm versus the ankle. If the ABI is ≤ 90%, further vascular work-up should be considered.

8. What should be done with a pulseless and deformed extremity?

The extremity should be gently realigned, the pulses should be re-evaluated, and the extremity should be splinted.

9. When should long bone fractures be stabilized?

Several studies have shown that long bone fractures should be stabilized within the first 24 hours. Such studies also demonstrate decreased rates of sepsis, acute respiratory distress syndrome (ARDS), pneumonia, and mortality in patients who had early skeletal stabilization.

10. Describe fat embolism syndrome.

The systemic release of intramedullary fat droplets and the cellular responses to them cause this syndrome. Patients with long bone fractures may develop a syndrome manifested by mental status changes, petechiae, and decreased O_2 saturation. Treatment is respiratory support. The syndrome is prevented by early skeletal stabilization.

11. What is the incidence of deep venous thrombosis (DVT) in patients with multiple trauma and lower extremity or pelvic fractures?

Depending on the screening method, the incidence of DVT in such patients is between 40% and 80%. Early patient mobilization and prophylactic measures, such as sequential compression stockings and subcutaneous low–molecular-weight heparin, have reduced its incidence. The use of vena cava filters to reduce the incidence of fatal pulmonary embolism in selected high-risk patients has gained popularity.

12. How is a patient's cervical spine best immobilized for transport?

In patients with a suspected cervical spine injury, the neck should be immobilized in a Philadelphia-type collar and further supported by sandbags and taping the head to a spine board. A Philadelphia-type collar limits approximately 40% of rotary motion and 60% of flexion/extension motion.

13. List the clinical signs suggestive of a cervical spinal cord injury in an unconscious patient.

In an unconscious patient in whom the mechanism of injury was a fall or a motor vehicle accident, incidence of cervical spine injury is 5–10%. Clinical signs include:

 • Flaccid areflexia, especially with flaccid rectal tone
 • Diaphragmatic breathing
 • Ability to flex but not extend the elbow
 • A response to painful stimulus above but not below the clavicle
 • Hypotension with bradycardia
 • Priapism

14. How is spinal shock characterized?

Shortly after spinal cord injury the cord may appear completely functionless, even though some areas are not completely destroyed. This produces flaccidity and areflexia instead of spasticity and hyperreflexia. Days to weeks later, spinal shock resolves; in areas of permanent loss, spasticity replaces the flaccidity. The return of the bulbocavernosus reflex (anal sphincter contraction with a gentle tug on the Foley catheter) frequently signifies the end of spinal shock.

15. Describe neurogenic shock.

Injury to the descending sympathetic pathways in the spinal cord results in loss of vasomotor tone and sympathetic innervation to the heart, which in turn results in vasodilitation and pooling of the blood in the extremities and viscera. The patient fails to become tachycardic or may become bradycardic as a result of loss of sympathetic innervation to the heart. The hallmark of neurogenic shock is bradycardia in the presence of hypertension.

BIBLIOGRAPHY

1. Alexander RH, Proctor HJ: ATLS Student Manual, 3rd ed. Chicago, American College of Surgeons, 1993.
2. Bone LB, Johnson KD, Weigelt J: Early versus delayed stabilization of femoral fractures: A prospective randomized study. J Bone Joint Surg 71A:336, 1989.
3. Bosse MJ, et al: Adult respiratory distress syndrome, pneumonia, and mortality following thoracic injury and a femoral fracture treated either with intramedullary nailing with reaming or with a plate. A comparative study. J Bone Joint Surg 79A:799, 1997.
4. Hansen ST Jr, Swiontkowski MF: Orthopaedic Trauma Protocols. New York, Raven, 1993.

17. BONE TUMORS

Brian E. Brigman, M.D., and James R. Neff, M.D.

1. What is the difference between a sarcoma and a carcinoma?

A sarcoma (*Sar* = Greek for "fleshy") is a malignancy arising in mesenchymal tissue (fibrous tissue, muscle, bone, adipose). A carcinoma arises from an epithelial cell origin. Sarcomas typically metastasize hematogenously, whereas carcinomas typically metastasize through the lymphatic system.

2. How common are primary malignant tumors of bone?

They are rare. About 2000 new primary malignant tumors of bone (excluding multiple myeloma) are diagnosed in the United States yearly.

3. What factors predispose someone to a malignant tumor of bone?

Radiation treatment	p53 mutations	Multiple hereditary exostoses
Chemotherapeutic treatment	Retinoblastoma	Langer-Giedion syndrome
Neurofibromatosis	Maffuci syndrome	Defect-11 syndrome
Paget's disease	Ollier's disease	Gardner's syndrome
Li-Fraumeni syndrome		

4. How are tumors of the musculoskeletal system staged?

Enneking developed a system of staging for musculoskeletal tumors based on biologic aggressiveness, anatomic site, and metastases. Biologic aggressiveness, or Grade (G), is an assessment of histologic grade, radiographic classification, and clinical course. Tumors are stratified into benign (G0), low-grade malignant (G1), and high-grade malignant (G2) categories based on these criteria. Anatomic site (T) places tumors into intracompartmental (T1) and extracompartmental (T2) groups. Intracompartmental tumors are contained within an anatomic compartment that serves as a natural barrier to tumor extension. These natural barriers include cortical bone, articular cartilage, joint capsule, and fascia. Extracompartmental tumors span at least one of these natural barriers. Tumors that have either regional or distant metastases are labeled M1, and those with no metastases are designated M0.

Benign lesions (G0) are staged into one of three groups. Benign stage 1 lesions are latent, static lesions. Benign stage 2 lesions are progressive, and may expand a fascial or cortical margin but do not broach it. Benign stage 3 lesions are aggressive and have breached compartments or have metastasized.

Malignant lesions without metastases are grouped into stage I (G1) or stage II (G2). Malignant lesions of either grade with local or distant metastases are grouped into stage III. Each of these malignant stages is further stratified based on anatomic site. Intracompartmental lesions are staged "A," and extracompartmental lesions are staged "B."

STAGE	IA	IB	IIA	IIB	IIIA	IIIB
Grade	G1	G1	G2	G2	G1 or G2	G1 or G2
Site	T1	T2	T1	T2	T1	T2
Metastases	M0	M0	M0	M0	M1	M1

5. Name some benign (G0), low-grade malignant (G1), and high-grade malignant (G2) bone lesions.

BENIGN (G0)	LOW-GRADE MALIGNANT (G1)	HIGH-GRADE MALIGNANT (G2)
Nonossifying fibroma	Parosteal osteosarcoma	Classic osteosarcoma
Osteoid osteoma	Periosteal osteosarcoma	Telangiectatic osteosarcoma
Osteoblastoma	Secondary chondrosarcoma	Primary chondrosarcoma
Enchondroma	Clear cell chondrosarcoma	Dedifferentiated chondrosarcoma
Osteochondroma	Adamantinoma	Fibrosarcoma
Chondroblastoma	Hemangioendothelioma	Malignant fibrous histiocytoma
Aneurysmal bone cyst	Chordoma	Ewing's sarcoma
	Giant cell tumor	

6. Discuss the principles for biopsy of musculoskeletal tumors.

Biopsy of musculoskeletal tumors should generally be relegated to the surgeon responsible for the final management of the tumor. An improperly placed biopsy incision may compromise the final outcome of treatment. Needle biopsy has the advantages of less morbidity and lower cost, but may not provide sufficient tissue for a diagnosis and is subject to sampling error. Excisional biopsy may be considered with small, benign appearing lesions. Open incisional biopsy should be planned with the definitive surgical procedure in mind, because the biopsy tract will be considered contaminated and necessarily will be removed en bloc with the tumor at the time of tumor excision. Transverse incisions should be avoided, and the biopsy should traverse the minimum number of compartments. Neurovascular structures should be avoided. The biopsy specimen should be taken from the periphery of the soft-tissue extension of the tumor. If there is no soft-tissue extension, a small round or oval window in the cortex should be fashioned to decrease the risk of pathologic fracture. A tourniquet should be used and meticulous hemostasis must be obtained.

7. Do sarcomas have a capsule?

Sarcomas do not have a true capsule. As they grow radially they compress adjacent tissue into a pseudocapsule. This pseudocapsule contains the zone of compression and a surrounding reactive zone made up of neovascular tissue and an inflammatory infiltrate.

8. Describe orthopaedic oncologic surgical margins.

There are four types of musculoskeletal surgical margins. An **intralesional margin** has a plane of dissection through the tumor; by definition, tumor is left behind. A **marginal margin** has a plane of dissection through the reactive zone of the pseudocapsule and may have left microscopic tumor behind. A **wide margin** is through completely normal tissue outside of the reactive zone and potentially may leave "skip" metastases behind. A **radical margin** is a complete excision of the affected compartment.

9. Which tumors make bone?

Only three tumors make bone. Osteoid osteoma and osteoblastoma are benign bone-forming tumors. A malignant bone-forming tumor is an osteosarcoma.

10. What is an osteoid osteoma? How does it present?

An osteoid osteoma is a benign osteoblastic lesion characterized by a well-demarcated central nidus of ≤ 1.5 cm surrounded by dense reactive bone. It typically occurs in the metaphyseal regions of long bones or in the posterior elements of the spine in patients aged 5–30 years. Patients present with pain that increases over time. It is typically worse at night and is characteristically relieved by salicylates or other NSAIDs. Lesions in the posterior elements of the spine can produce a painful scoliosis.

11. What are the treatment options for osteoid osteoma?

Surgical treatment by en bloc excision of the nidus or intralesional curettage has been the mainstay of treatment. A percutaneous radiofrequency ablative treatment has recently been described but is not a viable option for lesions in the spine. Medical treatment with NSAIDs is also an option.

12. Describe the difference between an osteoid osteoma and an osteoblastoma.

An osteoblastoma is larger than an osteoid osteoma and often does not have a rim of reactive bone around it. Both are common in the posterior element of the spine. Treatment of osteoblastoma is surgical excision.

OSTEOCHONDROMA AND ENCHONDROMA

13. Name the benign cartilage-forming tumors of the musculoskeletal system.

Osteochondroma, enchondroma, chondroblastoma, and chondromyxoid fibroma.

14. What is an osteochondroma? How does it present?

An osteochondroma is a benign, cartilage-capped cortical exostosis in the metaphyseal or epiphyseal region of bone. The most common sites are distal femur, proximal tibia, proximal humerus, distal radius, and distal tibia. Osteochondromas are thought to arise as the result of aberrant growth plate cartilage and grow through enchondral ossification until the growth plate from which they arose stops growing. They exist in sessile and pedunculated forms, and in each case the cortical margins of the osteochondroma are continuous with the cortical margin of the underlying bone. Osteochondromas are painless and are usually symptomless unless they are palpable. Occasionally neurovascular compression by an osteochondroma causes symptoms. A painful osteochondroma may signify a fracture of the lesion or malignant degeneration, typically to a low-grade chondrosarcoma. Malignant degeneration occurs in < 1% of osteochondromas. An autosomal dominant hereditary form (multiple hereditary exostoses) represents about 10% of patients with osteochondroma.

15. What is the treatment of osteochondroma?

Surgical excision is necessary only if the lesions become symptomatic or disfiguring.

16. What is an enchondroma?

An enchondroma is a benign island of mature cartilage within a bone, typically in the metaphyseal area. When located on the surface of the bone, it is termed a *periosteal chondroma*. It is the most common primary tumor of bone in the hand, but any bone can be affected. Enchondromas are usually asymptomatic.

17. What is the treatment for enchondroma?

Observation is the mainstay of treatment. If lesions grow or are painful, then en bloc excision or curettage is indicated.

18. What are Ollier's disease and Mafucci syndrome?

Ollier's disease is an eponym for multiple enchondromatosis. Lesions are often unilateral and may result in a dysplastic appearance to bones. There is a 30% risk of sarcomatous degeneration to chondrosarcoma in patients with Ollier's disease.

Maffuci syndrome is multiple enchondromas with associated soft-tissue angiomas. There is a 100% risk of sarcomatous degeneration to chondrosarcoma in patients with Maffuci syndrome.

Both Ollier's disease and Mafucci syndrome patients carry an increased risk of visceral malignancy, including gastrointestinal adenocarcinoma and astrocytoma.

CHONDROBLASTOMA AND GIANT CELL TUMOR

19. What is a chondroblastoma?

A chondroblastoma is a benign tumor characteristically located in the epiphysis or in an apophysis. Chondroblastomas typically affect people in their second decade of life. They are often painful and may limit joint motion. Histologically, the stromal cells of chondroblastomas are polyhedral with clear halos around the nuclei resulting in the characteristic "chicken wire" appearance. About 2% of chondroblastomas are metastatic to the lungs.

20. What is the treatment for chondroblastoma?

Intralesional curettage with bone grafting or cementage yields an approximate 10% recurrence rate.

21. What other tumor has a predilection for the end of a long bone?

Giant cell tumor.

22. What is the cell of origin for giant cell tumor, Ewing's sarcoma, and adamantinoma?

The cell of origin for each is unknown.

23. The histologic slide has giant cells on it. Doesn't that mean it is a giant cell tumor?

No. Many tumors, ranging from benign osteoid osteoma to malignant osteosarcoma, may contain giant cells.

24. Who gets giant cell tumors?

Giant cell tumor typically affects patients between 20 and 60 years of age. It is one of the few tumors that occur more commonly in women than in men. About one-half occur around the knee. Patients usually present with pain in the affected area. About 2% of giant cell tumors are metastatic to the lung.

25. What is the treatment for giant cell tumor?

Intralesional curettage with cementing or bone grafting gives local control in about 80% of patients.

CHONDROSARCOMA

26. What is a chondrosarcoma? How does it present?

A chondrosarcoma is a malignant, cartilage-forming tumor. It occurs in patients ≥ 30 years of age. Common sites include the pelvis (30%), proximal and distal femur, ribs, proximal humerus, and proximal tibia. Patients typically present with pain or a mass. Pelvic lesions are often misdiagnosed or diagnosed late.

27. What is the difference between a primary and secondary chondrosarcoma?

A primary chondrosarcoma arises de novo in a previously normal bone. A secondary chondrosarcoma arises from preexisting benign cartilage lesion, such as an enchondroma or osteochondroma. Primary chondrosarcomas may be low- or high-grade tumors. Secondary tumors are almost always low grade.

28. What is the most common stage of chondrosarcoma at presentation?
IA.

29. What is the treatment for chondrosarcoma?
Most lesions are low grade; therefore, chemotherapy is not necessary. Excision with a wide margin is standard treatment.

OSTEOSARCOMA

30. What is an osteosarcoma? How does it present?
An osteosarcoma is a malignant tumor that produces osteoid. Osteosarcomas are typically found in metaphyseal locations. More than one-half occur about the knee. Patients present with pain, a mass, or occasionally a pathologic fracture. It typically affects patients in their second or third decade, although there is a second peak of incidence in patients > 60 years old, usually with secondary osteosarcoma. Approximately 1000 new cases of osteosarcoma are diagnosed in the United States yearly.

31. What is the most common stage of osteosarcoma at presentation?
IIB (70%). About 20% are stage III.

32. What is a secondary osteosarcoma?
A secondary osteosarcoma develops in abnormal bone and is usually associated with irradiated bone, Paget's disease, or fibrous dysplasia. Secondary osteosarcomas are typically high-grade malignancies.

33. What are the radiographic findings of osteosarcoma?
Plain films often reveal permeative lesion with cortical destruction. Codman's triangles of bone appear as tumor extension elevates periosteum from the underlying bone. Cortical soft-tissue extension may produce radiating spicules of bone, resulting in the characteristic "sun ray" appearance.

34. What other imaging studies should be ordered?
At a minimum, an MRI of the region to assess soft-tissue extension and rule out skip lesions and a CT scan of the chest to rule out metastatic disease to the lungs should be obtained. Techniques to evaluate for extrapulmonary metastases include ^{99}Tc scintigraphy or rapid whole body STIR MRI.

35. What is the treatment for osteosarcoma?
Patients with high-grade tumors are subjected to a high-dose chemotherapeutic protocol, undergo wide or radical tumor excision, and may be subjected to a second chemotherapeutic protocol. Low-grade osteosarcomas (periosteal and parosteal) usually do not require chemotherapy.

36. What are the surgical options for osteosarcoma about the knee?
The initial decision is between amputation and limb salvage surgery. Involvement of the neurovascular bundle makes limb salvage difficult. If limb salvage is a viable option, several reconstruction methods are available following tumor excision. Fusion of the knee joint, reconstruction of the knee with a metal prosthesis, or allograft reconstruction are possible. In young children, these options are less appealing because of the resulting leg length discrepancy at maturity. In these patients an amputation, expandable prosthesis or Van Nes rotationplasty are options. A Van

Nes rotationplasty fuses the shortened femur to the shortened tibia after rotation of the tibia 180°
to allow the ankle joint to function as a knee joint in a prosthesis.

37. What is the common metastatic pattern found with osteosarcoma?

Like most sarcomas, osteosarcoma most often metastasizes hematogenously. The lungs, by
far, are the most common site of metastases, but metastatic disease can be found in liver, brain,
bones, kidneys, and regional lymph nodes.

38. What is the prognosis for osteosarcoma?

The prognosis has improved dramatically since the onset of adjuvant chemotherapeutic treatment. Today, 5-year disease-free survival rates in surgically accessible tumors usually range from
70%–80% following limb salvage surgery.

39. Are there any factors other than stage and adequacy of resection that affect prognosis?

Yes. Tumor size (patients with smaller tumors fare better) and response to chemotherapy
(patients with tumors responding to chemotherapy fare better). In a recent meta-analysis of prognostic factors, tumor necrosis in response to chemotherapy was the only variable that remained
significant following multivariate analysis.

40. What are MDR-1 and p-glycoprotein?

The MDR-1, or multidrug resistance −1 gene, codes for a 170 kDa membrane protein called
p-glycoprotein. This protein functions as an energy-dependent efflux pump which decreases the
intracellular concentration of many cytotoxic agents. This gene and its product play a part in the
resistance to chemotherapy expressed by some osteosarcomas and other tumors.

EWING'S SARCOMA

41. What is Ewing's sarcoma? How does it present?

Ewing's sarcoma is a primitive small and round blue cell tumor possibly related to primitive
neuroectodermal tumors. Patients are usually in their first two decades of life. They present with
pain and a mass at the site of the tumor, and they may have constitutional symptoms including
fever, anemia, leukocytosis, and an increased sedimentation rate. The tumor is characteristically
diaphyseal in location and affects the femur most commonly, but is seen in other long bones and
in pelvis in about 20% of cases.

42. What is the radiographic appearance of Ewing's sarcoma?

Ewing's sarcomas typically present as a permeative lesion with cortical destruction and a
soft-tissue mass. A periosteal reaction of layers of bone, the so-called "onion skin" appearance,
may be present.

43. What genetic derangement is noted in Ewing's sarcoma?

The translocation of chromosome 11 with chromosome 22 [t(11;22)(q24;q12)] is found consistently in Ewing's sarcoma.

44. What is the treatment for Ewing's sarcoma?

The treatment is in evolution. Until recently, radiation treatment alone was used. Problems
with recurrence, eventual leg length discrepancy, secondary sarcomas in irradiated limbs, and advances in chemotherapy and surgical techniques have led to protocols of neoadjuvant chemotherapy followed by wide resection and further chemotherapy. Location of the tumor (patients with
distal tumors fare better) and its response to chemotherapy (patients with tumors responding to
chemotherapy fare better) correlate with long-term survival.

45. What is the most common site of occurrence of adamantinoma?

The tibia.

MULTIPLE MYELOMA

46. What is multiple myeloma? How does it present?

Multiple myeloma is a tumor made up of malignant monoclonal plasma cells. It usually affects patients > 40 years old. Patients often present with malaise, bone pain, or a pathologic fracture.

47. What are the radiographic findings?

The classic radiographic appearance is multiple lytic "punched out" areas in bone. These lesions often do not show uptake of isotope on bone scan, making a skeletal survey the most important radiographic test.

48. What are the laboratory findings associated with multiple myeloma?

A serum protein electrophoresis usually reveals a monoclonal immunoglobulin spike in the α or γ region. Light chain immunoglobulins, or Bence-Jones protein, may be found in the urine. Hypercalcemia may be noted. Bone marrow aspirate reveals sheets of "clock-faced" plasma cells.

49. What is the treatment for multiple myeloma?

Multiagent chemotherapy, radiation, and surgical fixation of impending fracture. The average survival is < 2 years.

METASTATIC CARCINOMA

50. What is the most common malignant lesion in bone?

Metastatic carcinoma is by far the most common malignancy in bone.

51. Where do the majority of metastases to bone originate?

Breast, prostate, lung, kidney, and thyroid.

52. What are the most common sites for bony metastases?

Thoracic and lumbar spine, pelvis, femur, rib, proximal humerus, and skull.

53. How common are metastases to the hand?

Acral metastatic disease is very rare. When it does occur, it is usually from lung carcinoma.

54. How are bony metastases treated?

If the primary tumor is unknown, it should be identified. Treatment of metastatic disease is aimed at controlling pain and maintaining function. Local radiation may provide pain relief. Surgical fixation is indicated for impending fractures.

55. What are criteria for an impending fracture?

More than 50% destruction of diaphyseal cortex, a lesion > 2.5 cm in diameter, or persistent pain following irradiation.

BIBLIOGRAPHY

1. Aurias A, Rimbaud C, Buffe D, et al: Chromosomal translocations in Ewing's sarcoma. N Engl J Med 309:496–497, 1983.
2. Bieling P, Rehan N, Winkler P, et al: Tumor size and prognosis in aggressively treated osteosarcoma. J Clin Oncol 14:848–858, 1996.
3. Bridge JA, Schwartz HS, Neff JR: Bone sarcomas. In Abeloff MD, Armitage JO, Lichter AS, Niderhuber JE (eds): Clinical Oncology, 2nd ed. Orlando, FL, Harcourt Brace, 2000, Chapter 75.
4. Enneking WE, Spanier SS, Goodman MA: A system for the surgical staging of musculoskeletal sarcoma. Clin Orthop Rel Res 153:106–120, 1980.
5. Davis AM, Bell RS, Goodwin PJ: Prognostic factors in osteosarcoma: A critical review. J Clin Oncol 12:423–431, 1994.

6. Harrington KD: Impending pathologic fractures from metastatic malignancy: Evaluation and management. Instr Course Lect 35:357–381, 1986.

7. Kneisl JS, Simon MA: Medical management compared with operative treatment for osteoid osteoma. J Bone Joint Surg 74A:179–185, 1992.

8. Mankin HJ, Mankin CJ, Simon MA: The hazards of the biopsy, revisited. J Bone Joint Surg 78A: 656–663, 1996.

9. Picci P, Sangiorgi L, Rougraff BT, et al: Relationship of chemotherapy-induced necrosis and surgical margins to local recurrence in osteosarcoma. J Clin Oncol 12:2699–2705, 1994.

10. Rosenthal DI, Hornicek FJ, Wolfe MW, et al: Percutaneous radiofrequency coagulation of osteoid osteoma compared with operative treatment. J Bone Joint Surg 80A:815–821, 1998.

11. Skrzynksi MC, Biermann JS, Montag A, Simon MA: Diagnostic accuracy and charge-savings of outpatient core needle biopsy compared with open biopsy of musculoskeletal tumors. J Bone Joint Surg 78A:644–649, 1996.

12. Winkelmann WW: Rotationplasty. Orthop Clin North Am 27:503–523, 1996.

13. Wunder JS, Bell RS, Wold L, Andrulis IL: Expression of the multidrug resistance gene in osteosarcoma: A pilot study. J Orthop Res 11:396–403, 1993.

14. Wurtz LD, Peabody TD, Simon MA: Delay in the diagnosis and treatment of primary bone sarcoma of the pelvis. J Bone Joint Surg 81A:317–325, 1999.

II. Congenital and Developmental Disorders

18. CONNECTIVE TISSUE DISORDERS (SKELETAL DYSPLASIA)

Deepak V. Chavda, M.D.

1. Who pioneered the work on skeletal dysplasias?

Sir Thomas Fairbank of Edinburgh, Scotland, pioneered the work on skeletal dysplasia in his 1951 book, *An Atlas of General Affections of the Skeleton.*

2. How are the skeletal dysplasias classified?

Most orthopedists follow the classification developed by Rubin, which is based on anatomic distribution of bone changes. Two of the most common forms are multiple epiphyseal dysplasia and spondyloepiphyseal dysplasia.

3. Define the terms dysplasia, dwarfism, midget, dysostosis, malformation, and deformity.

Dysplasia is now the preferred term for dwarfism and is used when the developmental changes in the skeleton are generalized.

Dwarfism denotes a pathologic diminution in stature (below the tenth percentile). Dwarfism is further divided into the proportionate (**midget**) and disproportionate (short-limb or short-trunk) types. The short-limb variety is further subdivided according to the site of maximal shortening: rhizomelic (in the proximal portion), mesomelic (in the middle), and acromelic (in the distal portion).

Dysostosis denotes the developmental changes affecting a single bone or segment of the skeleton.

Malformation means a primary abnormality of development.

Deformity denotes a change in the structure of a previously normal bone.

4. What is multiple epiphyseal dysplasia (MED)?

MED, one of the more common bone dysplasias, is characterized by irregularity in development of the epiphysis. Late appearance or mottling of the ossification centers, knobby joints, stubby digits, and minor shortening of stature is present, with little or no vertebral involvement. The condition is extremely rare (prevalence: 11 per million index cases) and shows no gender predilection.

5. What is chondrodysplasia?

Chondrodysplasia is a heterogeneous group of rare conditions characterized by stippling of the epiphyses, disordered longitudinal bone growth, mental retardation, and cataracts. It is also referred to as chondrodystrophia fetalis ossificans, chondrodystrophia punctata, calcificans punctata, dysplasia epiphysealis punctata, stippled epiphyses, chondrodystrophia calcificans congenita, and Conradi's disease.

6. What is Stickler's syndrome?

Stickler's syndrome is characterized by epiphyseal changes similar to those of MED. The feature that differentiates Stickler's syndrome from MED is severe progressive myopia with retinal detachment and blindness. Patients may have conductive hearing loss and cleft palate. Spinal deformities include minimal platyspondyly and anterior wedging of the vertebrae, causing thoracic kyphosis (as in Scheuermann's disease). Stickler's syndrome is inherited as autosomal dominant.

7. What is dysplasia epiphysealis hemimelia (DEH)?

DEH is characterized by asymmetric abnormal cartilage proliferation and subsequent enchondral ossification in an epiphysis of a tarsal, carpal, or flat bone. It is limited to the medial or lateral half of a single limb. Other synonyms include tarsomegaly, tarsoepiphyseal aclasis, and benign epiphyseal osteochondroma. Its etiology is unknown.

8. What is the most common type of dwarfism?

The most common type of dwarfism is achondroplasia, a short-limbed disproportionate disorder that results from defective formation of enchondral bone. Formation of intramembranous bone is unaffected. The clinical syndrome consists of short limbs, a large, bulging cranium (especially the forehead), a low nasal bridge, a narrowed spinal canal in the lumbar region, and distinctive pelvic changes. It is autosomal dominant in inheritance, although 80–90% of cases are due to spontaneous new mutations. The most disabling clinical problems are thoracolumbar kyphosis or lumbar spinal stenosis. The latter affects up to 50% of achondroplasts.

Its presence in antiquity is evident from the depiction of the Egyptian goddess Ptah as an achondroplast and from the discovery of an achondroplastic skeleton from the early Egyptian period. In the Middle Ages, court jesters were often achondroplastic dwarfs. Even today they serve in circuses and theaters where they are incorrectly called "midgets."

9. Is lengthening of the lower limbs in patients with achondroplasia and hypochondroplasia a good option?

Yes and no. By using callus distraction (callotasis) surgical technique, it is possible to gain approximately 7 cm in both the femur and tibia. Functioning of the lengthened limbs improves, but malalignment of the mechanical axis of the bones may be present. The rate of complications following the procedure is much higher in children with underlying bone disorders compared with children with normal bone.

10. What is spondyloepiphyseal dysplasia?

Spondyloepiphyseal dysplasia is a group of disorders causing short-trunk disproportionate dwarfism. They are generally autosomal dominant, although the tarda form is x-linked recessive. Clinical features include precocious arthritis, coxa vara, atlantoaxial instability, retinal detachment, and myopia.

11. What is pseudoachondroplasia?

Pseudoachondroplasia is a short-limbed form of dwarfism that involves both the epiphyses and metaphyses. The prevalence is about 4 cases per million population. Clinically it can be distinguished from achondroplasia by the normal face and skull and the absence of interpedicular narrowing of the lumbar vertebrae. Precocious arthritis is a major problem.

12. What is marble bone disease?

Marble bone disease, also called osteopetrosis, is characterized by failure of bone resorption due to functional deficiency of the osteoclasts with persistence of calcified chondroid and primitive bone. On radiographs it appears as a striking opacity of the bones, lack of cortical endosteal margins, and failure of bone remodeling. The only effective treatment is bone marrow transplantation.

13. What is spotted bone disease?

Spotted bone disease, also called osteopoikilosis, is characterized by dense ovoid or circular spots in cancellous bone, usually found in clusters in the metaphyseal or epiphyseal regions of long bones. These 3–5 mm densities do not affect the cortex or the contour of the bone, and may be present at birth. The common locations are carpals, tarsals, ends of large tubular bones, or around the acetabulum. Spotted bone disease does not cause symptoms, and no treatment is required.

14. What is Caffey's disease?

Caffey's disease, or infantile cortical hyperostosis, is a rare, self-limiting condition of early infancy characterized by swelling of soft tissues, cortical thickening of the underlying bones, and hyperirritability. This disorder was first noted by Roske in 1930; however, it was thoroughly described by Caffey and Silverman in 1945.

15. What is osteogenesis imperfecta (OI)?

OI is in fact several genetically and clinically heterogeneous syndromes characterized by skeletal fragility. Other manifestations are dentinogenesis imperfecta, blue sclerae, deafness, and ligamentous hyperlaxity. Clinical features include multiple fractures, knee deformities, and scoliosis. It may be difficult to distinguish the tarda form of OI from child abuse.

16. Which clinical finding is a strong predictor of future walking ability in patients with OI?

The ability to sit by the age of ten months is a good predictor of future walking ability (75% of patients). No patients with OI who have delayed and dependent sitting walk.

17. What are clinically significant features of Marfan syndrome?

The clinically significant features of Marfan syndrome include disproportionately long, thin limbs, generalized joint laxity, dislocation of the lenses, dissecting aortic aneurysm, prolapsed cardiac valves, and increased prevalence of hernias. The syndrome was originally described in 1896 by Marfan, a French pediatrician. He termed the condition"dolichostemelia," meaning "long, thin limbs." Photographs of Abraham Lincoln suggest that he was afflicted with Marfan syndrome.

18. What is Ehlers-Danlos syndrome?

Ehlers-Danlos syndrome is a group of syndromes caused by defective collagen metabolism and characterized by skin changes of hyperextensibility, fragility, and easy bruisibility with resultant "cigarette paper" scarring, extreme ligamentous laxity of the joints, and bone fragility with osteopenia. There is no specific treatment for this disorder.

19. Define dyschondroplasia, Ollier's disease, and Maffucci's syndrome.

Dyschondroplasia is a rare, nonhereditary developmental defect characterized by the presence of circumscribed masses of cartilage arranged in a linear fashion in the interior of bones.

Multiple enchondromata is due to harmartomatous (developmental, not neoplastic) proliferation of cartilage cells that originate within the bones and from the cambium layer of the periosteum. When the lesions are predominantly unilateral, the eponym **Ollier's disease** is used. Multiple enchondromata with multiple hemangiomas is termed **Maffucci's syndrome**.

20. Describe fibrodysplasia (myositis) ossificans progressiva (FOP).

FOP is a rare disease transmitted in an autosomal dominant inheritance pattern. Defects in the skeletal patterning are present, particularly affecting the big toes. Progressive endochondral or enchondral ossification of the large striated muscles in a specific order ultimately leads to prolonged and severe disability. Painful swelling of the muscles (myositis) further leads to ossification at a mean age of 4.6 years (range 0–16 years). The muscles of the neck and upper spine are the first to be involved, followed by muscles around the hips, other major joints, and jaws. The rate and extent of involvement and disability has no relationship with the age of onset.

21. How is pseudomalignant heterotopic ossification (PHO) different from FOP?

PHO is a rare, self-limited connective tissue disorder of unknown origin. It usually occurs in the second or third decade (only occasionally during childhood). It may mimic soft tissue sarcoma (e.g., extraosseous osteosarcoma) or FOP. PHO affects the limbs (80% of patients) and often spares the big toes. It is possible that PHO is forme fruste of FOP.

22. What are the clinical and radiographic findings in early degenerative changes in the hip of diastrophic dysplasia patients?

Clinical: Rapid and progressive development of flexion contracture and restriction of rotational movements of hips

Radiographic: Flattening and inferomedial bulking of the femoral head
                    Double-hump deformation
                    Delayed (more than 12 years) appearance of the proximal femoral ossific nuclei

BIBLIOGRAPHY

1. Daly K, Wisbeach A, Sanpera I Jr, Fixsen JA: The prognosis for walking in osteogenesis imperfecta. J Bone Joint Surg 78-B:77–80, 1996.
2. Kaplan FS, Gannon FH, Hahn GV, et al: Pseudomalignant heterotopic ossification differential diagnosis and report of two cases. Clin Orthop 346:134–140, 1998.
3. Morrissy RT, Weinstein JN: Lovell and Winter's Pediatric Orthopaedics, 4th ed. Philadelphia, J.B. Lippincott, 1996.
4. Naudie D, Hamdy RC, Fassier F, Duhaime M: Complications of the limb-lengthening in children who have an underlying bone disorder. J Bone Joint Surg 80-A:18–24, 1998.
5. Smith R: Fibrodysplasia (myositis) ossificans progressiva. Clinical lessons from a rare disease. Clin Orthop 346:7–14, 1998.
6. Smith R: Osteogenesis imperfecta—Where next? (editorial) J Bone Joint Surg 79-B:177–178, 1997.
7. Tachdjian MO (ed): Pediatric Orthopaedics, 2nd ed. Philadelphia, W.B. Saunders, 1990.
8. Vaara P, Peltonen J, Poussa M, et al: Development of the hip in diastrophic dysplasia. J Bone Joint Surg 80-B:315–320, 1998.
9. Yasui N, Kawabata H, Kojimoto H, et al: Lengthening of the lower limbs in patients with achondroplasia and hypochondroplasia. Clin Orthop 344:298–306, 1997.

19. METABOLIC AND ENDOCRINE DISORDERS

David E. Brown, M.D.

1. How many types of cartilage are there?
1. Hyaline cartilage (articular surfaces, growth plate/physis)
2. Fibrocartilage (menisci)
3. Elastic cartilage (ear)

2. What are the zones of the growing epiphysis?
Beginning at the epiphyseal side, the four zones are (1) zone of growth, (2) zone of cartilage transformation, (3) zone of ossification, and (4) metaphysis. Some authors still use an older terminology that consists of five zones: (1) resting, (2) proliferative, (3) maturation, (4) provisional calcification, and (5) primary spongiosa.

3. What are the biologic effects of calcitonin?
Calcitonin, a peptide hormone produced chiefly by thyroid C-cells, results in lowering of serum calcium, inhibition of osteoclastic bone resorption, shrinking of osteoclasts, and mild stimulation of osteoblasts.

4. What are the effects of parathyroid hormone (PTH)?

PTH causes the kidney to increase reabsorption of calcium and excretion of phosphate. In bone osteoclastic resorption is stimulated, releasing calcium and phosphate. The net effect is an increase in serum calcium and a decrease in serum phosphorus.

5. What is a "brown tumor"?

Hyperparathyroidism, primary or secondary, leads to typical changes in bone. Histologic section reveals numerous osteoclasts on the bone surface with characteristic tunneling or dissecting resorption of bony trabeculae (also known as cutting cones). Also evident are resorption of pericellular bone by osteocytes (osteocytic osteolysis), increased woven bone, and marrow replacement by dense fibrous appearing tissue. When the diagnosis of hyperparathyroidism is delayed, such areas become quite large, resulting in a radiolucent lesion in the diaphysis of long bones, jaw, or skull that appears brown because of old and recent hemorrhage. Microscopic examination shows numerous giant cells in the fibrous cellular stroma. These "brown" tumors show dramatic regression both radiologically and histologically when hyperparathyroidism is controlled.

6. What is the daily requirement of calcium?

Adult	400–500 mg
Child	700 mg
Adolescent	1,000–1,300 mg
Pregnant women	1,500 mg
Lactating women	2,000 mg
Postmenopausal women	1,500 mg
Major fracture	1,500 mg

7. How much calcium is contained in 8 ounces of milk?

Eight ounces of milk contains 250 mg of calcium.

8. Where is the main storage of calcium and phosphorus in the body?

The skeleton contains 90% of calcium and 80% of phosphorus in the body.

9. What is cretinism?

Congenital or infantile hypothyroidism, which is called cretinism, is recognized by dwarfism and mental retardation. It is more common in girls (male-to-female ratio = 1:3). Other clinical features are dry skin, scanty and coarse hair, enlarged tongue, expressionless face, narrowed palpebral fissures, enlarged abdomen, umbilical hernia, and generalized lethargy. When diagnosed and treated early, prognosis is good for normal bone and mental development. Untreated cretins have increasing mental retardation with age and eventually succumb to infection.

10. What are the four causes of rickets?

1. Vitamin D deficiency   3. Chronic renal insufficiency
2. Renal tubular insufficiency   4. Hypophosphatasia

11. What is rickets?

Rickets is a disease process characterized by inadequate calcification of bone matrix (osteoid) in the immature skeleton. Osteomalacia is the same process in adults. Because of the growth of the immature skeleton, the disease process is more severe in children.

12. What are the clinical findings of rickets?

Muscular weakness
Lethargy
Protuberant abdomen
Craniotabes (enlargement of the forehead)
Thickening of weight-bearing joints (deformity of metaphyseal-epiphyseal junction)

13. What are the x-ray findings in rickets?
Thickened epiphyseal plate
Brush border of metaphysis
Flaring of metaphysis (trumpeting)
Thickening of osteochondral articulations of ribs (rachitic rosary)
Diminished cortical density
Coarse trabecular pattern, widely spaced and irregular

14. How does renal tubular disease cause rickets?
Renal tubular disease leads to increased renal clearance of phosphate and occasionally to excessive loss of calcium. Serum calcium is normal, whereas phosphate is low (1–3 mg/dl). The result is abnormal mineralization of osteoid. Because large doses of vitamin D (50,000–500,000 IU/day) are required, this group of disorders is called vitamin D-resistant rickets. It is one of the most common metabolic bone diseases of children.

15. What are the late deformities associated with vitamin D-resistant rickets?
Genu varum/valgum   Anterolateral bowing of tibia
Coxa vara   Protrusio acetabuli
Anterior bowing of femur   Kyphoscoliosis

16. How does chronic renal failure cause rickets?
The exact mechanism is unknown, but several factors may play a role, including (1) high levels of PTH, (2) acidosis, and (3) hypocalcemia, factors that alter calcium/phosphorus homeostasis and thus result in abnormal mineralization.

17. How does renal rickets differ from dietary rickets?
In renal rickets the high levels of PTH result in less osteoid and increased osteoclastic resorption of bone. There may be osteosclerosis at the base of the skull. Slipped epiphyses are common in renal rickets. Skeletal maturation is delayed.

18. What are the blood chemistry findings in the four common categories of rickets?

	DIETARY	RESISTANT	RENAL	HYPOPHOSPHATASIA
Phosphate	Low	Low	High	Normal
Calcium	Normal, low	Normal	Normal, low	Normal, high
Creatinine	Normal	Normal	High	Normal, high
Alkaline phosphatase	High	High	High	Very low

19. What is hypophosphatasia?
Hypophosphatasia is a genetically determined error of metabolism with low alkaline phosphatase activity and increased urinary excretion of phosphoryl ethanolamine.

20. How does the radiographic appearance differ from other forms of rickets?
Radiographs show severe osteoporosis and marked widening of the physis. Fractures are common. In milder cases the radiographic findings are difficult to distinguish from dietary rickets.

BIBLIOGRAPHY

1. Canale ST (ed): Campbell's Operative Orthopaedics, 9th ed. St. Louis, Mosby, 1998.
2. Doppelt SH: Vitamin D, rickets, and osteomalacia. Orthop Clin North Am 15:671–686, 1984.
3. Eastell R, Riggs BL: Calcium homeostasis and osteoporosis. Endocrinol Metab Clin North Am 16:829–842, 1987.
4. Mankin HJ: Rickets, osteomalacia, and renal osteodystrophy: An update. Orthop Clin North Am 21:81–96, 1990.

20. CEREBRAL PALSY AND NEUROMUSCULAR DISEASE

Marcia E. Bromley, B.S., and Paul W. Esposito, M.D., FAAP

CEREBRAL PALSY

1. Define cerebral palsy.

Cerebral palsy is a nonprogressive insult to the central nervous system during the perinatal period. A broad definition is necessary to address the multiple causes and vast array of clinical presentations.

2. Describe the classification system for cerebral palsy.

1. Diplegia—lower extremities involved more than upper extremities, but both are affected.
2. Hemiplegic—left-sided or right-sided involvement.
3. Paraplegic—lower extremities only affected.
4. Quadriplegic—all four extremities involved, plus head, neck, and trunk.
5. Tetraplegic—three extremities involved.

3. What are the types of involvement in cerebral palsy?

1. Spastic—hyperreflexic stretch reflexes
2. Athetoid—involuntary movements, passive resistance to motion, and/or posturing
3. Mixed—combination of both motion disorder and spasticity

4. Why is athetoid cerebral palsy less common than in the past?

Most cases of athetoid cerebral palsy were caused by kernicterus (the depositing of bilirubin in the basal ganglia) due to Rh incompatibility. Screening for Rh incompatibility, Rho-gam, and bilirubin-lights are greatly responsible for the decreased incidence of athetoid cerebral palsy.

5. What are the common causes for the various types of cerebral palsy?

Diplegia is associated with premature infants, who often sustain periventricular hemorrhage. Preventing premature births may avoid this problem. **Hemiplegia** is caused by a variety of insults, including trauma, infection, and cerebrovascular accidents. **Quadriplegia**, the most severely involved form, results from an anoxic event that causes global injury.

6. When do children with cerebral palsy walk?

In children with **hemiplegia**, ambulation frequently occurs at 12–16 months (the time at which the normal child walks). Children with **diplegia** will be delayed somewhat, but walking is usually initiated by age 4 years. In those with **quadriplegic** cerebral palsy, onset of ambulation depends on the extent of involvement. If walking is not initiated by age 7 years, the child will not walk.

7. Do all patients show spasticity early in life?

No. In fact, the more severely affected children are hypotonic or "floppy" early on; only later, when developmental delay is more evident, do they develop signs of spasticity.

8. Does central core disease (CCD) appear clinically the same as cerebral palsy?

No. CCD, like cerebral palsy, is a nonprogressive process but also is a myopathy that presents at birth with hypotonia and delayed motor milestones. Patients with CCD, however, do not exhibit spasticity. They may exhibit pes cavus, kyphoscoliosis, foot deformities, congenital hip dislocation, and joint contractures, but up to 40% of people with CCD are asymptomatic. The disorder is caused by a defective gene that creates abnormal proteins in the z-band of the muscle fiber, as opposed to cerebral palsy, which is a central nervous system disorder. CCD is an autosomal dominant trait with variable penetrance. The defective gene is also the site for malignant hyperthermia regulation; consequently, such patients often suffer from malignant hyperthermia (in fact, some patients are not diagnosed with CCD until after having had an episode of malignant hyperthermia).

9. How is cerebral palsy diagnosed?

Most patients present to the orthopedist after the diagnosis of cerebral palsy has been made, especially if the patient is a member of a high-risk group. Some children, however, are referred because they are not not walking by 18 months of age. Such children retain primitive reflexes and show signs of spasticity. In some cases, computed tomography (CT) and magnetic resonance imaging (MRI) scans may define the underlying cause. Congenital myopathies and other neurologic processes that do not progress to spasticity may have severe underlying hypotonia associated with developmental delays and, therefore, must be ruled out before diagnosis.

10. What early problems should the orthopedist look for in a child with cerebral palsy?

In the child with significant spasticity, the hips may dislocate as early as 18 months of age. Therefore, patients should have their hips examined and a pelvic radiograph every 6 months. Early detection of hip subluxation and dislocation, followed by surgical release of the adductor muscles and/or the iliopsoas muscles, frequently prevents the late development of a painful and stiff dislocated hip. After the age of 5 years, the child's course becomes less predictable and the treatment becomes generally more complicated.

11. What are the clinical signs of hip subluxation or dislocation?

1. Limited abduction, especially with rapid stretch (grab test)
2. Asymmetric knee height with the pelvis level and the knees flexed (Galeazzi sign)
3. Windswept posture (one hip adducted and the opposite side abducted)
4. Asymmetric leg length
5. Hip flexion contractures

12. What is the rationale for treating severely involved patients with dislocating hips?

Even children with severe, total-body involvement have a significant chance for a long life. A dislocated hip can be very painful, make nursing care more difficult, and, as a result, significantly affect the quality of life. A dislocated hip also may contribute to pelvic obliquity and scoliosis, which can make even wheelchair ambulation impossible.

13. Should a patient with spastic quadriplegia and a severe scoliosis have surgery for correction of the spinal curvature?

This matter is still debated among orthopedists today. Most agree that pain and loss of function, as measured by decreased ambulation or sitting ability, are indications for surgery. Still some orthopedists believe that the cost, complication rate, and extent of the surgery outweigh the surgical benefits. Benefits of spine stabilization may include improved sitting balance, ease of patient care, decreased pain, increased pulmonary function, and increased level of function. Drawbacks cited are the high cost of the surgery and the high risk of complications such as death, paralysis, wound infection, instrumentation problems, pulmonary complications, and decubitus ulcers.

14. What types of lower extremity deformities are most commonly seen in cerebral palsy?

1. Hip flexion/adduction
2. Equinus of the ankle
3. Knee flexion contracture
4. Hip adduction and flexion contracture
5. Contractures of the rectus fenorus

15. What does tendon lengthening do for spastic contractures?

Muscle contractures frequently do not resolve with stretching or bracing alone. The lengthening procedure attempts to balance muscle forces across the joints and increase the muscle excursion, thereby placing the joints in a more functional position. They do not, however, alter the spasticity of the muscles.

16. What is selective dorsal rhizotomy, and who are the best candidates for the procedure?

Selective dorsal rhizotomy involves a multiple-level lumbar laminectomy, with isolation of the dorsal nerve rootlets and selective sectioning of only those rootlets that cause spastic reflex action when electrically stimulated intraoperatively. This procedure, in effect, reduces spasticity in the patient and allows for better muscle control. The best candidates appear to be approximately 4-year-old, spastic diplegic, ambulatory children with excellent strength whose spasticity interferes with function.

17. Is there a medical treatment for spasticity in cerebral palsy?

Yes. Treatment of spasticity by intrathecal baclofen has become relatively common. A microinfusion pump placed in the subcutaneous tissues delivers the baclofen via percutaneous catheter to the intrathecal space at a rate determined by the patient's response to the medication. The rate is adjusted until the spasticity improves to an acceptable degree. Intrathecal baclofen pumps do not work for all dystonic patients, however, and other surgery may still be necessary.

18. Can patients with cerebral palsy benefit from injection of botulinum toxin?

Botulinum toxin type A injection clearly has been shown to be a safe means of at least transiently but significantly improving spasticity and function in selective muscles. Its use is limited by its lack of permanency and its toxicity, which is dose-related.

19. What is familial spastic paraplegia?

Familial spastic paraplegia is an autosomal dominant disorder that mimics cerebral palsy. Only the lower extremities are involved, however, and in the absence of a family history, the physician is obligated to look for other causes, such as birth trauma to the spinal cord. Complete lack of upper extremity involvement is not typical of cerebral palsy.

20. What factors differentiate the idiopathic and familial toe walkers from the child with mild spastic diplegia?

The idiopathic toe walker has a normal birth history, walked at the appropriate time, and has no signs of neurologic involvement (spasticity). Frequently a strong family history of toe walking is present. All other causes must be excluded before a diagnosis of mild spastic diplegia is made.

21. Are there any indications for surgery in the upper extremity in children with severe spastic cerebral palsy?

The goals of upper extremity surgery vary based on the severity of contractures, which may cause pain, difficulties in positioning, and hygiene problems, typically in spastic quadriplegics. Tendon releases may relieve these contractures if done prior to the development of severe joint contractures. If arthritis of the wrist has developed, arthrodesis of the wrist may be necessary to alleviate pain.

22. Are there any options to improve upper extremity function in children with spastic hemiplegia?

The arm and hand may be placed in a position for improved function; however, the limiting factors are proprioceptive sensation and the ability of the child to cooperate and operate with a rehabilitation program. Hemiplegic children frequently have a thumb in palm adduction deformity, which may be improved by either injection with botulinum toxin or surgical lengthening of the adductor pollicis. Pronation/flexion deformities of the wrist may be improved with procedure section transfer of the flexor carpi ulnaris or pronator quadratus. Many other procedures are available but surgical decision-making is crucial. Improvement in comfort and cosmesis is more common than improvement of function.

MYELODYSPLASIA

23. What are the different types of myelodysplasia?
1. **Meningocele** involves only the meninges. Patients usually have normal neurologic function.
2. **Myelomeningocele** involves neural elements that are part of an exposed sac and usually are not covered with skin. Arnold-Chiari brainstem involvement and hydrocephalus are also found.
3. **Lipomeningocele** is characterized by a lipoma in sacs, with neural elements intertwined. The skin usually is intact, and patients usually are neurologically sound at birth except for foot deformities and/or bowel and bladder dysfunction. Neurologic function deteriorates with growth unless the disorder is treated.

24. What are the common causes of death in children with untreated myelomeningocele?
1. Central nervous system infection
2. Progressive hydrocephalus

25. What are the common causes of deteriorating function in patients with myelomeningocele?
1. Progressive hydrocephalus secondary to shunt malfunction
2. Hydromyelia secondary to shunt malfunction
3. Spinal cord tethering with growth
4. Arnold-Chiari malformation

26. List the common presenting symptoms in older children with shunt malformation and/or hydromyelia.

Irritability	Progressive foot deformity
Decreased motor level	Progressive scoliosis
Worsening bowel or bladder function	Weakness of the upper extremities

27. What is the expected cause of an intraoperative anaphylactic reaction in a patient with neuromuscular problems such as myelomeningocele?
Children with cerebral palsy are at an increased risk for developing an anaphylactic reaction to latex. Patients who have undergone multiple surgical procedures or the placement of a ventriculoperitoneal shunt are considered high-risk for latex allergy and should be considered for preoperative latex-sensitivity testing. When obtaining the history of a child with cerebral palsy, all physicians should look carefully for sensitivity (i.e., urticaria, facial edema, bronchospasm) to latex products such as balloons, rubber balls, and rubber gloves. Eighteen to 40% of patients have been reported to be latex-sensitive. Many hospitals insist on latex-free environments for such patients to avoid the consequences of a previously undiagnosed hypersensitivity to latex.

MUSCULAR DYSTROPHY

28. In classic Duchenne muscular dystrophy, are patients typically male or female?
Duchenne dystrophy is a sex-linked, recessive trait; therefore, patients are typically male.

29. What are the presenting findings in Duchenne dystrophy?
1. Symmetric and progressive proximal muscle weakness
2. Deteriorating gait after delayed ambulation
3. Progressive toe walking
4. Pseudohypertrophy of the calf
5. Hard or rubbery feeling muscle
6. Elevation of serum CPK levels

30. What are the goals of treatment in muscular dystrophy?

1. To keep the patients ambulatory as long as possible.
2. To prevent contractures that interfere with ambulation.
3. To begin immediate postoperative ambulation if surgery is necessary.
4. To fuse the spine with rigid fixation to maintain a sitting balance after the patient no longer ambulates and mild scoliosis develops. (If fusion is delayed until scoliosis is severe, restricted pulmonary function will not allow a safe postoperative course, and the patient may become ventilator-dependent.)

31. What is the cause of death in most patients with Duchenne dystrophy?

Pulmonary failure or cardiomyopathy.

BIBLIOGRAPHY

1. Albright AL, Barry MJ, Painter MJ, Shultz B: Infusion of intrathecal baclofen for generalized dystonia in cerebral palsy. J Neurosurg 88:73–76, 1998.
2. Banta JV, Lonstein JE, Lubicky JP: Resolution: A 15-year-old with spastic quadriplegia and a 60° scoliosis should have a posterior spinal fusion with instrumentation. Dev Med Child Neurol 40:278–283, 1998.
3. Bell DF, Moseley CF, Koreska J: Unit rod segmental spinal instrumentation in the management of patients with progressive neuromuscular spinal deformity. Spine 14:1301–1307, 1989.
4. Corry IS, Cosgrove AP, Duffy CM, et al: Botulinum toxin A compared with stretching casts in the treatment of spastic equinus: A randomized prospective trial. J Pediatr Orthop 18(3):304–311, 1998.
5. Delfico AJ, Dormans JP, Craythorne CB, Templeton JJ: Intraoperative anaphylaxis due to allergy to latex in children who have cerebral palsy: A report of six cases. Dev Med Child Neurol 39:194–197, 1996.
6. Dormans JP, Templeton JJ, Edmonds C, Davidson RS: Intraoperative anaphylaxis due to exposure to latex (natural rubber) in children. J Bone Joint Surg 76A(11):1688–1691, 1994.
7. Evans RA: Orthopedic aspects of neuromuscular disorders in children. Curr Opin Pediatr 5:379–383, 1993.
8. Gamble JG, Rinsky LA, Bleck EE: Established hip dislocations in children with cerebral palsy. Clin Orthop 253:90–99, 1990.
9. Lazareff JA: Limited selective posterior rhizotomy for the treatment of spasticity secondary to infantile cerebral palsy: A preliminary report. Neurosurgery 27:535–538, 1990.
10. Loke J, MacLennan DH: Malignant hyperthermia and central core disease: Disorders of calcium release channels. Am J Med 104:470–486, 1998.
11. Papariello SG, Skinner SR: Dynamic electromyography analysis of habitual toe-walkers. J Pediatr Orthop 5:171–175, 1985.
12. Scrutton D: The classification of cerebral palsy. Dev Med Child Neurol 35(7):647–648, 1993.
13. Thomas C: Nemaline rod and central core disease: A coexisting z-band myopathy. Muscle Nerve 20:893–896, 1997.
14. Water PM, van Heest A: Spastic hemiplegia of the upper extremity in children. Hand Clin 14(1): 119–134, 1998.
15. Wong V: Use of botulinum toxin injection in 17 children with spastic cerebral palsy. Pediatr Neurol 18:124–131, 1998.

21. MISCELLANEOUS CONGENITAL DISORDERS

Brian E. Brigman, M.D., and Paul W. Esposito, M.D., FAAP

1. What are the orthopedic manifestations of Down syndrome?

Down syndrome affects 1 in 660 live births with a higher incidence with increasing maternal age. Trisomy 21 accounts for 95% of the cases. Common orthopedic sequelae include occipitoatlantal or atlantoaxial instability, hip subluxation-dislocation, patella subluxation-dislocation, and flexible planovalgus, all possibly related to the ligamentous laxity common in patients with Down syndrome. Other relatively common problems include scoliosis, spondylolisthesis, and slipped capital femoral epiphysis. Patients with Down syndrome have characteristically flat acetabula and flared iliac wings. A polyarticular arthropathy occurs in about 10% of Down syndrome patients, usually affecting the feet.

2. What is arthrogryposis?

Arthrogryposis is a group of nongenetic congenital contracture syndromes of unknown origin. Characteristically the upper extremities, if involved, are adducted and internally rotated at the shoulder. The elbows are extended and the wrists and fingers flexed with the thumb in palm. The lower extremities typically are noted for having flexed, abducted, and externally rotated hips; knees may be in flexion or extension, and clubfeet are common.

3. What is the treatment of choice for congenital muscular torticollis?

Congenital muscular torticollis is a painless contracture of the sternocleidomastoid muscle. Affected infants tilt their head toward and rotate their chin away from the affected sternocleidomastoid muscle. It is usually discovered in the first two months of life. The cause is thought to be ischemia to the muscle. Stretching of the affected muscle (lateral rotation and side bending) is effective about 90% of the time if started before 1 year of age. If stretching is not successful, surgical lengthening or release of the sternocleidomastoid should be considered to prevent facial deformity.

4. What is Klippel-Feil syndrome?

Klippel-Feil syndrome is a group of deformities that result from failure of segmentation of cervical vertebrae. Classically, patients have a low posterior hairline, short neck, and limited range of motion in the neck, especially with lateral bending. Klippel-Feil syndrome is associated with Sprengel's deformity, scoliosis, urinary tract anomalies, congenital heart disease, and hearing loss.

5. What is Sprengel's deformity?

Sprengel's deformity is characterized by an elevated and medially rotated scapula. It results from an interruption in the normal caudal migration of the scapula. In 30% of patients with Sprengel's deformity the scapula is bound to the cervical spine by fibrous tissue, cartilage, or an omovertebral bone. All patients with Sprengel's deformity will have loss of abduction and forward flexion; those with an omovertebral bone generally have less than 90° of abduction. Stretching exercises are not useful. Functional or cosmetic deformities can be treated with surgery.

6. What is von Recklinghausen's disease?

Neurofibromatosis (NF) affects 1 in 3000 newborns. NF is autosomal dominant with 100% penetrance, but about one-half of all cases are spontaneous mutations. Classic NF, or von Recklinghausen's disease (also called peripheral NF or NF1), makes up 85% of cases. Central NF, or NF2, is characterized by bilateral acoustic neuromas.

7. How do I diagnose NF?

The Consensus Development Conference on Neurofibromatosis of the National Institutes of Health concluded that diagnosis of NF1 is dependent on **two or more** of the following criteria:

1. Six or more café au lait macules at least 5 mm in greatest diameter in prepubertal children and at least 15 mm in greatest diameter in adults
2. Two or more neurofibromas of any type or one plexiform neurofibroma
3. Freckling in the axillary or inguinal regions
4. Optical glioma
5. Two or more Lisch nodules (Irish hamartoma)
6. A distinctive osseous lesion, such as sphenoid dysplasia or thinning of long bone cortex without pseudarthrosis.
7. A first-degree relative (parent, sibling, or offspring) with von Recklinghausen's disease identified by the above criteria.

8. What are the orthopedic manifestations of NF?

Pseudarthrosis of long bones, typically the tibia, but also the ulna, radius, and clavicle, is the most common orthopedic manifestation of NF. Pseudarthrosis of the tibia starts with anterolateral bowing of the tibia in infancy with a fracture when the patient begins walking.

Scoliosis and limb overgrowth are common in NF. Limb overgrowth can range from disproportional overgrowth of a single digit to one or more extremity.

9. What is the treatment for pseudarthrosis of the tibia?

Spontaneous union is rare. Bracing or casting is not effective. Plating and bone grafting have success rates less than 50%. Successful treatment with free vascularized bone grafts, external fixation and intramedullary rods has been described. Multiple operations are often needed, and shortening, angulation, and stiffness are common. About 5% of patients eventually require amputation, which may be below the knee (above pseudarthrosis), or, counterintuitively, a below pseudarthrosis ankle disarticulation (Syme's amputation).

10. How do you distinguish benign bowing of the tibia from potential pseudarthrosis of the tibia?

Posteromedial bowing of the tibia is usually benign and does not lead to fracture or pseudarthrosis. A possible long-term sequela is limb length discrepancy. Anterior or anterolateral bowing of the tibia is associated with progressive deformity, fracture, and pseudarthrosis of the tibia.

11. Name another disease process often associated with café au lait spots.

Fibrous dysplasia. Café au lait spots are tan macules located in the basal layer of the epidermis. They are typically absent during infancy and appear by age 9. Café au lait spots associated with neurofibromatosis have smooth margins (so-called "coast of California"), whereas those associated with fibrous dysplasia have jagged edges ("coast of Maine").

12. What defects are associated with VACTERLS?

The nonrandom, but unexplained, association of system defects previously known as VATER is now called VACTERLS. It includes:

- **V**ertebral anomalies, including failures of segmentation (vertebral bars and blocks), congenital scoliosis, and occult intraspinal pathology
- **A**nal anomalies, including imperforate anus or anal atresia
- **C**ardiac abnormalities
- **T**racheo**E**sophageal fistula
- **R**enal anomalies (single kidney)
- **L**imb anomalies, usually radially based, ranging from hypoplastic thumb to radial clubhand
- **S**ingle umbilical artery

13. What are the mucopolysaccharidoses?

The mucopolysaccharidoses are the largest group of lysosomal storage diseases. Lysosomes are enzymes that degrade intracellular molecules into smaller units for cellular metabolism or utilization. Defective activity of any of these enzymes leads to blockage in the breakdown process and intracellular accumulation of semi-degraded compounds. The mucopolysaccharidoses are subdivided into at least 12 types (see table, next page).

Incidence is about 1 in 10,000. Hurler (MPS I) and Morquio (MPS IV) are the most common. All are autosomal recessive with the exception of the X-linked recessive MPS II or Hunter disease. Orthopedic manifestations include stiff joints, thought to be related to deposition of mucopolysaccharide in the capsule and periarticular structures. Radiographic findings often include oval vertebral bodies with anterior beaking; wide, flat ilia; large acetabula, coxa valga, and an unossified femoral head.

The Mucopolysaccharidoses

TYPE	NAME	ENZYME DEFICIENCY	ACCUMULATED SUBSTANCE
MPS I	Hurler/Scheie	α-L-iduronidase	HS/DS
MPS II	Hunter	Iduronate-2-sulfatase	HS/DS
MPS IIIA	Sanfilippo A	Heparan sulfate sulfatase	HS
MPS IIIB	Sanfilippo B	α-N-acetylglucosaminadase	HS
MPS IIIC	Sanfilippo C	α-glucosaminide-N-acetyltransferase	HS
MPS IIID	Sanfilippo D	Glucosamine-6-sulfatase	HS
MPS IVA	Morquio A	N-acetyl galactosamine-6 sulfate sulfatase	KS/CS
MPS IVB	Morquio B	β-D-galactosidase	KS
MPS IVC	Morquio C	Uncertain	KS
MPS V	Formerly Scheie— No longer used		
MPS VI	Maroteaux-Lamy	Arylsulfatase B, N-acetylgalactosamine-4 sulfatase	DS/CS
MPS VII	Sly	β-D-glucuronidase	CS/HS/DS
MPS VIII		Glucoronate-2-sulpitatase	CS/HS

HS = heparan sulfate; DS = dermatan sulfate; KS = keratin sulfate; CS = chondroitin sulfate

BIBLIOGRAPHY

1. Goldberg MJ: Syndromes of orthopaedic importance. In Morrissy RT, Weinstein SL (eds): Lovell and Winter's Pediatric Orthopaedics, 4th ed. Philadelphia, Lippincott-Raven, 1996, pp 255–304.
2. Pizzutillo PD: Cervical spine: Pediatric. In Frymoyer JW (ed): Orthopaedic Knowledge Update 4. Rosemont, IL, American Academy of Orthopaedic Surgeons, 1993, pp 405–412.
3. Shaughnessy WJ: Shoulder: Pediatric. In Frymoyer JW (ed): Orthopaedic Knowledge Update 4. Rosemont, IL, American Academy of Orthopaedic Surgeons, 1993, pp 277–284.

III. The Shoulder

22. SUBACROMIAL SYNDROMES

David E. Brown, M.D.

1. What is the incidence of rotator cuff tears in humans?

Cadaver dissections reveal high rates of rotator cuff tears. Under age 70, the prevalence of tears is 30%; for ages 71–80 it is nearly 60%; and over 80 years, nearly 70%.

2. What is the incidence of rotator cuff tears in asymptomatic shoulders?

Magnetic resonance imaging (MRI) of asymptomatic shoulders demonstrated a prevalence of rotator cuff tears of 34%. Prevalence increases with advancing age.

Incidence of Rotator Cuff Tears in Asymptomatic Shoulders

AGE	%PARTIAL-THICKNESS TEAR	%FULL-THICKNESS TEAR
19–39	4	0
40–60	24	4
60+	26	28

3. What is the etiology of rotator cuff tears?

The exact etiology is unknown. A 1989 study revealed that in younger patients who had a documented rotator cuff tear, few had had a traumatic event, which suggests that the process was secondary to repetitive microtrauma, degeneration, and/or impingement. Older patients tended to have mild chronic impingement symptoms but then sustained an episode of trauma, after which larger tears of the cuff were found.

4. What are the significant features of the physical examination of subacromial syndromes?

Active and passive range of motion, shoulder strength, and areas of tenderness should be noted. Examination of shoulder stability is important, particularly in younger individuals. The presence of pain during forward elevation while the examiner stabilizes the scapula is the primary impingement sign. Pain during active abduction of the arm (with the arm in internal rotation) is a secondary impingement sign.

5. How is the strength of the supraspinatus and infraspinatus tested?

The supraspinatus is tested with the shoulder abducted to 90°, flexed 30°, and then maximally internally rotated. Downward pressure exerted by the examiner is resisted primarily by the supraspinatus. The infraspinatus is tested with the shoulder abducted at the side while the elbows are fixed 90°. The examiner resists active external rotation.

6. What are the most common differential diagnoses of exertional shoulder pain?

- Subacromial syndromes (rotator cuff tears, tendinitis, impingement)
- Shoulder instability
- Cervical radiculitis
- Acromioclavicular degenerative disease
- Thoracic outlet syndrome
- Suprascapular nerve entrapment

7. What are the causes of subacromial syndromes?
- Repetitive overhead use
- Trauma
- Forward sloping acromion or hooked or curved acromion
- Os acromiale
- Shoulder instability
- Technique errors during overhead shoulder sports

8. What is the treatment of subacromial syndromes?
1. Modification of activities, avoiding repetitive overhead use or technique errors
2. Ice and nonsteroidal antiinflammatory drugs (NSAIDs)
3. Therapeutic exercises and stretching
4. Subacromial injections
5. Surgical decompression and repair of rotator cuff tears

9. What are the three types of acromial morphology and their incidence?

Acromial Morphology

TYPE	INCIDENCE HEALTHY SUBJECTS	SUBJECTS WITH DOCUMENTED ROTATOR CUFF TEARS
Type I (flat acromion)	17%	3%
Type II (curved acromion)	44%	27%
Type III (hooked acromion)	39%	70%

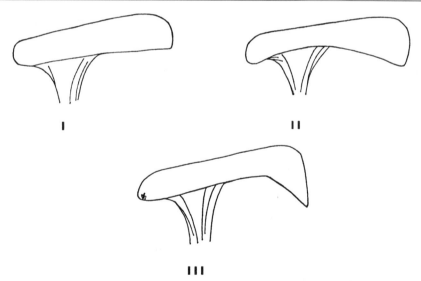

The three types of acromion morphology (as described by Bigliani).

10. Which radiographic tests are used to evaluate for rotator cuff tears? How useful are they?

Ultrasonography, single- and double-contrast arthrography, and magnetic resonance imaging (MRI) have been used to evaluate rotator cuff tears. Ultrasonography can confirm the presence of a significant rotator cuff tear; however, it is extremely dependent on the individual ultrasonographer. One study found only 30% accuracy compared with surgical confirmation. Arthrography is approximately 85% sensitive and specific in the diagnosis of complete cuff tear, but not highly accurate in the diagnosis of partial cuff tear. MRI appears to be 95% sensitive and specific in the diagnosis of complete tears. Intrasubstance degeneration, chronic tendinitis, and partial tearing are imaged by MRI with an accuracy rate of 85%.

11. What is the technique for supraspinatus repair?
- Perform acromioplasty (open or closed)
- Debride end of tendon to fresh tissue
- Mobilize tendon laterally. May need to:
  —Release coracohumeral ligament
  —Release capsule (incision above labrum)
- Use locking suture technique of choice
- Secure to greater tuberosity

12. What are the methods of securing the supraspinatus to the humeral head?
The two most common methods of repair are pulling the tendon into a bone trough medial to the greater tuberosity (sutures are brought through drill holes placed from the trough through the lateral humeral complex) and direct repair using suture anchors. The suture anchors are placed at the intended sight of repair. The anchor is placed into the edge of the subchondral bone adjacent to the articular surface. Direct repair with suture anchors has been shown to be significantly stronger. It is preferable to use **both** repair techniques.

13. What are the results of rotator cuff repair?
Using direct repair or local tendon transposition techniques, surgery has yielded good results in approximately 90% of patients. Pain relief and strength improvements generally follow successful repair. Return of range of motion has been shown to correlate with the timing of surgical repair. Repair within 3 weeks of injury yields the best return of range of motion.

14. What is the treatment of massive irreparable rotator cuff tears?
Treatment for this entity is controversial. Some authors advocate arthroscopic subacromial decompression and wide debridement of the cuff tear as a means of affording pain relief. In shoulders with normal passive motion and normal deltoid function, humeral prosthetic hemiarthroplasty has relieved pain. Recently, latissimus dorsi transfer has been reported to provide excellent pain relief with marked improvement in flexion and external rotation, yielding approximately 80% of normal shoulder function.

15. What are the causes of failure after rotator cuff repair?
- Persistent impingement
- Acromioclavicular joint pain
- Cervical spondylosis
- Re-rupture of the cuff
- Workers' compensation injury (secondary gain)

16. Describe the surgical technique of acromioplasty.
Complete acromionectomy is not indicated; partial inferior and anterior acromionectomy is sufficient. Removal of anterior acromial protuberance, including all acromion anterior to the acromioclavicular joint, is required. The coracoacromial ligament is resected. Resection of inferior acromioclavicular joint osteophytes is required. Complete excision of the distal clavicle is necessary only for severe acromioclavicular arthritis. Such procedures may be performed by either open or arthroscopic methods.

17. What are the results of open versus arthroscopic acromioplasty?
No difference in long-term surgical results is evident; both methods yield 85–90% good results. Arthroscopic acromioplasty has been shown in one study to allow return of shoulder function 4 months earlier than open methods.

18. What is the function of the long head of the biceps tendon?

The tendon has an important contribution as a humeral head depressor. Loss of its function may result in superior migration of the humeral head, which may aggravate or cause rotator cuff impingement.

19. What are the indications for biceps tenodesis?

Indications include significant degeneration or rupture of the tendon found at the time of a shoulder reconstructive procedure. Isolated biceps tenodesis has a high incidence of unsatisfactory long-term results when performed solely for bicipital pain.

20. What is the treatment of frozen shoulder syndrome?

Most patients show gradual reduction of pain and return of motion for periods up to 18 months. The syndrome itself may be self-limited. Treatment usually consists of physical therapy for range of motion, antiinflammatory medication, and subacromial or intraarticular corticosteroid injections. Patients who fail to improve with such methods may be candidates for manipulation under anesthesia, arthroscopic debridement, or decompression. Diabetics appear to have poor results from surgery.

21. What is the treatment of proximal biceps rupture?

Most patients do well with conservative management. Gradual return of range of motion and shoulder strength through physiotherapy is expected. Surgical repair by biceps tenodesis affords little improvement in strength. Distal biceps tendon ruptures are generally repaired surgically.

BIBLIOGRAPHY

1. Arntz CT, Matsen FA, Jackins S: Surgical management of complex irreparable rotator cuff deficiency. J Arthroplasty 6:363, 1991.
2. Bassett RW, Cofield RH: Acute tears of the rotator cuff: The timing of surgical repair. Clin Orthop 175:18, 1983.
3. Burk DL, Karasick D, Kurtz AB, et al: Rotator cuff tears: Prospective comparison of MR imaging with arthrography, sonography, and surgery. Am J Roentgenol 153:87, 1989.
4. Burkhart SS: Arthroscopic treatment of massive rotator cuff tears: Clinical and biomechanical rationale. Clin Orthop 267:45, 1991.
5. DiGiovanni J, Marva G, Park JY, et al: Hemiarthroplasty for glenohumeral arthritis with massive rotator cuff tears. Orthop Clin North Am 29:477–489, 1998.
6. Gartsman G: Arthroscopic acromioplasty for lesions of the rotator cuff. J Bone Joint Surg 72A:169, 1990.
7. Gerber C: Latissimus dorsi: Transfer for the treatment of irreparable tears of the rotator Cuff. Clin Orthop 275:152, 1992.
8. Iannotti JP, Zlatkin MB, Esterhai JL, et al: Magnetic resonance imaging of the shoulder: Sensitivity, specificity, and predictive value. J Bone Joint Surg 73:17, 1991.
9. Lehman C, Cuomo F, Kummer FJ, Zuckerman JD: The incidence of full thickness rotator cuff tears in a large cadaveric population. Bull Hosp Jt Dis 54:30–31, 1995.
10. Lyons AR, Tomlinson JE: Clinical diagnosis of tears of the rotator cuff. J Bone Joint Surg 74B:414, 1992.
11. Norwood LA, Barrack R, Jacobson KE: Clinical presentation of complete tears of the rotator cuff. J Bone Joint Surg 71:499, 1989.
12. Panni AS, Milano G, Lucania L, et al: Histological analysis of the coracoacromial arch: Correlation between age-related changes and rotator cuff tears. Arthroscopy 12:531–540, 1996.
13. Post M, Silver R, Singh M: Rotator cuff tear: Diagnosis and treatment. Clin Orthop 173:78, 1983.
14. Reed SC, Glossup N, Ogilvie-Harris DJ: Full-thickness rotator cuff tears. A biomechanical comparison of suture versus bone anchor techniques. Am J Sports Med 24:46–48, 1996.
15. Sher JS, Uribe J, Posada A, et al: Abnormal findings on magnetic resonance images of asymptomatic shoulders. J Bone Joint Surg 77:10–15, 1995.
16. Snyder SJ, Pachelli AF, Del Pizzo W, et al: Partial thickness rotator cuff tears: Results of arthroscopic treatment. Arthroscopy 7:7, 1991.
17. Tibone JE, Elrod B, Jobe FW, et al: Surgical treatment of tears of the rotator cuff in athletes. J Bone Joint Surg 68:887, 1986.

23. SHOULDER INSTABILITY

CDR *David P. Adkison*, M.D., MC USNR, *and*
LT *Elizabeth A. Moran*, M.D., MC USNR

1. What are the primary stabilizers of the shoulder joint?

Stability is both passive and active. Passive stability is present even in the absence of muscle forces (i.e., under anesthesia) and is a function of (1) a dished glenoid with normal labral compliance; (2) a competent, sealed capsule with limited shoulder joint volume; and (3) functionally intact and balanced capsule ligaments. Active stability is primarily a muscular function: (1) the rotator cuff muscles resist deltoid shear and other subluxating forces at the humeral head; (2) the superficial muscle layer (deltoid, biceps, triceps, pectoralis major, and latissimus dorsi) balance external torques around the shoulder; and (3) scapulothoracic muscles orient the shoulder on the body for optimal positioning.

2. What are the most important capsule ligaments? What directional ability do they impart?

Shoulder ligaments primarily function as "check reins" at the extremes of motion. The inferior glenohumeral ligament complex is the most important because it resists anterior/inferior shoulder translation when the arm is placed in abduction, external rotation, and extension. The middle glenohumeral ligament resists external rotation in the neutral shoulder and anterior translation in the shoulder abducted to 45°. The superior glenohumeral ligament resists inferior translation with the arm in neutral position. The coracohumeral ligament resists posterior/inferior humeral head translation.

3. Describe the course and branches of the axillary nerve.

The nerve arises from the posterior cord of the brachial plexus, courses down on the surface of subscapularis and then posteriorly into the quadrangular space. Here it is vulnerable, lying next to the humeral neck. It gives off an articular twig and then divides in two as it exits the quadrangular space. The deep branch supplies the deltoid; the superficial branch supplies teres minor and then sends a cutaneous branch to the lateral upper arm.

4. During midrange of motion, what provides glenohumeral stability?

During midrange of motion the capsular ligaments are lax and stability is created by the rotator cuff and biceps that maintain a **concavity-compression effect** around the joint. This is a dynamic action in which the rotator cuff compresses the humerus into the congruent glenoid cavity. Lesions that affect this congruency, such as a glenoid rim fracture or labrum detachment, result in a loss of normal concavity-compression.

5. Is the glenohumeral joint a congruent or incongruent articulation?

The glenohumeral joint articular surfaces are congruent, although the surface area of the humerus is much greater than that of the glenoid. The subchondral bone of the glenoid is less curved than the humerus, but the articular cartilage of the glenoid is thickest at the periphery. The thickness of the cartilage, along with the labrum, deepens the articulating portion of the glenoid and creates a highly conforming joint.

PATHOANATOMY

6. What is a Bankart lesion? Discuss the pathoanatomy of the IGHL failure and its contribution to joint laxity.

First described by Perthes, the Bankart lesion is the most common lesion in traumatic anterior shoulder dislocations and occurs in about 85% of cases. The Bankart lesion is a detachment of the anterior/inferior glenoid labrum from the bony glenoid rim. It represents an avulsion of the glenoid attachment of the inferior glenohumeral ligament. It has been found that before failing at the glenoid insertion, A significant amount of midsubstance strain (plastic deformation) of the IGHL has been found to take place before failing at the glenoid insertion, leading to the concomitant capsular laxity that may accompany Bankart lesion. Both lesions contribute to shoulder instability.

7. What is a Hill-Sachs lesion? How does it contribute to recurrent shoulder instability?

Caused by impaction of the dislocated humeral head on the glenoid rim, a Hill-Sachs lesion is an osteochondral depression in the posterior humeral head. It may play a causal role in cases of recurrent instability when large enough to decrease the humeral head's contribution to passive stability (this is reported to require a depression of about 50% of the articular surface.)

8. Define the eponyms TUBS and AMBRII, which have been coined to characterize types of shoulder instability. Also discuss how shoulder instability may be thought of as a spectrum of pathogenesis.

T   Traumatic
U   Unidirectional with
B   Bankart lesion responding to
S   Surgery

A   Atraumatic
M   Multidirectional with
B   Bilateral shoulder findings responding to
R   Rehabilitation and,
I   If surgery, perform an
I   Inferior capsular shift

The causes of a patient's instability often overlap. Symptoms may present after an acute traumatic event (unidirectional, less generalized laxity), after multiple episodes of repetitive microtrauma with or without a recent traumatic episode (bidirectional, increased focal laxity), or after no trauma at all (multidirectional, generalized laxity). A careful history and physical exam may sort out the etiology, but it must be kept in mind that a spectrum of instability exists and that overlap often occurs. Generalized laxity and traumatic capsular avulsion may coexist.

9. What are the most common mechanisms for production of anterior and posterior shoulder dislocations?

Most dislocations occur through an indirect force applied to the arm. **Anterior dislocations** (95% of all dislocations) are produced by an external rotation and/or hyperextension force applied to the shoulder that is already in about 90° of abduction, at the extreme of external rotation, and in varying degrees of extension. **Posterior dislocations** (5% of all dislocations) are caused by indirectly applied force to the arm when the shoulder is variably flexed, adducted, and internally rotated. The force is usually directed posteriorly along the axis of the arm. Posterior dislocations are associated with seizures, electrocutions, and lightning strikes.

10. Describe some of the preferred methods for reducing an anterior dislocation.

1. Apply gentle longitudinal traction with countertraction, which is safe and reliable; slow alternation between internal and external rotation is often required to achieve a reduction.

2. Place the patient prone with a wrist weight suspended from the unsupported shoulder. Rotate the scapula toward the humeral head by application of pressure to the scapular spine.

11. What is the recurrence rate for patients who sustain an anterior shoulder dislocation?

A 1987 prospective study by Hovelius reported recurrence rates over 5 years. Age at the time of initial dislocation was the most important prognostic factor, with recurrence rates of 55% in patients 12–22 years of age, 37% in those 23–29 years, and 12% in those 30–40 years. Immobilization for 3–4 weeks did not reduce recurrence rates.

12. Are any other injuries associated with anterior shoulder dislocations?

Axillary nerve palsy is uncommon in any age group. Rotator cuff tears occur frequently in those over age 40. Fractures of the greater tuberosity are common in the elderly. Major vascular injury to the axillary vessels is reported in those with atherosclerotic disease.

13. Which radiographic views are useful in evaluating shoulder instability?

Radiographs taken from perpendicular planes are required: a "true" AP radiograph (which demonstrates the inferior glenoid rim) and either an axillary or transcapular "Y" lateral view should be taken. Specialized views, such as the West Point view, for visualizing the inferior glenoid rim for suspected Bankart fracture may occasionally be needed.

14. Describe a typical rehabilitation plan for a first-time traumatic shoulder dislocation.

In contrast to traditional recommendations for immobilization of up to 6 weeks in young athletes, recent studies indicate that immobilization is required only until adequate pain relief is attained, which typically occurs after 1–3 weeks. Goals of rehabilitation are (1) restoration of a full painless range of motion, (2) avoidance of "provocative" positions for 6 weeks, and (3) strengthening the cuff and scapulothoracic muscles. Patients >45 years should have motion restored as quickly as tolerated because their incidence of stiffness is high and recurrence low.

15. List the indications for immediate surgery for traumatic shoulder instability.

- Failed or unstable closed reduction
- Soft tissue interposition by the rotator cuff, capsule, or biceps tendon
- Greater tuberosity fractures that remain displaced >1 cm after reduction
- Large glenoid rim fractures

16. Discuss the effect a glenoid rim fracture has on stability of the glenohumeral joint and how to treat it.

An anteroinferior glenoid rim fracture lessens the stabilizing effect of concavity-compression and may lead to instability. If the fracture fragment is > 25%, the fragment should be reduced and placed in its normal position. If the fragment is < 25%, re-establishing the capsular origin at the glenoid rim margin is most important, and the fragment may either be excised or left displaced.

17. What physical findings are typical of an unreduced posterior dislocation?

External rotation and elevation are limited. The anterior shoulder is flattened and the coracoid process may be prominent. This type of dislocation is the most commonly missed, usually because of inadequate physical and radiographic exams.

18. Describe the basis and techniques for the sulcus, apprehension, and relocation tests.

The **sulcus test** demonstrates the degree of inferior laxity; it is thought to be a test of the superior glenohumeral ligament and the coracohumeral ligament. It is performed by stabilizing the scapula with the arm hanging at the side. The humerus is then distracted inferiorly. A large gap occurs beneath the acromion. The sulcus test measures mid-range stability, i.e., capsular volume.

Apprehension tests are provocative in that they stress involved ligament structures in the position of instability, conceptually confirming end-range instability. For the inferior glenohumeral ligament, this means placing the arm in abduction, external rotation, and extension. This position may cause an abnormal anterior translation of the humeral head, thus producing either shoulder pain or a sense of impending subluxation.

By reducing or relocating the head into its normal position through manual pressure on the humeral head, the apprehension symptoms should be relieved.

19. What are the commonly performed shoulder stabilization procedures?

The **Bankart repair** and its modifications reattach the glenoid labrum to bone—in effect, a medial repair of the inferior glenohumeral ligament complex. When a shoulder has chronic instability, the ligaments may be incompetent interstitially as well, contributing to capsular laxity, necessitating adjustment of the ligament tension in order to restore ligament balance. This procedure is termed *capsulorraphy* or *capsular shift*. The adjustment is made medially, inferiorly, or laterally in the capsule. Lateral-based shifts are the most effective and reliable. Scores of other procedures have been described; they often work by limiting range of motion so that end-range laxity is not challenged. This approach is not currently in favor in the United States.

20. Describe the location and functional significance of the rotator interval.

The rotator interval is the seam between subscapularis and supraspinatus tendons. Functionally, this widening probably represents dysfunction in the coracohumeral and/or superior glenohumeral ligaments, because these ligaments lie on the deep surfaces of the involved muscles. It is often widened in multidirectional instability, and closure of the gap surgically will decrease inferior subluxation.

21. Which rotator cuff lesions are associated with chronic shoulder instability?

Complete-thickness tears may occur in older individuals with traumatic shoulder dislocations. Rotator cuff tendinitis and partial-thickness undersurface tears are very common in patients with chronic shoulder subluxation, whether traumatic or atraumatic. Shoulder subluxation often presents as an "impingement syndrome" and should be suspected in any overhead athlete or person with a history of traumatic instability who has what appears to be impingement pain.

22. Should patients with voluntary shoulder instability be operated upon?

Most voluntary subluxators or dislocators have underlying psychiatric problems that an orthopaedic surgeon cannot help. Patients who can dislocate voluntarily are poor surgical candidates. Any patient with generalized laxity, scapulothoracic instability, or mistracking should be placed in an aggressive rehabilitation program for a minimum of 6 months.

Some patients are positional dislocators. They are able to dislocate if they put their arm in a provocative position and demonstrate laxity and instability, which they generally do reluctantly. Such patients are good surgical candidates for reconstruction.

CONTROVERSIES

23. What is the role of arthroscopic repair in the surgeon's armamentarium for shoulder instability?

Long-term follow-up of athroscopic instability procedures have demonstrated failure rates between 20 and 40%. Open capsular repair studies have shown success rates of 90–95%. It is believed that an arthroscopic repair of a Bankart lesion does not address the possible concomitant ligamentous laxity, and even if the laxity is not specifically addressed during an open Bankart repair, subsequent scarring improves results. Evidence shows that the arthroscopic approach works best in a high-demand athlete who has unidirectional instability and no global laxity, generally following a traumatic episode with associated Bankart lesion.

The recent advancement of capsular-shrinking techniques might improve the arthroscopic outcomes, but long-term follow-up studies have not been performed. Improvement in suture anchor techniques that emphasize capsular advancement are increasing in success. Open capsular shift is currently the gold standard that all new techniques must be judged against.

24. How accurate is laxity testing in the awake and anesthetized patient? How useful is it in planning surgical procedures?

A wide range of normal laxity exists for all test methods, and the overlap between symptomatic and asymptomatic joints is considerable. Likewise, examiner skills when evaluating for shoulder laxity vary considerably. Side-to-side comparisons are helpful in some individuals, but are indeterminate in others, which probably represents our ability to detect pathologic motions or reproduce joint reaction forces necessary to recreate instability patterns.

BIBLIOGRAPHY

1. American Academy of Orthopaedic Surgeons: Orthopaedic Knowledge Update 5. Rosemont, IL, 1996.
2. American Academy of Orthopaedic Surgeons: OKU Shoulder and Elbow. Rosemont, IL, 1996.
3. Bigliani LU: The Unstable Shoulder. Monograph, American Academy of Orthopaedic Surgeons, Rosemont, IL, 1996.
4. Flatow EL, Warner JJP: Instability of the shoulder: Complex problems and failed repairs. J Bone Joint Surg 80A:122–140, 1998.
5. Rockwood CA, Matsen FA: The Shoulder, 2nd ed. Philadelphia, W.B. Saunders, 1998.

24. INJURIES OF THE SHOULDER IN THE THROWING ATHLETE

Kirk S. *Hutton*, M.D.

1. Why is the shoulder so often injured in the throwing athlete?

The glenohumeral joint has more range of motion than any other joint in the human body. Stability of this joint depends on intact muscles and ligaments rather than on bony supporting structures. The forces generated in the throwing shoulder are much greater than the forces generated in the shoulder musculature alone, and, therefore, cause significant stresses around this joint, making it susceptible to acute and chronic inflammatory conditions.

2. List the five phases of pitching.

(1) Wind-up, (2) early cocking, (3) late cocking, (4) acceleration, and (5) follow through.

From Blackburn TA: Baseball and softball. In Mellion MB, Walsh WM, Shelton GL: The Team Physician's Handbook, 2nd ed. Philadelphia, Hanley & Belfus, 1997, with permission.

3. How does throwing form affect the incidence of shoulder injuries in the throwing athlete?

Proper body mechanics require that the thrower use his or her body weight and large leg, trunk, and back muscle groups to generate kinetic energy across the shoulder in the direction of the thrown object. In general, shoulder injuries occur in one of two ways. Improper body mechanics during the wind-up and cocking phases place more dependence on the shoulder muscles to generate the required energy to propel the object, thus leading to fatigue of the shoulder muscles. After the thrown object is released, the retained energy in the throwing arm needs to be dissipated by reversing the initial process, i.e., using the large muscles in the lower limb and back to absorb this energy. An improper follow through results in retention of excessive energy in the soft tissues of the shoulder, subsequently causing tissue damage.

4. What type of injuries may occur in the throwing athlete?

Acute overuse injuries, such as rotator cuff tendinitis and biceps tendinitis, are common. Chronic injuries include impingement syndrome, rotator cuff tears, glenoid labrum tears, and shoulder instability. Inflammation from repetitive stress may injure the acromioclavicular and the sternoclavicular joints. Uncommon causes of shoulder pain in the throwing athlete include quadrilateral space syndrome, suprascapular nerve entrapment, axillary artery occlusion, axillary vein thrombosis, posterior capsular laxity, and glenoid spurs.

5. What are the common presenting symptoms of an athlete with shoulder pain?

The athlete generally reports anterior shoulder pain that becomes worse with increased throwing velocity in his or her throw, stating that he or she cannot obtain maximum velocity in workouts or in a game situation. Occasionally, posterior shoulder pain is present.

6. What are the important positive findings on physical examination of a thrower with shoulder pain?

Most athletes with shoulder pain have positive impingement signs. More important, however, are the signs of subtle instability, such as a positive apprehension sign and a positive relocation test. Posterior capsular tightness manifest by decreased internal rotation of the shoulder also is significant.

7. Describe the apprehension test.

The apprehension test is used to detect anterior instability of the glenohumeral joint, and involves bringing the involved shoulder into approximately 90° of abduction and externally rotating the shoulder. As external rotation increases, the athlete with anterior instability will feel as if the shoulder is going to "pop out." He or she will guard against further external rotation and become very apprehensive—thus, the apprehension test.

8. Describe the relocation test.

The first part of the relocation test is performed just like the apprehension test. With the patient lying supine, abduct and externally rotate the arm while applying gentle anterior pressure to the posterior aspect of the humeral head. In the athlete with anterior subluxation, this maneuver usually causes pain as opposed to the uncomfortable sensation that the shoulder may dislocate. The second part of the relocation test involves repeating the test, but then applying a posteriorly directed force to the humeral head. This maneuver maintains the head in the anatomic position. A positive test occurs if the athlete experiences relief of pain in maximal abduction and external rotation.

9. Why is it important to distinguish between impingement and instability?

A few years ago, it was believed that most young athletes with anterior shoulder pain had primary impingement. They underwent the standard anterior acromioplasty with repair of the rotator cuff as needed. Tibone et al. reported that the results of this operation in young throwing athletes were very inconsistent. They have now shown that such athletes usually have primary instability with secondary impingement. Thus, an anterior acromioplasty with excision of the coracoacromial ligament in this population may cause more instability of the shoulder and magnify the symptoms.

10. What is the treatment for primary instability and secondary impingement?

The initial treatment of athletes with this condition involves aggressive rehabilitation. The program should begin with "relative rest," i.e., cessation of the overhead activity that causes the pain. Stretching should be done carefully and only for muscle groups with obvious tightness. Stretching the anterior muscles and capsule in a patient with anterior instability may cause further laxity. Lastly, strengthening exercises concentrating on the rotator cuff and scapular rotators should be performed. The entire program should be continued for 6–12 months with appropriate supervision and documentation before considering any operative procedures.

11. What is the function of the scapular rotators?

Muscles included in the scapular rotator group are the trapezius, serratus anterior, and the rhomboids. Their main function in the throwing athlete is to aid in glenohumeral stability by placing the glenoid in an optimal position for the throwing event.

12. Name the rotator cuff muscles.

Supraspinatus, infraspinatus, teres minor, and subscapularis.

13. What is the function of the rotator cuff muscles?

The subscapularis is an internal rotator, whereas the infraspinatus and teres minor are external rotators of the glenohumeral joints. As a whole, the rotator cuff functions to center the humeral head in the glenoid, thus adding stability and maximum leverage to shoulder motions.

14. Do ligaments add to the stability of the shoulder?

Yes. The glenohumeral ligaments and the labrum add stability to the shoulder. In the overhead athlete, the inferior glenohumeral ligament is the most important, because it is the prime anterior stabilizer when the arm is abducted >90° and externally rotated.

15. How does anterior instability develop in the throwing athlete?

Anterior instability may develop after a high-energy trauma, but in the throwing athlete it more commonly starts as an overuse injury. Chronic overuse can stretch the static stabilizers of the shoulder, thus causing mild instability. Such instability leads to asynchrony in the firing of the scapular rotators and rotator cuff muscles, putting increased stress on the rotator cuff to contain the humerus in the center of the glenoid. As the rotator cuff muscles become weakened from the overload, the head of the humerus subluxes more anteriorly as the arm is abducted and externally rotated. Anterior subluxation then causes secondary impingement of the rotator cuff on the acromion and the coracoacromial ligament.

16. Are imaging studies helpful in the diagnosis of shoulder pain?

Yes. Plain x-rays should be taken to rule out bony pathology such as fractures and osteoarthrosis. Special x-ray views such as the axillary view and West Point may demonstrate signs of instability (spurring or erosion of the anterior glenoid or a Hill-Sachs lesion).

17. Which imaging modality may be the most useful tool in diagnosing the cause of shoulder pain?

Recent studies indicate that MRI is superior to ultrasound and CT arthrography in evaluating shoulder pain due to rotator cuff tears, subacromial impingement, coracoacromial arch stenosis, and osteoarthritis of the glenohumeral or acromioclavicular joint.

18. What other diagnostic tools are helpful?

Selective injections with lidocaine can help pinpoint the painful area in the shoulder. Diagnostic arthroscopy is superior to an open operative procedure because it provides excellent visualization of the glenohumeral joint and subacromial space, causes less soft tissue destruction, and has a shorter rehabilitation period. With newly developed techniques, arthroscopy also may be used to correct or repair many pathologic conditions in the shoulder. Arthroscopy also affords the clinician the opportunity to evaluate for the presence, degree, and direction of shoulder laxity while the athlete is under anesthesia.

19. Is surgery ever necessary?

Yes. if a throwing athlete with instability has faithfully completed 6–12 months of an aggressive supervised rehabilitation program and still cannot participate in throwing secondary to pain, a surgical procedure that addresses the anterior capsule and labrum should be performed. Athletes with documented rotator cuff tears, labrum lesions, or loose bodies should have such lesions repaired or excised.

20. What is a SLAP lesion?

A SLAP lesion is an entity originally described and classified by Stephen Snyder in 1990. SLAP (**S**uperior **L**abrum **A**nterior and **P**osterior) involves the superior labrum, the biceps anchor, and a portion of the glenohumeral ligament attachment.

21. Describe the mechanism of injury of a SLAP lesion.

Two commonly described mechanisms cause a SLAP injury. In an acute traumatic event, a **superior compression type injury** may represent a fall on an outstretched arm, causing the humeral head to ride superiorly and creating a compression and subsequent avulsion of the superior glenoid labrum. In a thrower, a repetitive microtrauma occurs from rotator cuff disease that results in a chronic or recurrent superior translation of the humeral head on the glenoid rim, thus causing a SLAP lesion.

The second mechanism is **inferior traction**. An acute traumatic event, usually involving carrying a heavy object that causes axial inferior traction on the arm and biceps tendon complex, may cause a SLAP lesion. In the thrower the mechanism is a repetitive microtrauma associated with the previously mentioned subtle anterior instability.

BIBLIOGRAPHY

1. Bisson LJ, Andrews JR: Classification in mechanisms of shoulder injuries in throwers. In Andrews JR, Zarins B, Wilk KE (eds): Injuries in Baseball. Philadelphia, Lippincott-Raven, 1998, pp 47–55.
2. Glousman R, Jobe F, Tibone J, et al: Dynamic electromyographic analysis of the throwing shoulder with glenohumeral instability. J Bone Joint Surg 70A:220–226, 1988.
3. Hurley JA: Shoulder arthroscopy: Its role in evaluating shoulder disorders in the athlete. Am J Sports Med 18:480–483, 1990.
4. Marone PJ (ed): Shoulder Injuries in Sports. Rockville, MD, Aspen Publishers, Inc., 1992.
5. Nelson MC, Leather GP, Nirschl RP, et al: Evaluation of the painful shoulder. J Bone Joint Surg 73A:707–715, 1991.
6. Rockwood CA, Mattsen FA (eds): The Shoulder, vols. 1 and 2, 2nd ed. Philadelphia, W.B. Saunders, 1998.
7. Snyder SJ, Karzel RP, Del Pizzo W, et al: SLAP lesions of the shoulder. Arthroscopy 6:274–279, 1990.
8. Tibone JA, Jobe FA, Kerlin RF, et al: Shoulder impingement syndrome in athletes treated by anterior acromioplasty. Clin Orthop 188:134–140, 1985.

25. ACROMIOCLAVICULAR AND STERNOCLAVICULAR JOINTS

Jeffrey P. Davick, M.D.

1. What type of joint is the acromioclavicular joint?

The acromioclavicular joint is a diarthroidal (synovial) joint with a fibrocartilaginous disc between the two bones (similar to a meniscus).

2. Name the important ligaments around the acromioclavicular joint.

The acromioclavicular ligament connects the distal end of the clavicle to the acromion, providing horizontal stability. The coracoclavicular ligament connects the coracoid to the clavicle. It is made of two bands that provide vertical stability, the conoid and the trapezoid.

3. Describe the most common mechanism of injury to the acromioclavicular joint.

The acromioclavicular joint is most commonly injured by a direct fall onto the point of the shoulder with the arm adducted.

4. List the types of acromioclavicular sprains.

Type I sprain—a partial injury to the acromioclavicular ligament with no instability or displacement. The coracoclavicular ligament remains intact.

Type II sprain—disruption of the acromioclavicular ligament. The coracoclavicular ligament remains intact, preventing significant superior displacement of the clavicle.

Type III sprain—disruption of both the acromioclavicular and coracoclavicular ligaments, allowing superior displacement of the clavicle.

Type IV sprain—an injury in which the clavicle is displaced not only superiorly but also posteriorly into the trapezius (buttonhole).

Type V sprain—the clavicle is displaced superiorly to the point at which the clavicle is in a subcutaneous position.

Type VI sprain—an extremely rare injury in which both the acromioclavicular and coracoclavicular ligaments are disrupted, with the clavicle displaced inferior to the acromion or coracoid. This is usually the result of a high-energy injury and should arouse suspicion for associated injuries (fractures of the shoulder girdle, brachial plexus injuries, or disruption of the sternoclavicular joint).

5. How is an incomplete type II sprain differentiated from a complete type III sprain?

Stress radiographs may be very helpful and are taken with 10–15 lb of weight **strapped** to the patient's wrist. (Patients should not hold the weights with their hands.) With the patient sitting or standing, an AP radiograph obtained with the weights will show superior displacement of the clavicle in the complete or type III acromioclavicular sprain. The distance between the coracoid and clavicle should be measured. A 40–50% increase in the distance between the coracoid and clavicle when compared to the uninjured side is indicative of a complete disruption.

6. How is an acute incomplete type I or type II acromioclavicular sprain treated?

Ice and immobilization are needed initially. Patients are usually most comfortable in an arm sling. Early range of motion and strengthening are recommended.

7. What type of treatment is recommended for an acute complete disruption (type III through type VI)?

Nonoperative treatment (as in types I and III) is used for patients with limited functional requirements and for uncomplicated type III injuries.

Operative treatment for a type III injury is controversial. Functional results (strength and range of motion) are the same with operative and nonoperative treatment.

Type IV sprains often require operative treatment because the clavicle is buttonholed through the trapezius and remains painful, especially with overhead activities.

Operative treatment is recommended for open injuries, type VI sprains, and when the clavicle is subcutaneous and in danger of eroding through the skin (type V).

Operative treatment consists of repair or reconstruction of the coracoclavicular structures. Pins across the acromioclavicular joint should be avoided; they tend to migrate to undesirable sites such as the mediastinum.

8. What is the recommended treatment for chronically painful acromioclavicular separations?

Excision of the distal clavicle is warranted, followed by reconstruction of the coracoclavicular structures if needed. Coracoclavicular position is maintained by heavy suture or a removable screw. The coracoacromial ligament is detached from the acromion and transferred to the clavicle to act as a new coracoclavicular ligament (the Weaver-Dunn procedure).

9. What type of joint is the sternoclavicular joint?

The sternoclavicular joint, similar to the acromioclavicular joint, is a diarthroidal (synovial) joint with a fibrocartilaginous disc (similar to meniscus) between the clavicle and sternum.

10. Name the important ligaments around the sternoclavicular joint.

The costoclavicular ligaments have anterior fibers that resist upward rotation of the clavicle, and posterior fibers that resist downward rotation of the clavicle. The sternoclavicular ligament is actually a thick portion of the capsule. Its anterior fibers resist upward displacement of the clavicle.

11. What is the usual mechanism of injury to the sternoclavicular joint?

The most common mechanism of injury is a motor vehicle accident. Significant forces are necessary to cause dislocation of the sternoclavicular joint. A direct blow to the clavicle most commonly causes a posterior dislocation of the sternoclavicular joint. An indirect force to the anterolateral aspect of the clavicle can cause an anterior dislocation of the sternoclavicular joint, whereas an indirect force to the posterolateral aspect of the shoulder will cause a posterior dislocation of the sternoclavicular joint.

12. What are the common findings on physical examination of a dislocated sternoclavicular joint?

With **anterior** sternoclavicular dislocation, the medial aspect of the clavicle is prominent and the asymmetry is obvious.

With a **posterior** sternoclavicular dislocation, the findings are subtle. The medial end of the clavicle may be less palpable but more tender when compared with the other side. Patients also may complain of shortness of breath or have difficulty swallowing.

13. Describe the best way to evaluate the sternoclavicular joint radiographically.

AP views of the sternoclavicular joint are often difficult to interpret. Special projections include the serendipity view, which involves a 40° cephalic tilt of the x-ray beam. The medial aspect of both clavicles is seen on this view. Superior displacement of the clavicle represents an anterior dislocation, whereas inferior displacement represent a posterior dislocation. CT scans easily delineate the position of the medial clavicle compared to the sternum. MRI also can be used to provide the same information as the CT scan, but it also shows the soft tissue anatomy and associated mediastinal structures.

14. What are the treatment recommendations for acute sternoclavicular sprains?

With mild sprains that are not dislocated, patients are treated symptomatically with a sling until they are comfortable, followed by early rehabilitation.

Anterior dislocation of the sternoclavicular joint is treated with closed reduction done under either intravenous sedation or general anesthesia. Open reduction has a high complication rate and is generally not necessary.

Acute posterior dislocation is repaired with closed reduction and usually performed under general anesthesia. A towel clip may be required to manually assist reduction of the sternoclavicular joint. An open reduction may be needed for a posterior dislocation, and such injuries should be reduced to avoid late complications from erosion into the underlying mediastinal structures.

15. What is the treatment recommended for chronically dislocated sternoclavicular joints?

For chronic anterior sternoclavicular dislocation, nonoperative treatment is generally preferred. Patients are usually minimally asymptomatic and the condition is primarily a cosmetic problem. For chronic posterior dislocation of the sternoclavicular joint, operative treatment may be necessary to prevent potential complications (erosion of the clavicle into the underlying mediastinal structures). Open reduction and stabilization are usually performed with the assistance of a thoracic surgeon.

BIBLIOGRAPHY

 1. Bergfeld JA, Andrish JT, Clancy WG: Evaluation of the acromioclavicular joint following first and second degree sprains. Am J Sports Med 6:153–159, 1978.
 2. Bjernfeld H, Hovelius L, Thorling J: Acromioclavicular separations treated conservatively. Acta Orthop Scand 54:747–745, 1983.

3. Cox JS: The fate of the acromioclavicular joint in athletic injuries. Am J Sports Med 9:50, 1981.
4. Dias JJ, Steingold RA, Richardson RA, et al: The conservative treatment of acromioclavicular dislocation: Review after five years. J Bone Joint Surg 69B:719–722, 1987.
5. Eskola A: Sternoclavicular dislocation: A plea for open treatment. Acta Orthop Scand 57:227–228, 1986.
6. Galpin RD, Hawkins RJ, Grainger RW: A comparative analysis of operative versus nonoperative treatment of Grade III acromioclavicular separations. Clin Orthop 193:150–155, 1985.
7. Glick JM, Milburn LJ, Haggerty JF, Nishimoto D: Dislocated acromioclavicular joint: Follow-up study of 35 unreduced acromioclavicular dislocations. Am J Sports Med 5:264–270, 1977.
8. Heinig CF: Retrosternal dislocation of the clavicle: Early recognition, x-ray diagnosis and management. J Bone Joint Surg 50A:830, 1968.
9. Larsen E, Bjerg-Nielsen A, Christensen P: Conservative or surgical treatment of acromioclavicular dislocation: A prospective, controlled, randomized study. J Bone Joint Surg 68A:552–555, 1986.
10. Lee KW, Debski RE, Shen CH, et al: Functional evaluation of the ligaments at the acromioclavicular joint during anteroposterior and superoinferior translation. Am J Sports Med 25:858–862, 1997.
11. Lemos MJ: The evaluation and treatment of the injured acromioclavicular joint in athletes. Am J Sports Med 26:137–144, 1998.
12. Levinsohn EM, Bunnell WP, Yuan HA: CT in the diagnosis of dislocations of the sternoclavicular joint. Clin Orthop 140:12–16, 1979.
13. MacDonald PB, Alexander JM, Frejuk J, Johnson G: Comprehensive functional analysis of shoulders following complete acromioclavicular separation. Am J Sports Med 16:475–480, 1988.
14. Mehta JC, Sachdev A, Collins JJ: Retrosternal dislocation of the clavicle. Injury 5:79–83, 1973.
15. Phillips AM, Smart C, Groom AF: Acromioclavicular dislocation. Conservative or surgical therapy. Clin Orthop 353:10–17, 1998.
16. Press J, Zuckerman JD, Gallagher M, Cuomo F: Treatment of grade II acromioclavicular separations. Operative versus nonoperative management. Bull Hosp Dis 56:77–83, 1997.
17. Rawes ML, Dias JJ: Long-term results of conservative treatment for acromioclavicular dislocation. J Bone Joint Surg Br 78:410–412, 1996.
18. Rockwood CA Jr, Groh GI, Wirth M, Grassi FA: Resection arthroplasty of the sternoclavicular joint. J Bone Joint Surg Am 79:387–393, 1997.
19. Weaver JD, Dunn HK: Treatment of acromioclavicular injuries, especially complete acromioclavicular separation. J Bone Joint Surg 54A:1187–1197, 1972.
20. Worman LW, Leagus C: Intrathoracic injury following retrosternal dislocation of the clavicle. J Trauma 7:416–423, 1967.

26. ARTHRITIS, ARTHROPLASTY, AND ARTHRODESIS OF THE SHOULDER

Edward V. Fehringer, M.D.

1. What is arthritis of the shoulder?

Arthritis of the shoulder is any disease process of the glenohumeral joint that causes destruction of the articular surface of the glenohumeral joint and results in pain and loss of motion.

2. What is the differential diagnosis for arthritis of the shoulder?

1. Rheumatoid arthritis
2. Osteoarthritis
3. Posttraumatic arthritis
4. Rotator cuff arthropathy
5. Avascular necrosis
6. Other (hemochromatosis, hemophilia, gout, calcium pyrophosphate deposition disease, and other seronegative arthropathies)

3. What are the most common causes of shoulder arthritis?

Rheumatoid arthritis is the most common arthritic condition of the shoulder that requires surgical intervention by an orthopedic surgeon. Osteoarthritis and posttraumatic arthritis are uncommon but not rare conditions.

4. What is the usual clinical presentation of a patient with rheumatoid arthritis affecting the shoulder?

Occasionally shoulder pain with loss of motion is the first presenting complaint that prompts the diagnosis of rheumatoid arthritis. Usually, however, the patient has a known diagnosis of rheumatoid arthritis. The onset of pain is insidious and transitory rather than constant and progressive.

5. What is the natural history of rheumatoid arthritis of the shoulder?

During painful inflammatory attacks, the patient holds the arm internally rotated against the chest in the protective position. Resulting inactivity causes stiffness in the joint capsule and adjacent soft tissues. Weakness of the rotator cuff and deltoid muscles ensues. The resulting loss of motion causes a deleterious effect on the nutrition of the articular surface of the humeral head and the glenoid, resulting in further progression of joint arthrosis. If the disease is left untreated, progressive attacks cause thinning of the rotator cuff and eventually rotator cuff tear.

6. Does rheumatoid arthritis affect the shoulder in different ways?

The four main types of involvement of the shoulder with rheumatoid arthritis are dry, wet, resorptive, and bursal.

Dry form: Patients present with marked stiffness and loss of joint space. Radiographs demonstrate sclerosis and areas of cyst formation in the bones with osteophyte formation. Minimal marginal erosions are present. Clinically patients with the dry form are stiffer and weaker than patients with other forms.

Wet form: Radiographs show evidence of exuberant granulations and marginal erosions that cause the end of the bone to become pointed. No osteophyte formation is seen, and the humeral head erodes into the glenoid in a variable manner.

Resorptive form: Presenting signs and symptoms are increased pain, loss of motion, and dramatic destruction and resorption of bone from both the humeral end and the glenoid.

Bursal form: Subacromial and subdeltoid bursas may become massively swollen. The subacromial bursa is filled with rice bodies. Attempts to aspirate fluid prove fruitless, occasionally causing the treating physician to suspect a solid neoplasm. The bursal form spares the glenohumeral joint.

7. What nonoperative treatments are available for rheumatoid arthritis of the shoulder?

Patients usually have been treated by rheumatologists and primary care physicians before referral to an orthopedic surgeon. Conservative treatments are directed at diminution of pain and preservation of motion. Physical therapy may be prescribed to restore motion after intermittent painful attacks that lead to loss of motion and "frozen" shoulder. Intraarticular injections of steroids diminish the acute inflammatory attacks and provide pain relief. Nonoperative treatment is not always the most conservative therapy. If joint motion is not maintained or if the disease process is not kept in check, rotator cuff disease may ensue with rupture of the rotator cuff tendons; subsequent arthroplastic reconstruction becomes more difficult and results less predictable.

8. What is the clinical presentation of the patient with osteoarthritis of the shoulder?

Patients complain of the insidious onset of dull aching pain in the shoulder with every range of motion. Symptoms progress to pain at rest and then to stiffness and loss of motion. Many patients give a history of previous fracture about the shoulder. Heavy laborers and competitive weightlifters are also at risk. Frequently patients have a known diagnosis of osteoarthritis of other joints, and many have undergone arthroplasty procedures for other joints. Radiographs demonstrate areas of sclerosis with subchondral cysts and osteophytes. Cysts form in the superior humeral head in the area of the greatest contact pressure when the shoulder is in maximal abduction. Osteophytes form inferiorly on the head and glenoid neck. The posterior aspect of the glenoid is the most severely affected, with bone erosion leading to loss of the normal 35° of glenoid anteversion.

9. What surgical options are available for treatment of shoulder arthritis?

Synovectomy, open or arthroscopic   Resection arthroplasty
Hemiarthroplasty and total shoulder arthroplasty   Arthrodesis

10. What is synovectomy of the shoulder? What are its indications?

Synovectomy refers to removal of the diseased synovial lining of the shoulder joint. It is performed in patients with rheumatoid arthritis of the shoulder to alleviate pain and to arrest temporarily the inflammatory disease process. Indications are inflammatory arthropathies of the shoulder. Synovectomy should be reserved for patients in the early stages of the disease in whom little articular or osseous destruction has occurred.

11. What are hemiarthroplasty and total shoulder arthroplasty? How do they differ?

Hemiarthroplasty is the surgical replacement of the diseased humeral head with a metallic implant. The metallic head is shaped similar to the humeral head. The humeral head is attached to a stem, which is inserted into the intramedullary cavity of the humerus and fixed with poly-methylmethacrylate (bone cement) or with a press-fit bony ingrowth interface. Current implants are made of either cobalt-chrome-molybdenum alloy or titanium, aluminum, and vanadium alloys. Total shoulder arthroplasty refers to replacement of the glenoid surface in addition to the humeral head. The glenoid component is made of an ultrahigh–molecular-weight polyethylene, which is fixed to the remaining glenoid with polymethylmethacrylate. Other designs include a polyethylene surface attached to a metal back that is coated with a porous metallic surface de-signed to promote bony ingrowth.

12. What are the indications for shoulder arthroplasty?

The main indication is uncontrolled pain secondary to arthritis in the shoulder. Relative indi-cations include progressive pain in the shoulder that can be controlled temporarily by conser-vative measures; impending rotator cuff destruction may hasten the recommendation for arthroplasty.

13. Is there a weak link in total shoulder arthroplasty?

Due to early loosening problems, the glenoid component is the weak link. Whether this is due to eccentric wear, component malposition, improper soft tissue tensioning, or all of these factors remains somewhat unclear.

14. What are the main considerations in selection of hemiarthroplasty versus total shoul-der arthroplasty?

Controversy exists at this point as to which to perform. Hemiarthroplasty is usually selected when the articular surface of the glenoid has been preserved or in which the rotator cuff is non-functional (e.g., avascular necrosis of the humeral head, posttraumatic arthritis after fracture, and cuff tear arthropathy [see question 25]). Debate persists as to whether or not to resurface the gle-noid. Generally, total shoulder arthroplasty is performed when the glenoid articular surface is worn; however, glenoid component loosening problems persist. Moreover, many patients with rheumatoid arthritis receive pain relief with simple hemiarthroplasty even when the articular sur-face of the glenoid is worn. Also, many patients with rheumatoid arthritis have sustained such dramatic erosion of the glenoid that the bone stock is inadequate for glenoid component place-ment. Total shoulder arthroplasty is a more technically demanding procedure, and should not be performed by someone who has not had adequate training in this area. Excellent results have been attained with both in terms of significant long-term pain relief as well as improvement in function. These results can also be achieved in young patients (those 50 years and younger). Rates of revision are typically higher for those who have had a hemiarthroplasty for the sequelae of trauma rather than rheumatoid arthritis. Risk of revision is also higher for younger patients and for those with a concomitant rotator cuff tear at the time of the initial surgery. Current and persis-tent issues of controversy include implant modularity, glenohumeral mismatch, and implant fixa-tion in addition to the role of glenoid replacement.

15. What are the contraindications to shoulder arthroplasty?

The only absolute contraindication is active infection. Relative contraindications include pa-tients with a neuropathic joint and young heavy laborers who are unwilling or unable to alter their lifestyle. Another relative contraindication is complete incompetence of the rotator cuff and deltoid, which renders the prosthesis highly unstable.

16. What are the different types of shoulder arthroplasty designs?

1. **Constrained design.** This original design resulted in an unacceptably high rate of glenoid loosening. The shoulder is one of the most unconstrained joints in the body and relies on muscular and soft-tissue balancing for stability. Constrained designs are currently unavailable.

2. **Unconstrained designs.** Because they are characterized by a nearly anatomic shape of the humeral head and glenoid surface, reconstruction of the shoulder with unconstrained design tends to recreate normal anatomy and biomechanics. The humeral component consists of an anatomically shaped articulating head made of metallic alloy and attached to a stem that is inserted into the humeral intermedullary canal. The humeral component is designed to maintain the integrity of the rotator cuff attachment at the anatomic neck. The glenoid is a flat dish made of polyethylene that is secured to the remaining glenoid with polymethylmethacrylate or a metal-backed porous ingrowth material.

3. **Semiconstrained designs.** These designs consist of a glenoid component with a superior polyethylene hood to help prevent superior subluxation of the humeral head. They are usually employed with a weak or incompetent rotator cuff or deltoid. Although theoretically appealing, even a small degree of constraint causes increased glenoid keel stresses, which theoretically hasten glenoid loosening.

17. What surgical approach is used for shoulder arthroplasty?

An extensile anterior approach (deltopectoral) to the shoulder exploits the internervous plane between the deltoid (axillary) nerve and the pectoralis major (medial and lateral pectoral) nerves.

18. What are the complications of shoulder arthroplasty?

1. **Proximal migration of the humeral component.** Proximal migration occurs in approximately 25% of cases and is not necessarily related to pain, loss of motion, rates of glenoid loosening, or rates of mechanical loosening. Improved glenoid designs and glenoid fixation have dramatically decreased the rate of mechanical loosening.

2. **Infection.** The infection rate of shoulder arthroplasty (0.5–3%) is consistent with that in other joints. Rates are higher in patients with rheumatoid arthritis because of their immunocompromised state.

3. **Instability.** Instability results from poor soft-tissue balance, muscle atrophy, or malposition of components.

19. What results can be expected from total shoulder arthroplasty?

Pain relief is the major result. Studies with follow-up for as long as 15 years report relief of pain in 90–95% of patients with osteoarthritis. Hemiarthroplasty yields pain relief in 85–90% of patients, but the pain appears to worsen with time. Patients with intact rotator cuffs obtain the best functional results; worse results are reported in patients with posttraumatic arthritis, who usually have preexisting rotator cuff and capsular scarring. Implant longevity is approximately equal to arthroplasties of other joints. Most studies indicated a revision rate of approximately 11% at 20 years.

20. Are there indications for primary hemiarthroplasty in fractures?

Both 4-part proximal humerus fractures with or without a dislocation as well as head-splitting fractures are indications for primary hemiarthroplasty. These fractures result in a complete disruption of the humeral head blood supply. Neither primary arthrodesis nor total shoulder arthroplasty is indicated, as the glenoid is likely normal. Cemented humeral head replacement is the treatment of choice.

21. Can a loose glenoid component be revised?

The glenoid bone stock is very limited. After symptomatic loosening occurs, rarely is enough bone left to accept a new prosthesis; therefore, removal of the glenoid component is indicated.

Uncemented components are bulky and require good bone stock and press fit to be useful. Resection arthroplasty can be used to treat sepsis but results in a flail shoulder. Arthrodesis following shoulder arthroplasty is difficult to achieve because of bone loss. Hemiarthroplasty with resection of the glenoid component and cement can improve pain with reasonable results. Scapular allograft is not indicated.

22. What is the likelihood of treating a patient with a classic osteoarthritic shoulder that has a full-thickness rotator cuff defect?

The incidence of full-thickness rotator cuff defects in osteoarthritis is $\leq 5\%$.

23. What is the role of soft tissue balancing in total shoulder arthroplasty?

Restoration of anatomy to near-normal status is extremely important to achieve a stable implant. To avoid sacrificing stability, it is not uncommon for soft tissues to be either over-tightened or insufficiently released.

24. Has there been an increase in component survivorship related to cementing techniques?

Meticulous attention to cement technique may improve the long-term survival of cemented shoulder arthroplasty components.

25. What is cuff tear arthropathy?

Cuff tear arthropathy refers to disease of the shoulder that is different from osteoarthritis and posttraumatic arthritis. Longstanding tears of the rotator cuff lead to disease of the humeral glenoid articular surface that is characterized by an irregular pebble stone appearance of the articular cartilage with collapse of the softened underlying bone. A massive tear of the rotator cuff results in dislocation and subluxation of the humeral joint, which appears as abnormal trauma on the articular surface. This process has also been referred to as "Milwaukee shoulder." The etiology is variable and not entirely understood. Surgical reconstruction is difficult because of the almost complete loss of the constraining force of the rotator cuff. This condition, when intolerable, has been treated with an oversized hemiarthroplasty component as well as with various forms of total shoulder arthroplasty. However, although the short-term results have been good, "overstuffing of the joint" (especially with an oversized component) has led to long-term postoperative stiffness and pain. As a result, the more recent trend has been to place a smaller, near-anatomic hemiarthroplasty with normal tensioning of the soft tissues.

26. What is shoulder arthrodesis? What are the surgical indications?

Shoulder arthrodesis is surgical resection of the glenohumeral surfaces and fusion. Relative indications for shoulder arthrodesis include young heavy laborers with osteoarthritis who are unwilling or unable to alter their lifestyle. Arthrodesis is occasionally recommended because of the fear of rapid mechanical loosening of an overused shoulder arthroplasty. Other indications include uncontrolled joint sepsis, complete loss of the rotator cuff and deltoid musculature, and salvage for failed total shoulder arthroplasty.

27. In what position should the shoulder be fused?

Shoulder arthrodesis should be performed so that the arm rests comfortably at the side without scapular winging and the hand can be brought easily to the mouth and front pocket. Twenty degrees of flexion, 30° of abduction, and 40° of internal rotation offer the best position for shoulder fusion.

28. What is resection arthroplasty? What are the surgical indications?

Resection arthroplasty is resection of the humeral head. One of the original techniques for treatment of intractable pain due to shoulder arthritis, this procedure is now rarely indicated, because it renders a flail shoulder and pain relief is unpredictable. Resection arthroplasty is most often used for intractable joint infection, infected nonunion of shoulder arthrodesis, and neoplastic processes of the shoulder.

BIBLIOGRAPHY

1. Arntz CT, Jackins S, Matsen FA: Prosthetic replacement of the shoulder for the treatment of defects in the rotator cuff and the surface of the glenohumeral joint. J Bone Joint Surg 75A:485–590, 1993.
2. Boyd AD Jr, Thomas WH, Scott RD, Thornhill TS: Total shoulder arthroplasty versus hemiarthroplasty: Indications for glenoid resurfacing. J Arthroplasty 5:329–336, 1990.
3. Cofield RD: Instruction course lectures. 34:268–277, 1985.
4. Figgie HE III, Inglis AE, Goldberg VM, et al: An analysis of factors affecting the long-term results of total shoulder arthroplasty in inflammatory arthritis. J Arthroplasty 123:130, 1988.
5. Friedman RJ: Arthroplasty of the Shoulder. New York, Thieme Medical Publishers, 1994.
6. Gartsman GM, Russell JA, Gaenslen E: Modular shoulder arthroplasty. J Shoulder Elbow Surg 6:333–339, 1997.
7. Green A: Current concepts of shoulder arthroplasty. Instr Course Lect 47:123–133, 1998.
8. Neer CS II: Shoulder Reconstruction. Philadelphia, W.B. Saunders, 1990.
9. Norris BL, Lachiewicz PF: Modern cement technique and the survivorship of total shoulder arthroplasty. Clin Orthop 328:76–85, 1996.
10. Rockwood CA Jr, Matsen FA III: The Shoulder, vols. 1 and 2, 2nd ed. Philadelphia, W.B. Saunders, 1998.
11. Sledge CB, Ruddy S, Harris ED Jr, Kelley WN (eds): Arthritis Surgery. Philadelphia, W.B. Saunders, 1994.
12. Sperling JW, Cofield RH, Rowland CM: Neer hemiarthroplasty and Neer total shoulder arthroplasty in patients fifty years old or less. Long-term results. J Bone Joint Surg 80A:464–473, 1998.

27. PEDIATRIC SHOULDER

Keith R. Gabriel, M.D.

1. You are called to the nursery to examine a newborn infant who does not spontaneously move one upper extremity. Visually the limb appears normal. What conditions should be included in the initial differential diagnosis?
- Birth palsy (brachial plexus palsy)
- Birth fracture

2. Erb's palsy involves primarily which roots of the brachial plexus?
Erb's palsy involves primarily the upper roots: C4–C6.

3. Which shoulder muscles are usually affected in Erb's palsy?
The shoulder external rotators (supraspinatus, infraspinatus, teres minor) and frequently the deltoid are affected. Occasionally the elbow flexors may be involved.

4. What is the characteristic positioning of the shoulder in Erb's palsy?
The characteristic positioning of the shoulder includes adduction and internal rotation.

5. Are there other types of birth palsy (brachial plexus palsy)?
Yes. The entire plexus may be involved, or only the lower roots, C8 and T1, may be injured (Klumpke's palsy). Erb's palsy is seen four times more frequently than other types.

6. What is the most common birth fracture?
The most common birth fracture involves the clavicle. Such fractures heal readily and are treated simply. Many infants are wrapped in a blanket, which may provide sufficient immobilization. Sometimes the sleeve of the baby's shirt is pinned or loosely sewn to the chest portion of the shirt. Any device (e.g., sling) that encircles the neck should be avoided.

7. During the nursery exam, you palpate what seems to be a clavicle fracture on the right side, but the infant moves the limb normally and does not protest or cry during the exam. A radiograph confirms a small gap in the middle third of the right clavicle. What do you suspect?

The likely diagnosis is pseudarthrosis of the clavicle. A birth fracture of the clavicle should be painful. Pseudarthrosis is a rare congenital condition that almost invariably occurs on the right. The diagnosis is confirmed if no healing reaction is seen on a radiograph at 2 weeks. Orthopedic intervention is usually deferred until age 3–5 years.

8. You are called to the nursery to see a newborn infant who does not spontaneously move the upper extremity. The infant seems to react with pain when you move the shoulder (glenohumeral) joint. Is it dislocated?

Almost certainly not. Shoulder dislocation, either congenital or traumatic, is rare. Birth fracture of the humerus, specifically a fracture through the proximal growth plate, is much more likely. Even when displaced, such fractures usually heal well. Treatment is the same as described for birth fracture of the clavicle.

9. You evaluate an infant with asymmetry at the base of the neck and scapulae. The infant moves the involved upper extremity and shows no sign of pain; yet shoulder abduction, active and passive, is limited compared with the other shoulder. What do you suspect?

The likely diagnosis is Sprengel's deformity (congenital elevation of the scapula). The involved scapula is usually small and displaced upward and forward. Orthopedic intervention depends on functional limitations, which are quite variable. Associated congenital anomalies (scoliosis, cervical fusions, cardiac and renal conditions) should be suspected.

10. A newborn infant has asymmetry of the front of the shoulder. Specifically, one side of the chest seems flat, as though a portion of the pectoralis musculature has not developed. Before talking to the family, what topic should you review?

The likely diagnosis is Poland's syndrome. Examine the infant for cardiac anomalies and syndactyly.

11. A 6-month-old infant seems fussy and has stopped using her shoulder. The child spontaneously moves the elbow, forearm, wrist, and hand. A reliable caretaker observed no trauma. What is your primary and urgent concern?

The urgent concern is infection. Both hematogenous osteomyelitis and septic arthritis may present insidiously. Fever is quite variable. The peripheral white blood cell count may not be elevated initially; the erythrocyte sedimentation rate and C-reactive protein are more sensitive, although nonspecific. Radiographic changes may take a week or more to develop. A high index of suspicion should be maintained.

12. A 13-year-old tennis player or baseball pitcher presents with activity-related pain in the dominant shoulder. The radiograph shows widening and irregularity of the proximal humeral physis. What is the diagnosis?

The disorder sometimes is called little leaguer's shoulder, although other overhead sports may be involved. It is treated symptomatically, and activity restrictions are usually sufficient. Permanent avoidance of the athletic activity is not necessary. The condition is self-limited with no known sequelae.

13. An adolescent swimmer complains of anterior shoulder pain after prolonged workouts. The radiographs are unremarkable. What is a possible diagnosis?

A possible diagnosis is impingement syndrome, sometimes called swimmer's shoulder. The musculotendinous structures of the rotator cuff are pinched repeatedly between the humeral head and the anatomic arch created by the anterior acromion, the acromioclavicular joint, and the coracoacromial ligament. In young athletes, impingement syndrome is usually treated by activity restrictions, physical therapy, and adjustment of the mechanics involved in the sport. In many young athletes, occult instability may be the primary cause of impingement symptoms.

14. What proportion of growth of the humerus is contributed by the proximal humeral physis?

About 80% of growth is contributed by the proximal humeral physis. Proportionately, this is the largest contribution that any growth plate makes to its respective long bone.

15. What bearing does the tremendous growth potential of the proximal humeral physis have on management of fractures of the proximal humerus in juvenile patients?

Moderate angulation or displacement is acceptable because of the tremendous potential for remodeling.

16. A pathologic fracture of the proximal humeral metaphysis in a juvenile patient is often the initial presentation of what benign bone tumor?

A pathologic fracture of the proximal humeral metaphysis is often the initial presentation of a unicameral cyst (simple bone cyst). The proximal humerus is the most common location of this benign tumor.

17. What is the only direct bony connection, or bony strut, between the chest and the shoulder?

The clavicle.

18. What is the most frequently fractured long bone in childhood?

The clavicle.

19. What is the usual treatment for fractures of the shaft of the clavicle?

Fractures of the shaft of the clavicle unite readily and are almost always treated by closed methods. Figure-of-eight bandages, slings, and combinations thereof are usually recommended.

20. What are the indications for open (operative) treatment of a clavicle fracture?

Open fractures must be treated with irrigation and debridement. Exploration may be needed if neurovascular compromise is suspected. A few clavicle fractures are grossly displaced, with the fracture fragments "buttonholed" through the platysma or trapezius; such fractures require open reduction.

21. Fractures and dislocations of the medial clavicle (sternoclavicular joint) are distinctly uncommon in children. When they occur, what is the usual direction of the displacement?

Displacement is usually anterior.

22. What may be the primary concern in a posteriorly displaced fracture-dislocation of the sternoclavicular joint?

The primary concern is compromise of mediastinal structures.

23. Shoulder separations (subluxation and dislocations of the acromioclavicular joint) occur commonly when an adult athlete falls directly onto the point of the shoulder. Would you expect the same injury in a juvenile soccer player?

No. Most distal clavicle or acromioclavicular joint injuries in children are fractures through the distal clavicular physis.

24. How often do you expect to treat children for traumatic dislocation of the shoulder?

Not often. Traumatic shoulder dislocation is uncommon before adolescence.

25. A child sustains traumatic dislocation of the shoulder, with no neurovascular compromise, and the dislocation is successfully reduced by closed reduction. Why should the prognosis still be guarded?

The recurrence rate is at least 50% when the initial dislocation occurs in childhood or adolescence.

BIBLIOGRAPHY

1. Bak K, Fauno P: Clinical findings in competitive swimmers with shoulder pain. Am J Sports Med 25:254, 1997.
2. Busch MT: Sports medicine. In Morrissy RT, Weinstein SL (eds): Lovell and Winter's Pediatric Orthopaedics, 4th ed. Philadelphia, Lippincott-Raven, 1996, pp 1181–1228.
3. Canale ST (ed): Campbell's Operative Orthopaedics, 9th ed. St. Louis, Mosby, 1998.
4. Kay SPJ: Obstetrical brachial palsy. Br J Plast Surg 51:43, 1998.
5. Ogden JA: Skeletal Injury in the Child, 2nd Ed. Philadelphia, W.B. Saunders, 1990.
6. Roberts SW, Hernandez C, Maberry MC, et al: Obstetric clavicular fracture: The enigma of normal birth. Obstet Gynecol 86:978, 1995.
7. Sanders JO, Rockwood CA, Curtis RJ: Fractures and dislocations of the humeral shaft and shoulder. In Rockwood CA, Wilkins KE, Beaty JH (eds): Fractures in Children, 4th ed. Philadelphia, Lippincott-Raven, 1996, pp 905–1022.
8. Schnall SB, King JD, Marrero G: Congenital pseudarthrosis of the clavicle: A review of the literature and surgical results of six cases. J Pediatr Orthop 8:316, 1988.
9. Tachdjian MO: Pediatric Orthopedics, 2nd ed. Philadelphia, W.B. Saunders, 1990.
10. Wagner KT, Lyne ED: Adolescent traumatic dislocations of the shoulder with open epiphyses. J Pediatr Orthop 3:61, 1993.

28. SHOULDER ARTHROSCOPY

Kirk S. Hutton, M.D.

1. What areas of the shoulder can be seen during routine shoulder arthroscopy?

Routine shoulder arthroscopy involves evaluation of the glenohumeral joint, including the rotator cuff, biceps tendon, articular surfaces, glenoid labrum, and other recesses where loose bodies may hide. Shoulder arthroscopy also includes evaluation of the subacromial bursa, bursal surface of the rotator cuff, coracoacromial ligament, anatomy of the acromion, and the acromioclavicular joint.

2. What types of procedures can be done arthroscopically in the shoulder?

Shoulder arthroscopy has evolved over recent years to involve many procedures that previously had been done open. It began as a strictly diagnostic procedure and progressed to the point where certain areas of the shoulder could be shaved and debrided. As arthroscopic techniques improved, surgeons performed arthroscopic subacromial decompressions/acromioplasties. Distal clavicle excisions also can be performed arthroscopically with the aid of high-speed burs. Recently, surgeons with advanced arthroscopic skills have performed anterior and posterior stabilizations using various suture and suture anchor techniques and heat-shrinking techniques. Glenoid labrum tears and rotator cuff tears are being completely repaired through the scope with the use of such techniques.

3. What are the indications for shoulder arthroscopy?

Arthroscopy may be used to aid in the diagnosis of any condition in which the preoperative diagnosis is unclear or incomplete. It also is indicated for the treatment of known pathology, such as impingement syndrome, shoulder instability, and rotator cuff pathology.

4. Does shoulder arthroscopy require any special equipment?

Yes. Many special instruments make shoulder arthroscopy easier to perform. In addition to the standard arthroscopic equipment, shoulder arthroscopy requires special guide rods (Wissinger rods and switching sticks) in order to move the portals. A longer arthroscopic probe also is helpful. Operative cannulas with diaphragms to prevent fluid leakage are necessary to reduce significant swelling that may occur during the procedure. Depending on the type of procedure, other specialized instruments may be needed, such as arthroscopic suture anchors and rotator cuff repair systems. An arthroscopic pump, although unnecessary, does help to gauge the pressure settings that aid in hemostasis.

5. What position should a patient be placed in for shoulder arthroscopy?

Two positions are routinely used. The most common position is the lateral decubitus position in which the patient is turned to lie on the nonoperative side and held in place with a bean bag or a type of kidney rest to stabilize his or her position. An axillary roll always is placed beneath the thorax to prevent pressure on the axillary artery. All bony prominences must be padded to prevent skin necrosis during the procedure. Once the body has been placed in this position, the arm may be held in place by a commercial traction unit or one made from pulleys in the operative suite. The position of the arm in the lateral decubitus position depends on the procedure, but in general approximately 20° of abduction and 5–10° of forward flexion is acceptable. The lateral decubitus position allows for easy access to the glenohumeral joint, the subacromial space, and also is an ideal position for performing a mini-open rotator cuff repair.

The lateral decubitus position. The patient lies on the nonoperative side throughout the procedure while the arm is held in place by a traction unit.

The second most commonly used position for shoulder arthroscopy is the beach-chair or semi-Fowler's position, which has the advantage of keeping all structures anatomically oriented. The patient is also in the appropriate position for an open anterior approach, if necessary. An assistant may be needed to place traction on the arm for certain procedures. The beach-chair position also allows for manipulation of the arm during surgery.

The beach-chair (semi-Fowler's) position. All structures are kept anatomically oriented to allow manipulation of the arm during surgery.

6. How is the examination under anesthesia conducted?

The examination under anesthesia is performed on the shoulder after the patient has received the general anesthetic. The range of motion and stability of the shoulder is tested, including anterior, posterior, and inferior translations. It is important to compare the operative with the nonoperative side to document a definitive notation of any type of instability before inserting the arthroscope into the shoulder. This very important part of the arthroscopic and presurgical procedure should be performed on every patient. The examination under anesthesia obviously removes a patient's response to painful motion of the shoulder and also takes away muscle contraction, possibly allowing detection of instability that was not diagnosed preoperatively due to patient guarding or pain.

7. What kind of anesthesia may help with shoulder surgery?

An interscalene block performed by the anesthesiologist may be a helpful regional block given before shoulder surgery. The block involves placing a needle between the anterior and middle scalene muscles and instilling local anesthetic in the area of the brachial plexus. A nerve stimulator helps to ensure the appropriate location of the block, but the paresthesia technique also may be used. It is important to perform the block on an awake patient to avoid potentially disastrous intraneural injections. The interscalene block not only decreases the amount of general anesthetic agent required during surgery, but also gives the patient 12–18 hours of postoperative pain relief.

8. Which portals are commonly used in shoulder arthroscopy?

The **posterior portal** is the most commonly used portal through which the arthroscope is first inserted into the glenohumeral joint. This portal is located 2–3 cm inferior and slightly medial to the posterolateral angle of the acromion and corresponds to the soft spot between the infraspinatus and teres minor muscles posteriorly. The anterior portal is commonly referred to as the working portal for glenohumeral arthroscopy.

The **anterior portal** may be established via an inside-out or an outside-in technique and should remain lateral to the coracoid process, entering the glenohumeral joint above the subscapularis tendon and under the biceps tendon. This area corresponds with the rotator interval in the glenohumeral joint. Numerous other accessory portals can be made anterolaterally and posterolaterally depending on the area of the glenohumeral or subacromial space that needs to be addressed surgically.

9. Which structures should be evaluated during routine shoulder arthroscopy?

Like any other surgical procedure, shoulder arthroscopy needs to be done in a systematic fashion. A technique should allow the surgeon to evaluate every structure within the shoulder and do it the same way every time. Snyder has published a useful 15-point glenohumeral joint evaluation and anatomy review that begins by visualizing from the posterior portal and evaluates the following structures:

1. Biceps tendon
2. Posterior labrum and capsule attachment
3. Inferior axillary recess and inferior capsular insertion to humeral head
4. Inferior labrum and glenoid articular surface
5. Supraspinatus tendon
6. Posterior rotator cuff insertion in the bare area of the humeral head
7. Articular surface of the humeral head
8. Anterior superior labrum, superior and middle glenohumeral ligament, and subscapularis tendon
9. Anterior/inferior labrum
10. Anterior/inferior glenohumeral ligament

The remaining five structures are visualized with the arthroscope in the anterior portal and include:

11. Posterior glenoid labrum
12. Posterior aspect of rotator cuff, including infraspinatus and supraspinatus
13. Anterior glenoid labrum and inferior glenohumeral ligament attachments to the labrum
14. Subscapularis tendon and recess, as well as middle glenohumeral ligament
15. Anterior surface of the humeral head with subscapularis attachment and biceps tendon passage

10. Is the intraarticular anatomy the same in every shoulder?

No. Many variations are found involving the glenoid labrum and the anterior glenohumeral ligaments that are important for the shoulder arthroscopist to recognize. Less experienced shoulder surgeons may think that some anatomic variants are abnormalities and attempt to repair these normal structures. Two common normal variants include a cordlike middle glenohumeral ligament and the Buford complex, which involves a cordlike glenohumeral ligament with no anterosuperior glenoid labrum.

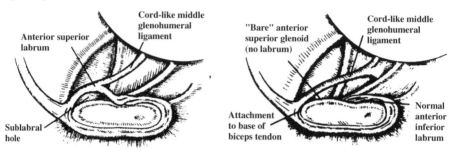

Left, The cordlike middle glenohumeral ligament may attach to the superior labrum, often with an underlying sublabral hole. (From Snyder SJ: Shoulder Arthroscopy. New York, McGraw-Hill, 1994, p 33, with permission.)

Right, The Buford complex is a rare but important anatomic formation to recognize. It is often mistaken for a pathologic labral detachment. (From Snyder SJ: Shoulder Arthroscopy. New York, McGraw-Hill, 1994, p 32, with permission.)

11. What is the difference between the subacromial bursa and the glenohumeral joint?

The subacromial bursa and glenohumeral joint are anatomically separate areas that are evaluated during routine shoulder arthroscopy. The glenohumeral joint is an area that involves the articular surface of the glenoid, the humeral head, and all other structures mentioned in Snyder's 15-point anatomic checklist for shoulder arthroscopy. The subacromial bursa is a completely separate area in which the arthroscope must be moved superior to the rotator cuff and in a space between the acromion and the superior surface of the rotator cuff. In the subacromial bursa, visualization is generally more difficult and the anatomy is less well defined. The structures involved in this area include the bursal surface of the rotator cuff, the undersurface of the acromion, the coracoacromial ligament, the subdeltoid bursa, and the AC joint. The arthroscopic subacromial decompression is performed in the subacromial bursa. Also, some arthroscopists perform an excision of the distal clavicle while working in the subacromial space.

12. What common abnormalities can be diagnosed during shoulder arthroscopy?

Shoulder arthroscopy is highly useful in the diagnosis and treatment of many shoulder problems. For example, full-thickness or partial-thickness tears of the rotator cuff can be diagnosed. Some surgeons classify rotator cuff tears as partial- versus full-thickness tears, whereas others further classify them as "A" tears, which involve tears on the articular surface; "B" tears, which are seen in the subacromial bursa; or "C" tears, which are complete tears of the rotator cuff. Other abnormalities that can be diagnosed include partial or full biceps tendon tears, glenoid labrum tears, and SLAP (superior labrum, anteroposterior) lesions (SLAP lesions are detailed in chapter 24). A Bankart lesion is another type of glenoid labrum tear that involves an avulsion of the anterior labrum and the glenohumeral ligaments away from the anterior neck of the glenoid. Degenerative changes of the humeral head and glenoid articular surfaces also can be diagnosed, as well as the presence or absence of osteochondral loose bodies, adhesive capsulitis, and other synovial disorders.

13. Describe the glenoid labrum.

The glenoid labrum is a fibrocartilaginous tissue that encircles the glenoid. The biceps tendon attaches to this area, as do the glenohumeral ligaments. The superior labrum often appears loosely attached and may have a meniscoidlike appearance. The glenoid labrum serves as attachment for the glenohumeral ligaments and biceps, and also adds stability to the shoulder by adding depth and concavity to the glenoid socket itself. The glenoid labrum can be damaged in many ways, such as a Bankart lesion from a dislocation or a SLAP lesion from the mechanisms documented in chapter 24, as well as degenerative changes from chronic rotator cuff disease or arthritis.

14. What common complications may occur from incorrect portal placement during shoulder arthroscopy?

Portal placement is highly crucial for proper shoulder arthroscopy. During placement of the posterior portals, the axillary nerve and the descending branch of the suprascapular nerve are at risk. The axillary nerve is approximately 6–7 cm distal to the posterolateral corner of the acromion and spine of the scapula. This distance is some 4–5 cm below the usual posterior portal placement; therefore, the axillary nerve should be safe. The suprascapular nerve is the most commonly injured nerve during shoulder arthroscopy and is located 1.5–2 cm medial to the edge of the glenoid below the area of the spinoglenoid notch. If the posterior portal is too medial, the suprascapular nerve can be injured. It is important to use a blunt trochar and identify the anatomic landmarks before placing this portal to avoid nerve injury.

While making the anterior portals, it is important to always stay lateral to the coracoid process. Structures at risk during anterior portal placement include the cephalic vein, axillary nerve, and musculocutaneous nerve. A common saying in shoulder arthroscopy with regards to the coracoid is that the lateral side is the "safe side," the medial side is the "suicide."

15. What other potential complications may occur during shoulder arthroscopy?

As with any surgical procedure, appropriate positioning and protection of the patient during the procedure is of paramount importance. Appropriate positioning of the head and neck avoids neck or brachial plexus stretch lesions. Padding all bony prominences prevents skin-pressure injuries. In the lateral decubitus position with the arm held in the arthroscopic traction device, stretch or traction injuries may occur to the arm if too much weight is applied over a prolonged period. Shoulder arthroscopy also involves the use of arthroscopic fluid to distend the joint or subacromial bursa; fluid extravasation and compartment syndromes may result if the pressure on the arthroscopic pump and the fluid system is not well managed. Compartment syndrome in the shoulder is very rare but has occurred; prevention is the best form of treatment. Small amounts of swelling and tissue edema should not cause worry, because the body gradually resorbs the arthroscopic fluid within 1–2 hours after the procedure.

16. What is a subacromial decompression? How is it performed?

A subacromial decompression is a procedure initially developed by Neer and performed in an open technique. Recently, shoulder surgeons have advanced to performing this arthroscopically in patients diagnosed with impingement syndrome, rotator cuff tendinitis, or subacromial bursitis. The subacromial decompression is performed in the subacromial bursa. It involves shaving and excising the thickened pathologic subdeltoid bursa, excision of the coracoacromial ligament, and use of a high-speed motorized bur to remove any bone spurs on the anterolateral portion of the acromion. The goal is to create more space in the subacromial subdeltoid bursa and eliminate the impingement process to relieve shoulder pain.

17. How much bone should be removed from the undersurface of the acromion during a subacromial decompression?

The goal of a subacromial decompression is to create a flat (type I) acromion. Bigliani has classified acromion morphology type I as a flat acromion without a slope; a type II acromion has a gentle curve; and type III acromion has a hook along the anterior aspect of the accordion. This anatomy may be seen when viewing from the lateral portal but is more commonly seen on the preoperative outlet x-rays. During the arthroscopic subacromial decompression procedure, a cutting-block type procedure is used in which the bur is placed from the posterior portal along the undersurface of the acromion to verify that no curve or anterior hook remains. Knowing the anatomy of the acromion preoperatively on the x-rays also tells the surgeon how much bone to remove to create a flat acromion.

BIBLIOGRAPHY

1. Beals TC, Harryman DT, Lazarus MD: Useful boundaries of the subacromial bursa. Arthroscopy 14:465–470, 1998.
2. Bigliani LU, Ticker JB, Flatow EL, et al: The relationship of acromial architecture to rotator cuff disease. Clin Sports Med 4:823–838, 1991.
3. Matthews DS, Terry G, Vetter WL: Shoulder anatomy for the arthroscopist. Arthroscopy 1:83, 1985.
4. Morrison DS, Port J: Basics of shoulder arthroscopy. In Hawkins RJ, Misamore GW (eds): Shoulder Injuries in the Athlete. New York, Churchill Livingstone, 1996, pp 87–101.
5. Phillips BB: Arthroscopy of upper extremity. In Canale ST (ed): Campbell's Operative Orthopaedics, 9th ed. St. Louis, Mosby, 1998, pp 1562–1594.
6. Snyder SJ: Diagnostic arthroscopy: Normal anatomy and variations. In Snyder SJ (ed): Shoulder Arthroscopy. New York, McGraw-Hill, 1994, pp 23–39.
7. Snyder SJ, Karzel RP, Del Pizzo W, et al: SLAP lesions of the shoulder. Arthroscopy 6:274–279, 1990.

29. FRACTURES OF THE SHOULDER

Kirk S. Hutton, M.D.

1. What mistake is commonly made when evaluating a patient with a suspected shoulder girdle fracture?

One of the most common mistakes made is not obtaining adequate x-rays. It is mandatory to have two orthogonal views of the glenohumeral joint, such as an AP and an axillary lateral view. When it is difficult to obtain an axillary lateral view, a tangential or scapular Y view will suffice.

2. Name a possible mechanism for a lesser tuberosity fracture.

A posterior glenohumeral dislocation is a known mechanism for causing a lesser tuberosity fracture. The subscapularis attaches to the lesser tuberosity and may cause a bony avulsion of the structure during a posterior dislocation. Posterior dislocations are common after electrocution injuries or with seizures.

3. Describe the major blood supply to the humeral head and proximal humerus.

The major blood supply to the humeral head is from the anterior humeral circumflex artery. The arcuate artery is a continuation of the ascending branch of the anterior humeral circumflex artery, which is the main portion that penetrates the bone and supplies the humeral head. It routinely enters the bone in the area of the intertubercular groove and gives branches to the lesser and greater tuberosities. A small contribution to the humeral head blood supply comes from branches of the posterior circumflex artery and from tendinous osseous and anastomosis from the vascular rotator cuff.

4. Which nerve injuries are commonly associated with fractures about the shoulder?

The most commonly injured nerve is the axillary nerve. The axillary nerve innervates the deltoid muscle as well as the teres minor muscle. It is relatively fixed to the posterior cord of the brachial plexus and to the deltoid; therefore, any abnormal downward pressure on the proximal humerus can result in a traction injury to this nerve. It is also susceptible to injury with any dislocation because it is relatively close to the inferior capsule of the glenohumeral joint. The suprascapular nerve, which innervates the supraspinatus and infraspinatus, also can be injured, but it is much less likely. Injury to the musculocutaneous nerve is very rare.

5. **What is the most commonly used classification system for proximal humerus fractures?**

In 1970 Charles Neer developed his four-part classification system, which is based on the anatomy and biomechanical forces around the proximal humerus. Four primary fragments involved in proximal humerus fractures are the greater tuberosity, lesser tuberosity, humeral head, and the humeral shaft. Over 80% of humerus fractures are considered nondisplaced, but any fracture with > 1 cm of displacement or any fracture fragment angulated > 45° in the Neer system is considered a displaced fragment. The fracture classification refers to the number of **displaced segments**, not to the number of fragments or lines.

6. **How are proximal humerus fractures treated?**

Eighty-five percent of proximal humerus fractures are minimally displaced or nondisplaced and may be treated with early functional exercises.

Two-part anatomic neck fractures are difficult to reduce closed. Open reduction and internal fixation are difficult because of inadequate bone purchase for screws. Most authors agree that hemiarthroplasty gives the most predictable results for displaced fractures.

Displaced two-part greater tuberosity fractures may cause impingement under the acromion. Displacement > 0.5 cm is associated with persistent pain. Open reduction and internal fixation are recommended with displacement > 1 cm.

Two-part surgical neck fractures require 3–4 weeks of sling immobilization if they are minimally displaced. Angulation often occurs after closed reduction without internal fixation. Several forms of internal fixation have been described, including percutaneous pin, intramedullary fixation, tension band wire, and plate fixation.

Three-part fractures in active, young patients are generally best treated with open reduction and internal fixation.

Four-part fractures are associated with avascular necrosis in up to 90% of patients. Immediate hemiarthroplasty has become the accepted method of treatment.

7. **Why is the treatment of three- and four-part proximal humerus fractures different from other fractures of the proximal humerus?**

Typically, three- and four-part proximal humerus fractures occur in older individuals with osteoporotic bone or in younger individuals who have sustained very high energy trauma. Because of disruption of blood supply, four-part humerus fractures have a very high incidence of avascular necrosis, which has been determined to be between 13 and 34%. These fractures, especially in the elderly, are best treated with a hemiarthroplasty. Three-part fractures in elderly patients with very osteoporotic bone may also require hemiarthroplasty when stable internal fixation is not adequate.

8. **What is the treatment of a humeral head impression fracture?**

Treatment of impression fractures of the articular surface of the proximal humerus varies according to the percentage of the humeral head involved, as well as the time of diagnosis. If the injury is diagnosed within 2–3 weeks and the humeral head involvement is < 20% of the articular surface, closed reduction may be adequate. If the head defect is > 45% or a dislocation has been missed for six months or more, Hawkins has recommended a hemiarthroplasty of the proximal humerus. Head defects of 20–45% require some type of open reduction and internal fixation or bony transfer, depending on the location of the defect.

9. **Why is a head-splitting fracture difficult to treat?**

Head-splitting fractures usually occur with a fracture of either tuberosity and involve significant damage of the blood supply to the articular surface. In a young patient with good bone stock, open reduction and internal fixation may be attempted, but this is very difficult and success is low. Most authors recommend treatment of a head split fracture with a hemiarthroplasty.

10. **Describe some common complications associated with proximal humerus fractures.**

Vascular complications are obviously associated with proximal humerus fractures, and the axillary artery accounts for approximately 6% of all arterial trauma. The most common site of injury to the axillary artery is near the origin of the anterior circumflex artery. Another complication associated with vascular injury, as previously mentioned, is avascular necrosis, especially in three- and four-part humerus fractures. Brachial plexus injuries, primarily the axillary nerve component, have been associated with proximal humerus fractures and may be as high as 6%. The axillary nerve is more commonly injured in dislocations or fracture dislocations. Nonunions and malunions also are a potential complication and must be treated accordingly. Frozen shoulder or adhesive capsulitis is probably a much more common complication and rates are probably higher than noted in the literature.

11. Are there any growth plates or epiphyseal lines around the scapula that may be confused with a scapular fracture?
    The os acromiale is probably the best known separate bone in the scapula that results from failure of coalescence of the adjacent ossification centers of the acromion process of the scapula. There are four ossification centers present about the acromion, but the most common site of nonunion is between the meso-acromion and the meta-acromion. An unfused apophysis of the acromion is present in approximately 2.7% of patients and is bilateral in 60% those cases.

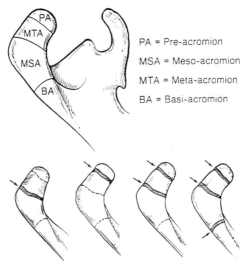

PA = Pre-acromion

MSA = Meso-acromion

MTA = Meta-acromion

BA = Basi-acromion

Ossification centers about the acromion with potential sites of nonunion, creating os acromiale.

12. What is a floating shoulder?
    A floating shoulder includes a scapular fracture combined with a proximal humerus fracture or a clavicle fracture. A floating shoulder causes a significantly unstable mid portion in the glenohumeral joint and represents a difficult treatment scenario, which usually requires open reduction and internal fixation of at least one component of the fracture.

13. Describe potential mechanisms of injury for scapular body fractures.
    The scapula is well protected, sandwiched between a thick muscle mass posteriorly and the thoracic cavity anteriorly. Because of its anatomic location, scapular fractures are uncommon, constituting only one percent of all fractures. A direct blow is probably the most common cause of injury of the scapular body, but sudden contractures of divergent muscles also may cause fracture. Electrical shock and seizures are included in this mechanism of injury. It should be remembered that of all scapular fractures, scapular body fractures have the highest incidence of associated injuries. Because of their mechanism of injury, up to 95% of scapular fractures are associated with other injuries.

14. Describe the associated injuries that may be found in conjunction with a scapular fracture.

Significant associated injuries can be seen in as many as 98% of individuals with scapular fractures because of the high energy force that is required to fracture the scapula. A pneumothorax may be seen in as many as 38% of individuals with scapular fractures, and the vast majority of these are delayed in onset anywhere from 1–3 days after the injury. Follow-up chest x-rays are mandatory when treating patients with scapular fractures. Other associated injuries include rib fractures, pulmonary contusion, brachial plexus injury, clavicle fractures, arterial injuries, as well as blunt abdominal and spinal cord injuries. It is the associated injuries that may cause the 10–15% mortality rate seen in patients with scapular fractures from blunt trauma.

15. How are scapular fractures evaluated radiographically?

True scapular anteroposterior (AP) and lateral views as well as a glenohumeral axillary projection should be done. The radiographs should be evaluated for fractures of the scapular body and spine, coracoid, glenoid, acromioclavicular joint, glenohumeral joint, and scapulothoracic articulation. Computed tomography (CT) is often necessary to further evaluate the extent of the fracture.

16. What is the classification of scapular fractures?

Scapular fractures are grouped into glenoid, acromion, coracoid, and scapular body fractures. Glenoid fractures may be further divided into glenoid rim, glenoid neck, and fractures through the glenoid cavity. Any fracture line that runs from the posterior scapular spine or acromion to the undersurface of the acromion and the spinoglenoid interval is considered an acromial fracture.

17. What is the most common treatment of scapular fractures?

Greater than 90% of all scapular fractures are treated nonoperatively. Symptomatic treatment includes sling and swathe for comfort. Range-of-motion exercises are initiated early. Return of full function will take several months. The prognosis, in general, is excellent.

Surgical indications for glenoid rim fractures include fractures that will result in persistent subluxation of the humeral head. Such fractures have ≥ 10 mm displacement with involvement of one-fourth of the anterior or one-third of the posterior glenoid rim.

Surgical indications for glenoid neck fractures include translational displacement ≥ 1 cm and/or angulatory displacement ≥ 40° in either the transverse or coronal planes. Significant displacement has been associated with loss of shoulder abduction, weakness, pain, and increased incidence of poor functional outcome.

Isolated fractures of the coracoid and acromion are generally treated nonoperatively as above. Surgical indications include significant displacement resulting in functional compromise.

18. What is the most common clavicle fracture?

Clavicle fractures are common injuries. They account for 5–10% of all instances of adult trauma. Middle third clavicle fractures account for 80% of all clavicle fractures.

19. What is the classification of clavicle fractures?

Allman divided clavicle fractures into three basic groups. Middle third clavicle fractures as classified as Group I and are the most common type. Group II fractures involve the lateral third of the clavicle and are the second most common. Group III fractures are medial third clavicle fractures.

Neer further subdivided the Group II (lateral third) fractures into five subtypes:

Subtype 1: minimally displaced interligamentous fractures

Subtype 2: displaced fractures with the fracture line medial to the coracoclavicular ligament insertion

Subtype 3: fractures that enter the acromioclavicular joint
Subtype 4: childhood injuries
These fractures are displaced, but the coracoclavicular ligament remains attached to a periosteal sleeve.

20. What is the treatment of a clavicle fracture?
Most clavicle fractures are treated with figure of eight harness or shoulder sling until pain begins to resolve. Surgical treatment comprises open reduction and internal fixation using Dynamic Compression Plating and screws. Indications for surgical intervention include neurovascular symptoms, skin breakdown due to bony prominence, and nonunion.

BIBLIOGRAPHY

 1. Bigliani LU, Flatow EL, Pollock RG: Fractures of the proximal humerus. In Rockwood CA, Matsen FA (eds): The Shoulder, 2nd ed. Philadelphia, W.B. Saunders, 1998, pp 337–389.
 2. Boublik M, Hawkins RJ: Clinical examination of the shoulder complex. J Orthop Sports Phys Ther 18:379–385, 1993.
 3. Butters KP: The scapula. In Rockwood CA, Matsen FA (eds): The Shoulder, 2nd ed. Philadelphia, W.B. Saunders, 1998, pp 391–427.
 4. Craig EV: Fractures of the clavicle. In Rockwood CA, Matsen FA (eds): The Shoulder, 2nd ed. Philadelphia, W.B. Saunders, 1998, pp 428–482.
 5. Crenshaw AH: Fractures of the shoulder girdle, arm, and forearm. In Canale ST (ed): Campbell's Operative Orthopaedics, 9th ed. St. Louis, Mosby, 1998, pp 2285–2296.
 6. Gerber C, Krushell RJ: Isolated rupture of the tendon of the subscapularis muscle. J Bone Joint Surg 73B:389–394, 1991.
 7. Hawkins RJ: Musculoskeletal Examination. St. Louis, Mosby Year-Book, 1995.
 8. Hawkins RJ, Hobeika PE: Impingement syndrome in the athletic shoulder. Clin Sports Med 2:391–405, 1983.
 9. Hawkins RJ, Mohtadi NG: Clinical Evaluation of shoulder instability. Clin J Sports Med 1:59, 1991.
10. Matsen FA, Arntz CT: Subacromial impingement. In Rockwood CA, Matsen FA (eds): The Shoulder. Philadelphia, W.B. Saunders, 1990, pp 623–646.
11. Matsen FA, Thomas SC, Rockwood CA: Anterior glenohumeral instability. In Rockwood CA, Matsen FA (eds): The Shoulder. Philadelphia, W.B. Saunders, 1990, pp 526–622.

IV. The Elbow and Forearm

---

30. ELBOW DISLOCATIONS AND INSTABILITY

Edward R. McDevitt, M.D., CAPT MC USN, and
P. Norman Ove, M.D.

---

1. What is an elbow dislocation?

An elbow dislocation is a disassociation of the joint that connects the humerus with the radius and the ulna.

2. How common are dislocations of the elbow?

Although the elbow is one of the most highly constrained or stabilized joints, dislocations of the elbow are not rare. Only dislocation of the shoulder and the proximal interphalangeal (PIP) joints of the fingers are more common.

3. How do most elbow dislocations occur?

Most occur in sporting events, usually in young people aged 15–25 years. Elbow dislocations also may occur in high-speed motor vehicle or motorcycle accidents.

4. What is the mechanism of injury in most elbow dislocations?

The usual mechanism of injury is a fall on an extended or hyperextended elbow.

5. How are elbow dislocations described?

Like all dislocations, elbow dislocations are described by the position of the distal segment in relation to the proximal segment. Where does the distal segment, the ulna, lie in relation to the proximal segment, the humerus? In >90% of cases, the dislocation is posterior or posterolateral. The ulna is posterior to the humerus in a posterior elbow dislocation.

6. Describe the other types of elbow dislocations.

Although the most common dislocation is posterior, elbow dislocations also may be anterior, medial, lateral, or divergent. Anterior dislocations are rare and are associated with a high degree of soft-tissue disruption. In a divergent dislocation, which is also rare but very serious, the radius and the ulna dislocate from the humerus in different directions. For a divergent dislocation to occur, the strong musculotendinous complex that binds the ulna and radius together must be completely disrupted.

7. What are the physical findings in an elbow dislocation?

Most patients are in extreme pain. They usually hold the affected forearm with the opposite hand. The elbow is usually held in slight flexion. The forearm appears slightly foreshortened compared with the normal forearm. The olecranon is usually palpable and prominent posteriorly. Swelling of the elbow is usually present and increases with time.

8. How is the presence of a fracture determined?

After documenting the neurovascular status, gently and slowly flex the elbow, carefully feeling for crepitus, which is usually present in a fracture but absent with an elbow dislocation. Obtain radiographs expeditiously.

9. What should be done if a fracture is associated with the elbow dislocation?

Fractures associated with elbow dislocations are not uncommon. Elbow dislocations without associated fractures are called simple dislocations, whereas those associated with associated fractures are called complex dislocations. The fractures most commonly associated with elbow dislocations involve the radial head, the coronoid process of the ulna, and the medial epicondyle. Most complex elbow dislocations are inherently unstable, and most of the associated fractures require surgery. Nevertheless, it is still imperative to reduce the dislocation of the elbow, whether or not an associated fracture is present.

10. What should be done for a patient with a suspected elbow dislocation?

In assessing the patient with an elbow injury, it is critical to check neurovascular function of the forearm and hand *before* an attempt is made to manipulate the joint back into place.

11. How does one check the neurovascular function?

First, check the sensation of pain and light touch distal to the elbow, documenting any paresthesia. Test the median, ulnar, and radial nerves for muscle strength distal to the elbow. Ask the patient to touch the thumb to the fifth finger to assess median nerve function. Ulnar nerve function can be assessed by testing the interosseous muscles, all of which are innervated by the ulnar nerve. Have the patient spread the fingers apart to test for interosseous function. The radial nerve can be assessed by having the patient extend the thumb, fingers, and wrist. Even children can be persuaded to attempt these three muscle tests. The brachial artery should be palpated at the elbow and compared with the unaffected side. The ulnar and radial arteries should be palpated at the wrist. All findings should be documented.

12. What neurovascular injuries are common in elbow dislocations?

In most elbow dislocations the neurovascular examination is unremarkable; the median and ulnar nerves and the brachial artery are most susceptible to injury.

13. What should be done if neurovascular injury is present?

After documentation of the injury, an attempt should be made promptly to reduce the dislocation. Often neurovascular injuries resolve with reduction. Carefully check the neurovascular status after relocation. An arteriogram should be obtained promptly if vascular injury is suspected.

14. Describe the procedure for reducing a dislocation of the elbow.

Elbow dislocations should be reduced as soon as possible. Team physicians covering sports with a high incidence of elbow dislocations are able to quickly and easily reduce the elbow shortly after the injury. If time has elapsed since the injury occurred and soft-tissue swelling is present, reduction is best accomplished under regional or general anesthesia. Intravenous anesthesia, with small doses of diazepam and morphine, is effective and usually allows reduction to be accomplished readily.

Before any reduction maneuver, the neurovascular status *must* be documented. If radiographs have been obtained, they should be examined carefully. Where is the ulna in relation to the humerus? Look for any associated fractures, especially at the coronoid process of the proximal ulna and the radial head. In most cases, the ulna is posterior to the humerus.

Many methods have been described for reduction of elbow dislocations. The easiest and most reliable involves gentle traction applied to the forearm with counteraction applied to the distal aspect of the humerus. The reduction maneuver can be accomplished with the patient either supine or prone. Many prefer the supine position, especially if intravenous anesthesia is used, because it is easier to assess the airway with this position.

If available, an assistant is useful. The assistant stands at the head of the patient, applying steady traction to the upper aspect of the humerus, while the physician applies gentle distal traction to the elbow. As the elbow is gently extended, any medial or lateral displacement of the ulna can be corrected by a counterforce applied to the side of the displacement. Keep one hand on the forearm, applying distal traction, and with the other hand correct the medial/lateral displacement. Then gently flex the elbow to accomplish the reduction. Often a loud "clunk" is palpated and heard. It is often helpful to use one hand to flex the elbow while the other hand pushes the bones back together. In a posterior dislocation, the ulna is posterior to the humerus. While applying a posterior force on the distal humerus with your thumb, wrap your other four fingers around the proximal aspect of the ulna and pull the ulna anteriorly. As you gently flex the elbow with one hand, your opposite hand gently wedges the humerus and the ulna together.

If no assistant is available, a closed reduction of the elbow with the patient in a prone position may be useful. The gravity method of reduction described by Parvin is a gentle method that can be used by the sole practitioner. The patient lies prone on the stretcher while gentle downward traction is applied with one hand to his or her wrist. After a few minutes of traction, the muscle spasm should subside. With your opposite hand apply a gentle upward pressure on the anterior distal humerus, lifting the arm as traction continues to be applied downward. The reduction should occur with an audible "clunk."

After reduction, carefully reassess neurovascular function. Gently flex and extend the elbow to ensure that the reduction is complete. Passive extension within 15–20° of full extension without subluxation implies a stable reduction. Apply a well-padded posterior splint with the elbow held at 90° of flexion. Obtain postreduction radiographs to ensure complete reduction of the dislocation and to rule out any new fractures.

15. What should be done if the elbow dislocation cannot be reduced?

The usual cause of an irreducible dislocation is entrapped fragments within the joint space, most often the fractured medial epicondyle. If the dislocation has not reduced after two gentle attempts under intravenous anesthesia, closed reduction under general anesthesia should be attempted. If the elbow is not reducible even after general anesthesia, open reduction is necessary.

16. Describe the treatment for a patient with an elbow dislocation after reduction.

Recent studies clearly show that prolonged immobilization (>4 weeks) is associated with poor results. Early active motion appears to be the key to successful rehabilitation after dislocation. If the patient demonstrates inherent stability with passive extension to 15–20° without recurrent dislocation, active motion is started within 1 week. Since 1986 at the United States Naval Academy, elbow dislocations without fracture have been treated with an immediate program of active range of motion instead of immobilization. Initial study of the midshipmen shows long-term stability with preservation of range of motion and return to full sports participation.

17. Is there any danger in starting an early active range-of-motion program?

No. Increased instability has not been demonstrated in patients who have been started on an early active range-of-motion program, which actually appears to result in less pain and suffering.

18. What are the late complications of elbow dislocations?

1. Recurrent dislocation of the elbow is extremely rare, but when it occurs, it is disabling.

2. Almost all patients with dislocations of the elbow have a mild loss of terminal extension. Loss of motion can be minimized through an early range-of-motion program.

3. Heterotopic ossification may occur after dislocation of the elbow, but is rarely severe enough to limit motion of the elbow.

BIBLIOGRAPHY

1. Broberg MA, Morrey BF: Results of treatment of fracture dislocations of the elbow. Clin Orthop 216:109–119, 1987.
2. Cohen MS, Hastings H: Acute elbow dislocation: Evaluation and management. J Am Acad Orthop Surg 6:15–23, 1998.
3. Hotchkiss RN, Green DP: Fractures and dislocations of the elbow. In Rockwood CA, et al (eds): Rockwood and Green's Fractures in Adults. Philadelphia, J.B. Lippincott, 1991, pp 779–793.

4. Josefsson PO, Gentz CF, Johnell O, et al: Surgical versus nonsurgical treatment of ligamentous injuries following dislocation of the elbow joint. Clin Orthop 214:165–169, 1987.
5. Josefsson PO, Gentz CF, Johnell O, et al: Dislocations of the elbow and intraarticular fractures. Clin Orthop 246:126–130, 1989.
6. Jupiter JB, Mehne DK: Trauma to the adult elbow and fractures of the distal humerus. In Browner BE, et al (eds): Skeletal Trauma. Philadelphia, W.B. Saunders, 1992, pp 1141–1145.
7. Mehlhoff TL, Noble PC, Bennett JB, et al: Simple dislocation of the elbow in the adult: Results after closed treatment. J Bone Joint Surg 70A:244–249, 1989.
8. Moehring HD: Traumatic dislocations of the shoulder girdle and elbow. In Chapman MW (ed): Operative Orthopedics, 2nd ed. Philadelphia, J.B. Lippincott, 1993, pp 470–476.
9. Parvin RW: Closed reduction of common shoulder and elbow dislocations without anesthesia. Arch Surg 75:972–975, 1957.
10. Ring D, Jupiter JB: Current concepts review: Fracture-dislocation of the elbow. J Bone Joint Surg 80:566–580, 1998.
11. Ross G, McDevitt ER, et al: Treatment of simple elbow dislocation using a rapid motion protocol. Am J Sport Med May–June 1999.
12. Stanley EA, Mehlhoff TL: Elbow and forearm: Trauma. In Orthopedic Knowledge Update 4. Rosemont, IL, American Academy of Orthopedic Surgeons, 1993, pp 321–322.

31. THROWING INJURIES AND OTHER ATHLETIC INJURIES OF THE ELBOW

P. Norman Ove, M.D., and
Edward R. McDevitt, M.D., CAPT MC USN

1. What is the first step in diagnosing an elbow injury?

Examination should begin with a thorough history, including mechanism of injury, location of pain, activities that aggravate or relieve symptoms, and history of prior injuries or treatment. Only then should the examiner proceed with the physical examination.

2. How should one perform the physical examination of the elbow?

Examination should begin with inspection of the elbow and its relationship to the body and comparison of the elbows for swelling or differences in size, shape, or carrying angle. Examination then proceeds with maneuvers that may be more painful. Compare active and passive range of motion, strength, and stability to varus, valgus, and anteroposterior stresses. One may then palpate the anterior, posterior, medial, and lateral aspects of the elbow for tenderness, crepitus, or deformity.

3. List the differential diagnosis for an athlete presenting with anterior elbow pain.

Biceps tendinitis   Anterior capsular strain or tear
Biceps rupture   Median nerve compression syndrome

4. What specific elbow motion should be tested when biceps tendinitis or rupture is suspected?

The biceps is an elbow flexor and forearm supinator. Both conditions can be expected to cause pain and weakness with resisted elbow flexion and supination.

5. Will active elbow flexion and supination be possible after a complete rupture of the biceps tendon?

Yes. The brachialis is the prime flexor of the elbow, and the supinator in the forearm still provides supination. Supination and flexion strength are decreased by 20–50%.

6. What other findings help to diagnose a distal biceps tendon rupture?

Typically the biceps tendon is not palpable, but this finding may be observed by swelling. Often a deformity in the distal arm is present at the site where the muscle belly has retracted proximally. Ecchymosis in the antecubital area is also suggestive of acute rupture.

7. Should radiographs be obtained?

Yes. They usually are normal, but they may reveal avulsion fragment or degenerative changes at the radial tuberosity.

8. Which is more common—distal or proximal rupture of the biceps tendon?

Only 3% of ruptures occur at the elbow; 97% occur in the shoulder, often in association with chronic rotator cuff impingement.

9. Do symptoms usually precede acute biceps rupture at the elbow?

Yes. As with Achilles tendon rupture, athletes commonly report preexisting chronic tendinitis. Degenerative changes in the tendon may make it more susceptible to a tear from a traumatic event.

10. Describe the treatment of biceps tendinitis.

As with all overuse syndromes, the first mode of treatment is to decrease the aggravating activity and to rest the inflamed tissue. Ice for acute inflammation or heat for chronic conditions and nonsteroidal antiinflammatory drugs (NSAIDs) are helpful and usually well tolerated by athletes. Recalcitrant cases may require splinting for 1–2 weeks.

11. Do steroids help biceps tendinitis? Is any risk involved?

Steroid injection around the inflamed tendon may be of benefit in recalcitrant cases but increases the risk of subsequent tendon rupture. Injections should be used sparingly and with caution.

12. What are the predisposing factors for tendon rupture?

History of prior symptoms	Male sex
Steroid injections	Age >30 years

13. What is the treatment of distal biceps rupture?

The treatment of complete rupture in the athletic population is surgical reattachment of the tendon to the bicipital tuberosity of the radius. After surgery the elbow is immobilized in flexion and supination for 6–8 weeks.

14. How is anterior capsule strain differentiated from biceps injury?

Anterior capsule strain is usually related to hyperextension as opposed to flexion-supination. Ecchymosis and deep tenderness to palpation may be present, but tenderness is usually more diffuse rather than isolated around the biceps tendon.

15. What more significant injury must be ruled out when anterior capsular strain is suspected?

With a hyperextension mechanism the possibility of a spontaneously reduced elbow dislocation should be considered.

16. Should radiographs be obtained in hyperextended elbow injuries?

Yes. Fracture and/or dislocation should be ruled out. With an anterior strain, bony avulsion flecks from the capsular margins may be seen. Later radiographs may reveal heterotopic calcification in the anterior tissues.

17. How long should the injury be splinted or immobilized? Why?

Immobilization should be minimal—perhaps 1 day, if needed for comfort. Prolonged splinting greatly increases the likelihood of developing a flexion contracture at the elbow. Early active range-of-motion exercises are essential to regain full motion.

18. Why should passive range-of-motion (PROM) therapy be avoided or used cautiously?

PROM therapy, especially if painful, leads to further tissue trauma that may result in heterotopic ossification. Gentle, pain-free PROM by a qualified therapist or trainer may be permissible.

19. Give another name for median nerve compression syndrome at the elbow.

Pronator syndrome.

20. How do the symptoms of pronator syndrome differ from those of other causes of anterior elbow pain?

Pain is usually just distal to the elbow in the proximal forearm, may be associated with numbness in the volar forearm or median distribution in the hand, and is often aggravated by resisted pronation activities.

21. What four structures may be responsible for pronator syndrome?

- Ligament of Struthers/supracondylar process
- Lacertus fibrosus
- Pronator teres
- Flexor digitorum superficialis (FDS) arcade

22. What provocative tests may help to identify which structure is responsible?

The following maneuvers should reproduce pain or numbness:
- Supracondylar process—elbow flexion of 120–135°
- Lacertus fibrosus—resisted forearm supination
- Pronator teres—resisted forearm pronation
- FDS arcade—resisted long finger flexion

23. How is pronator syndrome treated?

Most cases respond to modification of activities and physical therapy modalities for stretching and strengthening. Surgical decompression may be required for recalcitrant cases.

24. List the differential diagnosis for an athlete presenting with posterior elbow pain.

1. Triceps tendinitis
2. Triceps rupture (or olecranon fracture)
3. Olecranon impingement syndrome
4. Olecranon bursitis

25. What are the common findings in athletes with triceps tendinitis?

- Posterior elbow pain
- Tenderness at the triceps insertion or in the distal part of the tendon
- Resisted elbow extension causes increased pain

26. Should radiographs be obtained?

Yes. Degenerative calcifications or traction spurs may be present. Of greater importance, stress fracture of the olecranon should be excluded.

27. What findings indicate rupture of the triceps mechanism rather than overuse tendinitis?

Tear of the triceps or olecranon fracture is usually associated with an extremely forceful contraction or a fall on the elbow. Other common findings include severe pain and swelling in the posterior elbow and an inability to extend actively. A palpable defect may be present at the site of tendon or bony disruption.

28. Are radiographs useful?

Yes. In addition to excluding an olecranon fracture, radiographs reveal bony avulsion fractures in 80% of triceps tendon avulsions.

29. In what position should a nondisplaced olecranon fracture be immobilized?

Treatment of tendon ruptures and olecranon fractures should be surgical. The pull of the triceps muscle is significant, and even in full extension a well-aligned fracture will become displaced.

30. Define hyperextension overload syndrome of the elbow.

Also called olecranon impingement syndrome or boxer's elbow, this condition is an overuse syndrome caused by repetitive valgus extension overload of the elbow. It is common in the throwing motions, which cause the olecranon process to impinge against the medial wall of the olecranon fossa. Athletes commonly complain of pain during the extension phase of throwing and catching or locking in or near extension.

31. What physical findings may suggest the hyperextension overload syndrome?

Typical findings include posterior tenderness or swelling, lack of full extension, pain with forced valgus in full extension, and palpable loose bodies.

32. Are radiographs helpful?

Yes. Anteroposterior, lateral, and axial radiographs may reveal spurring or fracture of the olecranon tip, loose bodies, or hypertrophy of the olecranon.

33. What is the role of arthroscopy in olecranon impingement syndrome?

A loose body or an olecranon osteophyte usually can be removed arthroscopically. Both loose bodies and spurs at times may be quite large, and removal may require a small posterior arthrotomy.

34. What is the leading differential diagnosis for traumatic or chronic olecranon bursitis? How should it be ruled out?

Septic olecranon bursitis is usually much more painful and more impressive on examination but may be confused with the nonseptic conditions in the early stages. It can be ruled out by aspirating the bursa through a sterile field and checking a Gram stain and culture for bacteria.

35. How does treatment of the two types of olecranon bursitis differ?

Chronic bursitis, caused by repetitive trauma or irritation to the bursa, should be treated with NSAIDs and protective padding. Both chronic and acute traumatic bursitis can be decompressed by aspiration, compression, and splinting for a short period. Septic olecranon bursitis should be treated by surgical incision, drainage, and antibiotics.

36. List the differential diagnosis for an athlete presenting with medial elbow pain.
- Medial epicondylitis/flexor-pronator strain
- Ulnar collateral ligament sprain
- Cubital tunnel syndrome
- Little leaguer's elbow

37. What is golfer's elbow?

Golfer's elbow is an overuse syndrome caused by repetitive tension overloading of the flexor-pronator muscle at or near its insertion on the medial epicondyle.

38. What are the likely symptoms and findings in patients with golfer's elbow?

Athletes complain of medial and proximal forearm pain aggravated by golfing, curling, and throwing curve balls. Diagnosis can be confirmed by reproducing the pain with resisted wrist flexion and forearm pronation.

39. What other medial elbow problem is common among pitchers?

Pitchers, quarterbacks, and racquetball and squash players frequently develop chronic sprains of the ulnar collateral ligament (UCL) caused by repetitive valgus stress across the elbow. Long-standing chronic cases may develop UCL laxity with elbow instability.

40. What are the findings in patients with UCL sprains?

The primary finding is tenderness over the anterior oblique portion of the UCL. With the elbow flexed, the UCL is palpable below (more posterior than) the flexor-pronator attachment to the medial epicondyle. Pain is increased by valgus stress of the elbow. More severe cases exhibit valgus laxity.

41. Are radiographs helpful?

In some cases radiographs may reveal calcifications or spurring along the UCL. The gravity stress view can be used to demonstrate UCL laxity.

42. How is little leaguer's elbow different from the other medial elbow overuse syndromes?

Because children and adolescents still have open growth plates, their joints are subjected to different injuries from those of adults. Repeated tensile stresses on the medial epicondyle can result in inflammation and partial separation of the apophysis. Occasionally an avulsion may occur after a single forceful muscle contraction.

43. What findings may be evident on radiographs?

In early milder cases radiographs are normal. In chronic cases radiographs may show widening or irregularity of the medial apophysis compared with the opposite side. In youngsters presenting with acute severe pain, radiographs may reveal avulsion fracture of the medial epicondyle.

44. What is the management of little leaguer's elbow?

Relatively acute cases should be treated with rest or even splinting for 1–2 weeks. In chronic cases pitching may have to be curtailed for 2–3 months to allow adequate rest. Proper coaching and throwing techniques are imperative to reduce the incidence and to prevent recurrence.

45. When is surgery indicated?

Surgery is **never** indicated for the overuse syndrome. However, in acute injuries with displacement of the epicondyle >2 mm or incarceration of the fragment within the joint, surgical reduction and fixation are required to restore joint congruity and ligament stability.

46. What medial elbow problem may present with vague aching in the forearm and tingling in the fourth and fifth fingers?

Such symptoms suggest cubital tunnel syndrome, an entrapment neuropathy of the ulnar nerve at or about the elbow. It may be the result of a cubitus valgus deformity, but in athletes it is more commonly due to trauma (confusion or subluxation of the ulnar nerve), muscle hypertrophy (especially of the flexor carpi ulnaris from excessive curls), or inflammation from adjacent tissue injury (UCL sprain).

47. List the findings suggestive of cubital tunnel syndrome.
- Positive Tinel's sign at the cubital tunnel
- Decreased sensation in the ulnar forearm and hand
- Increased pain and numbness with forced elbow flexion
- Weakness or atrophy of the first dorsal interosseous muscle (resisted index finger abduction)
- Weakness in grip strength

48. What other conditions must be considered? Name a test for each.
1. Cervical radiculopathy—foraminal compression (Spurling's sign)
2. Thoracic outlet syndrome (Adson's sign)
3. Ulnar nerve compression at the wrist (Tinel's sign at Guyon's canal)

49. What diagnostic test may confirm cubital tunnel syndrome?

Electromyography (EMG) and nerve conduction velocity (NCV) studies may demonstrate slowing of conduction velocity across the elbow.

50. Is surgical decompression necessary?

Surgical decompression may be necessary with a progressive neurologic deficit or with failure of nonsurgical management. Initial treatment should consist of rest, NSAIDs, protective padding, and avoidance of extreme flexion. If symptoms warrant, acute episodes may be treated with splinting at 30–45° of flexion for a few days or at night to relieve compression.

51. List the differential diagnosis for an athlete presenting with lateral elbow pain.

• Lateral epicondylitis
• Radial head fracture
• Radiocapitellar chondromalacia/osteochondritis dissecans
• Posterior interosseous nerve compression syndrome

52. What is tennis elbow? What causes it?

Tennis elbow or lateral epicondylitis is an overuse syndrome due to repetitive tension overloading of the wrist extensor origins at the lateral epicondyle. Such stresses are increased with pronation or resisted supination of the forearm. The problem is common in racquet sport athletes and is aggravated by vibration (strings too tight, off-center hits), faulty backhand and topspin mechanics, and a grip that is too small. Other wrist dorsiflexion and supination activities, such as hammering and using a screwdriver, are also common causes.

53. Besides point tenderness at the lateral epicondyle, what other finding should be present to diagnose tennis elbow?

Increased pain at the lateral epicondyle with resisted wrist dorsiflexion confirms inflammation of the origin of the extensor carpi radialis brevis (ECRB).

54. Are steroid injections beneficial in treating tennis elbow?

Yes. Most athletes, however, respond to rest, modification of technique and/or racquet, NSAIDs, and temporary use of a tennis elbow strap or even a wrist cock-up splint.

55. How does a tennis elbow strap work?

The elbow strap results in partial tenodesis of the ECRB at the proximal forearm, which reduces vibratory and tensile stresses at its origin on the epicondyle.

56. A fall on the outstretched arm that results in elbow pain is likely to cause what injury?

Compressive axial loading across the lateral elbow frequently results in a radial head fracture.

57. What is the posterior fat pad sign? What does it suggest?

The posterior fat pad sign is a radiolucency in the posterior elbow joint seen on the lateral radiograph. The posterior fat pad normally rests within the confines of the olecranon fossa and is not visible; however, it can be displaced out of the fossa by blood or other fluid within the joint. Hemarthrosis, which can be confirmed by aspiration, suggests an intraarticular fracture. Oblique views may be necessary to visualize nondisplaced fractures.

58. How are radial head fractures classified? How does classification relate to treatment?

Type I: step-off <3 mm and angulation of <30°; treated with brief splinting (1–2 weeks) and early range-of-motion exercises.

Type II: step-off >3 mm or angulation >30°; treated surgically with an attempt at open reduction and internal fixation.

Type III: comminuted; usually requires radial head excision.

59. A pitcher being treated for a UCL sprain also complains of lateral elbow pain. What other elbow problem should you suspect? Why?

Tension overloading of the medial structures during throwing and in racquet sports is frequently accompanied by compression overloading of the radiocapitellar joint laterally. Repeated stresses may cause diffuse articular damage (chondromalacia) or more specific lesions, such as osteochondritis dissecans, osteochondral fractures, or loose bodies.

60. What are the expected findings?

Affected athletes frequently cannot achieve extension. Palpation reveals tenderness at the radiocapitellar joint and crepitus with pronation and supination. Radiographs should be evaluated for decreased radiocapitellar joint space, articular spurring, defects or irregularities in the radial head or the capitellum, and loose bodies. Such lesions may require computed tomography (CT), magnetic resonance imaging (MRI), or arthroscopy for complete evaluation.

61. What other condition coexists in 5% of athletes with tennis elbow and often makes routine treatment unsuccessful?

Posterior interosseous syndrome may coexist with tennis elbow. It is a compression neuropathy of the posterior interosseous branch of the radial nerve at the point where it passes under the edge of (arcade of Frohse) or through the supinator muscle.

62. What structures does the posterior interosseous nerve (PIN) innervate? What findings would you expect on examination?

The posterior motor branch of the radial nerve supplies the extensor carpi ulnaris and the finger and thumb extensors, all of which may show signs of weakness. Radially innervated sensation is normal, because the radial wrist extensors arise proximal to the supinator. Tinel's sign may be positive about 4 fingerbreadths distal to the lateral epicondyle.

63. How does the possibility of concomitant PIN syndrome alter the treatment of tennis elbow?

The initial treatment is unaltered. For both conditions nonsurgical measures are usually successful. Alterations in technique and/or equipment are often helpful, although NSAIDs and a period of rest also may be needed. Occasional steroid injections may be useful. Surgical debridement and release of the inflamed ECRB tendon may be required for recalcitrant cases of tennis elbow. If surgery is contemplated, consideration also should be given to whether exploration and neurolysis of the PIN are warranted.

BIBLIOGRAPHY

1. Andrews JR: Bony injuries about the elbow in the throwing athlete. In Stauffer ES (ed): Instructional Course Lectures 34. St. Louis, Mosby, 1985.
2. Gabel GT, Morrey BF: Tennis elbow. In Cannon WT (ed): Instructional Course Lectures 47. St. Louis, Mosby, 1998.
3. Hoppenfield S: Physical Examination of the Spine and Extremities. Norwalk, CT, Appleton-Century-Crofts, 1976.
4. Hotchkiss RN: Fractures of the radial head and related instability and contracture of the forearm. In Cannon WT (ed): Instructional Course Lectures 47. St. Louis, Mosby, 1998.
5. Jobe FW, Nuber G: Throwing injuries of the elbow. Clin Sports Med 5:621, 1986.
6. Morrey F: The Elbow and Its Disorders. Philadelphia, W.B. Saunders, 1985.
7. Nirschl RP: Sports and overuse injuries to the elbow: Muscle and tendon trauma. Tennis elbow. In Morrey BF (ed): The Elbow and its Disorders, 2nd ed. Philadelphia, W.B. Saunders, 1993, pp 537–559.
8. Pecina M, Krmpotic-Nemanic J, Markiewitz A: Tunnel Syndromes. Boca Raton, FL, CRC Press, 1991.
9. Posner MA: Compressive neuropathies of the median and radial nerves at the elbow. Clin Sports Med 9:343, 1990.
10. Spinner M: Injuries to the Major Branches of Peripheral Nerves of the Forearm. Philadelphia, W.B. Saunders, 1978.
11. Yocum LA: The diagnosis and nonoperative treatment of elbow problems in the athlete. Clin Sports Med 8:439, 1989.
12. Zarine B, Andrews R, Carson WG Jr: Injuries to the Throwing Arm. Philadelphia, W.B. Saunders, 1985.

32. ARTHROSCOPY OF THE ELBOW

Thomas M. Heiser, M.D.

1. What are the indications for arthroscopy of the elbow?

Loose bodies   Adhesions
Olecranon osteophytes   Osteochondritis dissecans of the capitellum
Synovitis   Chondromalacia of the radial head

2. What are the contraindications for arthroscopy of the elbow?

The contraindications are bony ankylosis and severe fibrous ankylosis that prevent the introduction of the arthroscope into the elbow joint.

3. Describe the position of the arm when the patient is supine.

The entire arm is allowed to hang freely over the side of the table with the elbow at 90° and the hand pointed toward the ceiling, directed at a pulley. This elbow position allows the neurovascular structures in the antecubital fossa to be at maximal relaxation.

4. What size and angle of an arthroscope are most commonly used for elbow arthroscopy?

A 4-mm, 30°-angled arthroscope is optimal for visualization.

5. Name the medial, lateral, and posterior bony landmarks to be outlined before initiation of the procedure.

The medial landmark is the tip of the medial epicondyle; the lateral landmarks are the radial head and the lateral epicondyle; and the posterior landmark is the olecranon.

6. What are the five most commonly used portals for elbow arthroscopy?

The anteromedial, anterolateral, direct lateral, posterolateral, and straight posterior are the most commonly used portals.

7. Into which area should a needle be inserted to obtain maximal capsular distension?

The location is palpated between the lateral epicondyle, olecranon tip, and radial head.

8. Describe the position of the anterolateral portal.

The portal is located 3 cm distal and 2 cm anterior to the lateral epicondyle.

9. Describe the position of the anteromedial portal.

The anteromedial portal is located 2 cm anterior and 2 cm distal to the medial epicondyle, aiming directly toward the center of the elbow joint.

10. Describe the position of the direct lateral portal.

The direct lateral portal is the same spot at which the needle was inserted to distend the elbow joint capsule.

11. Describe the position of the posterolateral portal.

The posterolateral portal is 3 cm proximal to the olecranon tip immediately superior and posterior to the lateral epicondyle and lateral margin of the triceps muscle. This portal is established with the elbow in 20–30° of flexion by aiming toward the olecranon fossa.

12. Describe the position of the straight posterior portal.

The straight posterior portal is 3 cm proximal to the olecranon tip and 2 cm medial to the posterolateral portal, directly through the triceps tendon. This portal also should be established with the elbow in 20–30° of flexion.

13. From which portal are the capitellum and radial head best seen?
The anteromedial portal.

14. Through which portals can the coronoid process of the ulna be seen?
The anteromedial and anterolateral portals.

15. What two types of pathology are most commonly found in the posterior compartment of the elbow?
Loose bodies and olecranon osteophytes.

16. Which nerves are at risk at the medial aspect of the elbow?
The ulnar and median nerves.

17. Which nerve is at risk at the lateral aspect of the elbow?
The radial nerve.

18. What is a limitation of arthroscopy with the patient in a supine position?
The arm is unstable and tends to swing like a pendulum in response to pressure.

19. List advantages to positioning the patient prone for elbow arthroscopy.
Traction is eliminated, and gravity on the forearm tends to stabilize and assist in distension of the anterior compartment.

20. What rehabilitation instructions are given to the patient for the immediate postoperative period?
The patient should wear a sling for comfort and begin active-assistive range-of-motion exercises on the first postoperative day, progressing to full range of motion as tolerated.

BIBLIOGRAPHY

1. Andrews JR, St. Pierre RK, Carson WG: Arthroscopy of the elbow. Clin Sports Med 5:653–662, 1984.
2. Baumgarten TE, Andrews JR, Satterwhite YE: The arthroscopic classification and treatment of osteochondritis dissecans of the capitellum. Am J Sports Med 4:520–523, 1998.
3. Esch JC, Baker CL: Arthroscopic Surgery: The Shoulder and Elbow. Philadelphia, J.B. Lippincott, 1993.
4. McGinty JP: Operative Arthroscopy. New York, Raven Press, 1991.
5. Morrey BF: The Elbow and Its Disorders. Philadelphia, W.B. Saunders, 1993.
6. Phillips BB, Strasburger SE: Arthrofibrosis of the Elbow. Arthroscopy 14:38–44, 1998.
7. Woods G: Elbow arthroscopy. Clin Sports Med 6:557–564, 1985.

33. ARTHRITIS OF THE ELBOW

Edward V. Fehringer, M.D.

1. What are the three major types of arthritis that involve the elbow?
In order of frequency: rheumatoid, posttraumatic, and osteoarthritis.

2. Describe the epidemiology and presenting history.
Most patients (except those with rheumatoid arthritis) present between the third and eighth decades of life and have a history of previous severe fracture or dislocation of the elbow, repetitive trauma to the elbow, or an occupation that requires heavy physical exertion with the upper extremities, such as squeezing a hammer or operating a jackhammer.

3. What are the findings of the physical examination?

A flexion contracture is usually present with additional loss of flexion. Bony crepitance is palpable with flexion/extension and pronation/supination. Tenderness is elicited on forced extension and flexion at the terminal ranges of motion.

4. What is the radiographic appearance of osteoarthrosis of the elbow?

Anteroposterior and lateral views of the elbow typically demonstrate osteophytes of the olecranon and coronoid as well as the coronoid and olecranon fossa. Loose bodies are frequently present.

5. List the surgical procedures available for osteoarthrosis of the elbow.

1. **Elbow arthroscopy** with synovectomy and removal of loose bodies is indicated when an identifiable loose body restricts range of motion and causes pain. Synovectomy in the rheumatoid elbow is indicated only in the early stages of disease.

2. **Anterior capsulectomy** is indicated when severe flexion contracture has developed, but the arthrosis is not severe.

3. For **open decompression** of impinging areas, various procedures have been described.

4. **Interposition/distraction arthroplasty**

5. **Total elbow arthroplasty**

6. **Excisional arthroplasty**

7. **Arthrodesis**

6. Are there differences in the presenting complaints of patients with rheumatoid arthritis, osteoarthritis, and posttraumatic arthritis of the elbow?

Pain is the common complaint, but each type may experience stiffness, weakness, or instability. Typically, patients with rheumatoid arthritis complain of pain with instability in the joint, which, in 90% of cases, is exacerbated by involvement of the ipsilateral shoulder and wrist. The patient afflicted with osteoarthritis complains of loss of motion with pain, which restricts the ability to work and to perform activities of daily living.

7. What is the radiographic presentation of rheumatoid arthritis?

There are four distinct stages: stage 1, normal radiograph, with the possibility of osteoporosis with active synovitis; stage 2, symmetric joint narrowing, normal architecture; stage 3, distinct alteration of subchondral architecture that may be relatively mild (type A) or extensive (type B); and finally, stage 4, gross destruction of most or all of the articular architecture. This stage is characterized clinically by instability and, sometimes, severe, extensive pain.

8. What is the natural history of rheumatoid arthritis in the elbow?

1. Synovitis is the first, prominent pathologic process. Biomechanics remain normal. Osteoporosis is present but without gross articular destruction.

2. Joint narrowing occurs with progressive worsening of the osteoporosis.

3. Joint architecture is distorted with loss of contour of the joint. Osteoporosis worsens, subchondral cysts form, and clinical complaints of instability begin.

4. Finally, gross joint destruction results in loss of articular surfaces and gross instability of the joint.

9. What are the surgical options for treatment of rheumatoid arthritis of the elbow?

1. Synovectomy with or without radial head excision
2. Interposition arthroplasty
3. Joint replacement

Stage, age, and other joint involvement determine the choice.

10. What has been the experience of arthroscopic synovectomy?

It is technically demanding and difficult to perform a complete synovectomy without causing neurovascular injury. Early success has been achieved with somewhat diminished 3-year satisfactory results. It is unclear whether it is superior to open synovectomy. Arthroplasty surgeons tend to prefer replacement over synovectomy because of the more predictable long-term results.

11. What are the indications, advantages, and disadvantages of radial head resection?

Resection is recommended for pain relief when a radiocapitellar joint is involved and the ulno-humeral involvement is relatively mild or moderate. This procedure is recommended for pain relief and not for increased motion. Motion postoperatively is highly variable, with 50% of cases unchanged, 30% improved, and 20% exacerbated. Follow-up at 5 years shows an approximately 75% success rate. Radial head resection is not offered as a long-term solution to the rheumatoid patient because the disease process most likely will progress in the joint.

12. What is the current role of Silastic radial head replacement in elbow surgery?

Although Silastic radial head replacement is advocated by a few authors, the increasing concern about silicone particulate synovitis and lymphadenitis with a subsequent autoimmune response has lessened the enthusiasm. The procedure is currently not recommended by most elbow surgeons.

13. What is interposition/distraction arthroplasty of the elbow? What are its indications?

Interposition arthroplasty refers to resecting the diseased articulating surfaces and filling the joint with interposed materials, thereby relieving pain. Many materials have been tried in the past, such as ivory pegs, lanolin, and celluloid. Most recently, materials such as muscle flaps, fascia, skin, gel foam, and fat have been used. External fixators are placed at the elbow to allow distraction across the joint as healing occurs. The distraction technique is not universally accepted and because of its technical complexity is used by relatively few surgeons. Interposition arthroplasty is preferred in a heavy laborer. Disadvantages include unpredictable pain relief and unpredictable effects on instability. This procedure is used in select patients who want to avoid elbow arthrodesis or total elbow arthroplasty.

14. What is total elbow arthroplasty?

Total elbow arthroplasty involves replacement of the articulating surfaces of the distal humerus and the proximal ulna of the elbow. The radial head is not included in the reconstruction.

15. When is total elbow arthroplasty indicated?

Total elbow arthroplasty is indicated when arthrosis of the elbow has progressed to the point that the patient is unable to tolerate the pain and has failed conservative therapies or less invasive surgical treatment. Arthroplasty is indicated for treatment of rheumatoid and degenerative joint disease of the elbow, severe supracondylar and intracondylar fractures of the elbow in elderly patients, and intracondylar and supracondylar nonunions of the distal humerus.

16. What are the contraindications for total elbow arthroplasty?

Active infection in the joint is an absolute contraindication. Relative contraindications are young patients with an active lifestyle or heavy laborers unwilling or unable to alter their lifestyle.

17. What elbow arthroplasty designs are used currently?

There are two types of prosthetic joint designs in current use: unlinked (typically referred to as "unconstrained") surface replacements, and linked ("semiconstrained"). Excellent results have been achieved with both at different institutions with the main indications for elbow arthroplasty.

18. List the major complications of total elbow arthroplasty.

1. Loosening (largely overcome by the use of intramedullary stems and avoidance of fully constrained systems)

2. Instability, including dislocations, subluxations, or maltracking (predominantly with the nonconstrained designs)

3. Infection

4. Ulnar nerve injury

19. Identify the three main technical considerations in elbow arthroplasty.

1. Arthroplasty is usually performed through a posterior approach. The ulnar nerve must be explored and transposed anteriorly.

2. Careful attention must be given to soft-tissue balancing, especially with the minimally constrained design.

3. The ulnar aspect of the lateral collateral ligament must be repsired to prevent postoperative instability.

20. What are the results of total elbow arthroplasty?

Ninety percent of patients are highly satisfied with pain relief. Overall, motion is increased 90% in flexion, 0% in extension, and 60–70% in pronation and supination. Survivorship analysis predicts a failure rate of approximately 20% at 10 years.

21. Is there a role for total elbow arthroplasty in the acute fracture setting?

In selected elderly patients with comminuted distal humeral fractures, total elbow arthroplasty is an option.

22. Do patients with rheumatoid arthritis fare better in terms of results from arthroplasty?

Patients with rheumatoid arthritis and low-demand elderly patients with distal humerus fractures or distal humeral mal- and nonunions typically have better long-term results because of the decreased rate of loosening.

23. What is excisional arthroplasty of the elbow? What are the relative indications?

Excisional arthroplasty is removal of the intraarticular osseous structures of the elbow joint. It is usually performed after a failed total elbow arthroplasty. Results are better when the condyles of the humerus are present. If a flail elbow results, usually the elbow becomes nonfunctional.

24. What are the indications for arthrodesis of the elbow?

Arthrodesis of the elbow is an unsatisfying operation for both the patient and the surgeon. It is usually performed for intractable sepsis about the elbow or when no other reconstruction technique is possible. There is no optimal position of flexion in which to fuse the elbow, and significant limitations in accomplishing activities of daily living usually follow arthrodesis of the elbow.

BIBLIOGRAPHY

1. Azar FM, Wright PE II: Arthroplasty of shoulder and elbow. In Canale ST (ed): Campbell's Operative Orthopaedics, 9th ed. St. Louis, Mosby, 1998, pp 497–513.
2. Figge HE III, Inglis AE, et al: Current concepts review: Total elbow arthroplasty. J Bone Joint Surg 70A:778–783, 1983.
3. Frymoyer JW (ed): Orthopedic Knowledge Update, No. 4. Chicago, American Academy of Orthopedic Surgeons, 1993.
4. Lee BP, Morrey BF: Arthroscopic synovectomy of the elbow for rheumatoid arthritis: A prospective study. J Bone Joint Surg 79A:770–772, 1997.
5. Morrey BF: Post-traumatic contracture of the elbow: Operative treatment, including distraction arthroplasty. J Bone Joint Surg 72A:601–618, 1990.
6. Morrey BF: Primary degenerative arthritis of the elbow: Treatment of ulno-humeral arthroplasty. J Bone Joint Surg 74B:409–413, 1992.
7. Morrey BF: Semiconstrained elbow replacement for distal humeral nonunion. J Bone Joint Surg 77B:67–72, 1995.
8. Morrey BF: The Elbow and Its Disorders. Philadelphia, W.B. Saunders, 1985.

9. Norris TR (ed): OKU Shoulder and Elbow. Chicago, American Academy of Orthopaedic Surgeons, 1997.
10. O'Driscoll SW: Elbow arthritis: Treatment options. J Am Acad Orthop Surg 1:106–116, 1993.
11. Sledge CB, et al: Arthritis Surgery. Philadelphia, W.B. Saunders, 1994.

34. COMPARTMENT SYNDROMES OF THE UPPER EXTREMITY

Vern J. Prochaska, M.D.

1. What is compartment syndrome?

Compartment syndrome is a combination of signs and symptoms resulting from increased pressure within a confined space. The increased pressure causes damage to the tissues in the compartment by decreasing circulation.

2. What are the five Ps of compartment syndrome?

Pain, pallor, paresthesias, paralysis, and pulselessness are the classic signs of compartment syndrome. Paralysis and pulselessness are late findings. If the process has progressed to this point, the limb is less likely to be salvageable.

3. What is the earliest and most sensitive finding in compartment syndrome?

Pain is usually the earliest sign and is often out of proportion to what may be expected from the extent of the injury. Pain with passive stretch of the muscle in the compartment is the most reliable clinical test.

4. Is compartment syndrome possible in a patient without pain?

A patient without pain still may have a compartment syndrome. Pain may be diminished or absent in the late stages as a result of nerve ischemia. A central neurologic deficit or unconsciousness should lower the threshold for prompt treatment.

5. Name the five most common causes of compartment syndrome.

The five most common causes are fracture, soft-tissue injury, arterial injury, prolonged limb compression, and burns.

6. What is Volkmann's contracture?

In 1881 Richard von Volkmann described the contracture and paralysis caused by tissue damage that occurs as a sequela of compartment syndrome. He blamed the ischemia on tight bandaging of the extremity. The term is often used synonymously with compartment syndrome, ischemic muscle damage, and the characteristic position of the hand after forearm compartment syndrome.

7. How is pressure in a compartment measured?

Several methods are available, and anyone dealing with patients at risk should be familiar with at least one. Whitesides popularized an infusion technique that uses supplies available in any hospital. Matsen advocates a similar technique but modifies it for continuous monitoring by using and infusion pump and a blood pressure transducer. Mubarak's wick catheter technique directly measures compartment pressures. In addition, a commercially available device made by the Stryker company is simple and reliable.

8. At what pressure does compartment syndrome exist?

Various upper limits are given by different authors. The most commonly recommended pressure threshold is 30 mmHg. Some add a time element and recommend 30 mmHg for 8 hours or 30 mmHg if the duration is unknown. The hypotensive patient tolerates less compartment pressure. Mubarak and Hargens have found that neuromuscular deficits occur when the intramuscular pressure rises to within 35–40 mm of diastolic blood pressure.

9. What is the treatment for compartment syndrome?

The treatment of compartment syndrome consists of complete and prompt fasciotomy of all compartments involved. A high index of suspicion should be maintained, and if compartment syndrome is seriously considered, a fasciotomy should be done. The morbidity from compartment release is much less than the morbidity from a missed compartment syndrome.

10. How many compartments are in the forearm?

The forearm consists of the volar compartment, dorsal compartment, and a compartment of the mobile wad (brachioradialis, extensor carpioradialis brevis, and extensor radialis longus). The three compartments of the forearm differ from those of the leg in that they are interconnected. Fasciotomy of the volar compartment may decompress the other two. This possibility should not be relied on, however, and any clinically involved compartment should be released.

11. What are the compartments in the hand?

There are 10 compartments in the hand: 1 for each of the 4 dorsal interosseous muscles, 3 for the volar interossei, 1 for the adductor pollicis, and 1 each for the thenar and hypothenar muscles.

12. Can compartment syndrome occur in a finger?

Yes. Although there is no muscle in the finger, nerves and soft tissue can become ischemic because of excessive swelling. The finger has a tight investing fascia that is relatively unyielding.

13. Which muscles are most often involved in compartment syndrome of the forearm?

The muscles closest to the bone are affected first. Therefore, the flexor digitorum profundus and flexor pollicis longus are most often involved, followed by the flexor digitorum superficialis and pronator teres.

14. What is the characteristic position of the hand in Volkmann's contracture?

In a classic Volkmann's contracture, the fingers and thumb are fixed in flexion with the wrist in slight flexion. The position of the hand and degree of flexion contracture depend on the extent of muscle damage.

15. What is the treatment of established Volkmann's contracture of the forearm?

Treatment of established contractures depends on the level of involvement but generally includes tendon release and tendon transfer to restore function.

BIBLIOGRAPHY

1. Eaton RG, Green WT: Epimysiotomy and fasciotomy in the treatment of Volkmann's contracture. Orthop Clin North Am 3:175, 1972.
2. Feliciano DV, Cruss PA, Spjat-Patrinely V, et al: Fasciotomy after trauma to the extremities. Am J Surg 156:533, 1988.
3. Garfin S, Mubarak S, Evans K, et al: Quantification of intracompartmental pressure and volume under plaster casts. J Bone Joint Surg 63A:449, 1981.
4. Green DP (ed): Operative Hand Surgery, 4th ed. New York, Churchill Livingstone, 1998.
5. Hargens AR, Mubarak SJ: Current concepts in the pathophysiology, evaluation and diagnosis of compartment syndrome. Hand Clin 14:371–383, 1998.

6. Lagerstrom CF, Reed RL II, Rowlands BJ, Fischer RP: Early fasciotomy for acute clinically evident post traumatic compartment syndrome. Am J Surg 158:36, 1989.
7. Mabee JR, Bostwick TL: Pathophysiology and mechanisms of compartment syndrome. Orthop Rev 22:175, 1993.
8. Matsen FA III: Compartment syndrome: A unified concept. Clin Orthop 113:8, 1975.
9. Ortiz JA Jr, Berger RA: Compartment syndrome of the hand and wrist. Hand Clin 14:405–418, 1998.
10. Rockwood CA Jr, Green DP, Bucholz RW (eds): Rockwood and Green's Fractures, vols. 1 and 2, 4th ed. Philadelphia, Lippincott-Raven, 1996.
11. Sundararaj GD, Mani K: Pattern of contracture and recovery following ischemia of the upper limb. J Hand Surg 10B:155, 1985.
12. Whitesides TE Jr, Haney TC, Morimoto K, Harada H: Tissue pressure measurements as a determinant for the need of fasciotomy. Clin Orthop 113:43, 1975.

35. NERVE ENTRAPMENTS OF THE ELBOW AND FOREARM

Jeffrey J. Tiedeman, M.D.

1. How are nerve injuries classified?

Seddon classified nerve injuries as neurapraxia, axonotmesis, and neurotmesis. **Neurapraxia** is caused by localized ischemic demyelination often from compression or contusion. **Axonotmesis** results in interruption of the axons and their myelin sheaths but the endoneurial tube remains intact. Stretching or compression is a common cause of axonotmesis. **Neurotmesis** is caused by anatomic disruption of the axons, the myelin sheath, and the endoneurial tube (e.g., from a laceration or severe stretching injury). Spontaneous recovery cannot be expected in neurotmesis; surgical repair or grafting is necessary to maximize function. Complete recovery of nerve function is not expected in adults with neurotmesis.

2. What is pronator syndrome?

Pronator syndrome is essentially a high carpal tunnel syndrome (CTS) because it represents another entrapment neuropathy of the median nerve. Like CTS, it may produce numbness and paresthesias in the median innervated digits, weakness in the thenar muscles, and pain in the wrist and forearm. Unlike CTS, pronator syndrome typically does not cause nocturnal symptoms. Tinel's sign is negative at the wrist, and although nerve conduction studies of the median nerve may be delayed, the delay does not occur at the wrist.

3. What structure can cause entrapment of the median nerve in pronator syndrome?

As the name indicates, the most common source of compression is the pronator teres muscle. Pronator teres compression can be elicited by resisted forearm pronation with the elbow extended. The lacertus fibrosus also has been implicated as a possible cause; compression is elicited by resisted flexion of the elbow with the forearm in supination. Lastly, the arch of the flexor digitorum superficialis also may be responsible for median nerve compression. This muscle is tested by resisted flexion of the proximal interphalangeal (PIP) joint of the middle finger.

4. Describe anterior interosseous syndrome.

Anterior interosseous syndrome is compression of the anterior interosseous nerve, which branches from the median nerve approximately 4–6 cm below the elbow. It functions entirely as a motor nerve and supplies the flexor pollicis longus (FPL), the FDP to the index and middle fingers, and pronator quadratus muscles. Despite its motor function, pain in the forearm is a commonly presenting problem.

5. Where is Gantzer's muscle?

Gantzer's muscle is an accessory head to the FPL muscle and may be responsible for compression of the anterior interosseous nerve.

6. What is the Kiloh-Nevin sign?

The Kiloh-Nevin sign, which is elicited by asking the patient to form an "O" with the tips of the thumb and index finger, is used to test terminal function of the digits against resistance. In a patient with anterior interosseous syndrome, fine-pinch posture is abnormal. The index finger is extended at the distal interphalangeal (DIP) joint as it makes contact with the pulp of the thumb (which is also hyperextended at the IP joint level).

7. What is a Martin-Gruber anastomosis?

A small minority of patients may have crosslinks among the three main nerves of the upper limb. The Martin-Gruber anastomosis is an anomaly in which motor nerve fibers normally carried entirely in the ulnar nerve enter the ulnar nerve from the median nerve via branches in the forearm. In patients with this anomaly, dysfunction or disruption of the ulnar nerve above the level of the anastomosis may not result in motor loss of muscles in the hand typically innervated by the ulnar nerve.

8. What is cubital tunnel syndrome?

Cubital tunnel syndrome refers to entrapment of the ulnar nerve in its passage around the medial aspect of the elbow. The ulnar nerve normally passes through the anatomic cubital tunnel, which is a fibroosseous ring formed by the medial epicondyle and the proximal part of the ulna; it is bridged by a specific fascial sheet known as Osborne's fascia.

9. The ulnar nerve supplies which structures?

The ulnar nerve provides motor supply to the flexor carpi ulnaris and one-half of the flexor digitorum profundus (FDP), the palmar and dorsal interosseous muscles, the hypothenar muscles, the ulnar two lumbrical muscles, the adductor pollicis, and the deep head of the flexor pollicis brevis (FPB). The ulnar nerve also supplies sensation to the small finger and the ulnar half of the ring finger. Through its dorsal sensory branch it also supplies sensation to the dorsal ulnar aspect of the hand.

10. What provocative tests are used to substantiate a diagnosis of cubital tunnel syndrome?

Tinel's sign is invariably positive over the ulnar nerve in the cubital tunnel, producing a tingling sensation that radiates to the ulnar two fingers. The elbow flexion test is performed by maximally flexing the elbow. Pain and paresthesias in the ulnar nerve distribution within 60 seconds constitute a positive test and are virtually diagnostic of cubital tunnel syndrome.

11. How is Froment's sign elicited?

The patient is asked to pull on a sheet of paper with the index finger and thumb while the examiner withdraws it strongly. The patient with normal function maintains maximal contact of the digital pulp with the paper by extending the IP joint of the thumb. In ulnar nerve dysfunction, the control of the metacarpophalangeal (MCP) joint is lost through paralysis or weakness of the adductor pollicis and the deep head of the FPB. Consequently, the MCP joint collapses into hyperextension and the IP joint flexes to compensate for the resulting lack of pinch strength.

12. What is radial tunnel syndrome?

Radial tunnel syndrome, or resistant tennis elbow, is entrapment or compression of the posterior interosseous nerve in the lateral aspect of the proximal forearm. Patients may present with motor weakness in the radially innervated muscles of the forearm, pain in the lateral aspect of the elbow region, or both. Because of its close proximity to the lateral epicondyle, this problem is sometimes difficult to differentiate from lateral epicondylitis or tennis elbow.

13. Which structures are typically responsible for posterior interosseous nerve compression?
The mnemonic **FREAS** is useful for remembering the structures that compress the posterior interosseous nerve:

F = Fibrous bands
R = Recurrent radial vessels (the leash of Henry)
E = Extensor carpi radialis brevis
A = Arcade of Frohse
S = Supinator (the distal border)

14. What is Wartenberg's syndrome?
Originally described as cheiralgia paresthetica, Wartenberg's syndrome is an entrapment neuropathy at the point where the sensory branch of the radial nerve emerges from beneath the edge of the brachioradialis tendon, 6–8 cm proximal to the radial styloid. The condition typically arises as a result of previous trauma or from repeated pronation and supination of the forearm.

15. What is Wartenberg's sign?
The inability to adduct the extended small finger to the extended ring finger is referred to as Wartenberg's sign. The patient's ring and small fingers will form a "V" that they are unable to close. It is a sign of ulnar nerve dysfunction with inactivity of the interossei and hypothenar muscles. The small finger remains abducted due to the unopposed activity of the extensor digiti minimi.

16. How does lateral antebrachial cutaneous neuropathy present?
The lateral antebrachial cutaneous nerve is the terminal sensory branch of the musculotaneous nerve. It supplies sensation over the radial half of the forearm from the elbow to the wrist. Compressive neuropathy may occur in persons who perform repeated overhead motions such as throwing (racquet sport athletes and swimmers). It is thought to occur from forced repeated pronation with the elbow extended. Compression occurs at the lateral margin of the biceps aponeurosis. A positive Tinel's sign may be elicited immediately lateral to the biceps tendon. Initial treatment consists of relative rest and/or corticosteroid injection at the site of the Tinel's sign. This should be coupled with elbow splinting in moderate flexion. Surgical release is occasionally necessary.

BIBLIOGRAPHY

1. Blacker GJ, Lister GD, Kleinert HE: The abducted little finger in low ulnar nerve palsy. J Hand Surg 1A:190–196, 1976.
2. Dellon AL: Review of treatment results for ulnar nerve entrapment at the elbow. J Hand Surg 14A:688–700, 1989.
3. Eversmann WW Jr: Entrapment and compressive neuropathies. In Green DP (ed): Operative Hand Surgery, 3rd ed. New York, Churchill Livingstone, 1993, pp 1341–1385.
4. Gelberman RH, Eaton R, Urbaniak JR: Peripheral nerve compression. J Bone Joint Surg 75A:1854–1878, 1993.
5. Idler RS: General principles of patient evaluation and nonoperative management of cubital syndrome. Hand Clin 12:397–403, 1996.
6. Lister GD: Compression. In Lister GD (ed): The Hand: Diagnosis and Indications, 3rd ed. New York, Churchill Livingstone, 1993, pp 283-322.

36. ELBOW AND FOREARM FRACTURES

David E. Brown, M.D.

1. What is the difference between a supracondylar fracture, a transcondylar fracture, and an intercondylar fracture of the distal humerus?

Supracondylar fractures occur in the distal humeral metaphysis above the joint capsule, and are completely extraarticular. **Transcondylar** fractures, more commonly seen in the elderly osteoporotic population, are a variation of the supracondylar fracture in that the fracture plane occurs within the capsule of the elbow. **Intercondylar** fractures, in which the fracture line splits the medial and lateral condyles, usually are associated within a supracondylar fracture.

2. How does treatment differ for the three types of fracture?

Supracondylar fractures usually occur from an extension injury. Nondisplaced fractures may be treated by splint alone, whereas displaced fractures usually require open reduction and internal fixation.

Transcondylar fractures occur in osteoporotic bone; thus fixation is difficult. Closed reduction with percutaneous pinning is often the best treatment choice. Poor bone quality makes rigid internal fixation difficult to achieve.

Intercondylar fractures, if nondisplaced, can be treated by cast immobilization. The much more common displaced and comminuted fractures require accurate open reduction and rigid internal fixation followed by early range-of-motion therapy. Bone grafting is advisable in comminuted fractures.

3. What is the classification system for intercondylar fractures?

Ryseborough and Radin developed a classification system that involves four types:

Type I: Completely nondisplaced with a transverse supracondylar fracture
Type II: Separation of fractures without rotation
Type III: Significant displacement and malrotation of the condylar fracture fragments
Type IV: Central comminution, regardless of the fracture pattern

4. What is the most common mechanism of radial head fracture?

The most common mechanism is a fall on the outstretched arm. Associated injuries include elbow dislocations and fractures of the distal radius and proximal humerus.

5. What is the classification system of radial head fracture?

Mason's classification system is the most widely used:

Type I: Nondisplaced fracture that is easily missed without sufficient clinical suspicion
Type II: Marginal radial head fracture with minimal displacement, depression, or angulation
Type III: Radial head fracture that is comminuted or more than minimally displaced
Type IV: Radial head fracture associated with elbow dislocation (no figure)

TYPE I   TYPE II   TYPE III

6. What is the treatment of radial head fracture?

Treatment depends on the fracture type. Types I and II generally are treated with short splint-ing and early therapy designed to achieve return of full range of motion. Such fractures are stable. However, type II fractures with > 2 mm of displacement and a mechanical block to extension should be treated with anatomic reduction and internal fixation.

7. How much angulation can be accepted in an adult diaphyseal radius or ulna fracture?

Cadaver studies indicate that malangulation of 0–10° results in little loss of rotational motion, whereas 10–15° may result in up to 20° of rotational loss. Malangulation > 20° restricts rotation by ≥50%.

8. What is the Essex-Lopresti lesion?

The Essex-Lopresti lesion is a comminuted fracture of the radial head, with disruption of the interosseous membrane and distal radioulnar joint. Thus, excision of the radial head leads to disastrous results, because the entire radius migrates proximally. Treatment involves open reduction and internal fixation or replacement arthroplasty of the radial head followed by ac-curate reduction and pinning of the distal radioulnar joint. The surgical pin is removed in 6 weeks once the interosseous membrane and distal radioulnar joint ligaments and capsule have healed.

9. Describe the two types of capitellum fractures.

Type I fractures occur in the coronal plane and usually involve the entire capitellum. They are usually displaced and rotated. Open reduction and rigid internal fixation are preferred. Excision of the fracture fragment also has been shown to give satisfactory results, although it is generally reserved for low-demand patients or patients in whom accurate reduction and rigid fix-ation cannot be achieved.

Type II capitellum fractures involve the articular cartilage and a small shell of subchon-dral bone. Thus, the chances of satisfactory healing after internal fixation are slight. Excision is advised.

10. What is the mechanism of olecranon fractures?
Olecranon fractures usually result from a fall directly onto the olecranon.

11. Describe the treatment options and recommendations for olecranon fractures.
   1. Splinting
   2. Open reduction and internal fixation with tension band wiring
   3. Excision of the fracture fragment if < 50% of the articular surface of the ulna is involved
   Rarely, nonoperative treatment is indicated. In nondisplaced fractures in low-demand patients, splinting in 40° of flexion may be satisfactory.
   Open reduction and internal fixation are advised for most fractures. The AO method of tension band wiring with either longitudinal K-wires or screws and figure-of-eight tension band wire is preferred for avulsion fractures and transverse fractures without comminution. Plate fixation is generally preferred for oblique fractures or comminuted fractures.

12. What are the common mechanisms of fractures of the shafts of the radius and ulna?
A fall on the outstretched hand or a direct blow.

13. What is the treatment of radial and ulnar shaft fractures in adults?
The treatment of choice is accurate anatomic reduction and rigid internal fixation, which are best achieved by following AO principles of interfragmentary compression. Compression plating should use at least a 5-hole plate.

14. What are the indications for bone grafting of diaphyseal fractures of the radius and ulna?
   1. Comminution of > ⅓ of the diameter of the shaft
   2. Segmental defects
   3. Fracture nonunion
   The bone graft should not be placed along the interosseous membrane. Grafting of the radius and ulna must be performed through a separate incision to minimize the risk of radioulnar synostosis.

15. When should the plates and screws be removed after internal fixation of forearm fractures?
Timing is controversial because of the risk of refracture of the diaphysis after plate removal. Many surgeons advise leaving the plates in place unless they are causing symptoms. The rate of refracture varies from 10–20% in published series. If the plates are to be removed, the fracture must be completely healed, and the arm must be protected from heavy activities for at least 6 weeks.

16. List the risk factors for refracture after plate removal.
   1. Early plate removal (< 18 months after surgery)
   2. Use of 4-mm rather than 3-mm compression plates
   3. Failure to protect the forearm after plate removal
   4. Marked comminution of the original fracture

17. What is a Monteggia fracture?
Dislocation of the radial head with a diaphyseal fracture.

18. What is a Galleazzi fracture?
Dislocation of the distal radioulnar joint with fracture of the diaphysis of the radius.

19. Give three other names for a Galleazzi fracture.
   1. Fracture of necessity (it is necessary to perform internal fixation with this fracture pattern)
   2. Piedmont fracture (Hughston and colleagues in the Piedmont Orthopaedic Society originally described the poor results from nonoperative management)
   3. Reverse Monteggia fracture

20. What is the treatment of Monteggia fracture?
1. Anatomic reduction of the radial head dislocation—usually closed
2. Open reduction and rigid internal fixation of the ulnar fracture

21. What is the treatment of Galleazzi fracture?
1. Anatomic reduction and rigid internal fixation of the radial fracture
2. Closed reduction of the distal radioulnar joint (DRUJ) dislocation
3. Postoperative immobilization in full supination to maintain reduction of the DRUJ reduction and rigid internal fixation.

22. What is a night-stick fracture?
A night-stick fracture is an isolated fracture of the diaphysis of the ulna resulting from a direct blow, so-called because it was originally described in victims of beatings with police nightsticks. If the fracture is nondisplaced, treatment by cast immobilization or functional bracing is successful. Fractures that are more than minimally displaced do best with anatomic reduction and rigid internal fixation.

23. What is the treatment of pediatric fractures of the humerus?
Nondisplaced fractures can be treated with splinting in approximately 110° of flexion for 3 weeks, followed by protected range of motion.

Most supracondylar fractures, however, are displaced and require accurate reduction. Although the fracture usually can be maintained after reduction by the above splinting method, there is risk of vascular compromise from immobilization of more severe injuries in flexion. Best results are achieved when reduction is followed by percutaneous pin fixation. The fracture then is immobilized in ≤ 90° of flexion, which allows improved perfusion and improved venous return.

24. What are the complications of pediatric supracondylar fractures?
1. Vascular compromise
2. Nerve injury from either stretching or direct trauma at the fracture site (the radial nerve is the most commonly injured, followed by the median nerve)
3. Fracture malunion that results in cubitus varus due to malrotation (small amounts of medilateral displacement or anteroposterior angulation are tolerated)
4. Volkmann's ischemic contracture (compartment syndrome of the forearm)

25. What is Baumann's angle?
Baumann's angle is the angle between a line drawn along the long axis of the humeral shaft and a transverse line through the growth plate of the capitellum. A normal Baumann's angle is 70–75°.

26. Describe the types of Monteggia lesions in children.
Type I: Anterior dislocation of the radial head; ulna fracture with anterior angulation
Type II: Lateral dislocation of the radial head with radial angulation of the proximal ulna fracture
Type III: Posterior dislocation of the radial head with posterior angulation of ulna fracture
Type IV: Anterior dislocation of the radial head with concomitant fracture of the proximal radial shaft. The ulnar fracture has anterior angulation.

27. What is the treatment of medial condyle fracture?
Treatment of this uncommon fracture depends on the degree of displacement. Nondisplaced or minimally displaced fractures are treated with splint or cast immobilization for 3–4 weeks. Displacement > 2–3 mm requires open reduction and internal fixation.

28. What is the treatment of lateral condyle fractures?
Lateral condyle fractures are usually Salter-Harris type IV fractures of the distal humeral physis. Nondisplaced fractures may be splinted, provided there is a close radiographic follow-up.

Fractures with > 1–2 mm of displacement require open reduction and internal fixation with smooth K-wires.

29. Which is more common, medial or lateral condyle fractures?
Lateral condyle fractures make up > 50% of all distal humeral physeal injuries.

30. What is the most common complication of lateral condyle fractures?
The most common complication is cubitus valgus deformity, usually due to nonunion or gross malunion of the fracture fragment. This complication may cause tardive ulnar nerve palsy, which should be addressed early because of the propensity for motor loss.

31. What is the treatment of radial neck fractures in children?
These Salter-Harris type II fractures are generally nondisplaced and can be treated with short-term immobilization and early range of motion. Significant displacement or angulation should prompt concern about a spontaneously reduced elbow dislocation.

32. How much angulation or displacement of the radial neck fracture is acceptable?
Up to 30° of angulation or 3 mm of displacement is acceptable.

33. What are the indications for radial head excision in children?
None. Excision of the radial head is commonly associated with cubitus valgus, proximal migration of the radius, and proximal radioulnar synostosis. Markedly comminuted radial head fractures are uncommon in children. The fracture generally occurs at the radial neck, thus leaving sufficient residual bone in the head to allow closed or open reduction or K-wire fixation of the fracture fragments.

34. What is a medial epicondyle fracture?
A medial epicondyle fracture is usually an avulsion fracture of the apophysis of the medial epicondyle. It occurs in adolescents, usually as the result of a forced valgus injury to the elbow. It is also seen in throwing athletes, because the flexor pronator mass is forcefully contracted at ball release. Nondisplaced fractures may be treated with immobilization. Any displacement in the dominant arm of a throwing athlete mandates anatomic reduction and internal fixation.

35. What is the treatment of diaphyseal fractures of the radius and ulna in children?
Treatment includes closed reduction and cast immobilization. Diaphyseal fractures heal more readily in children than in adults; children are more tolerant of short-term immobilization and more accepting of malangulation and translocation.

36. How much angulation or displacement is acceptable in a child?
The acceptable degree of angulation or displacement depends on the age of the child. In children up to 6 years of age, as much as 15° of angulation can be accepted. In older children, only 10° should be accepted. Even complete translocation (bayonet apposition) is tolerated in a child because of the tremendous healing potential of the pediatric periosteum.

BIBLIOGRAPHY

1. Badelon O, Bensahel H, Mazoa K, et al: Lateral humeral condylar fractures in children: A report of 47 cases. J Pediatr Orthop 8:31–34, 1988.
2. Beaty JH: Fractures and dislocations about the elbow in children. In Eilert RE (ed): American Academy of Orthopedic Surgeons Instructional Course Lectures, 41. Park Ridge, IL, American Academy of Orthopedic Surgeons, 1992, pp 373–384.
3. Case SL, Hennrikus WL: Surgical treatment of displaced medial epicondyle fractures in adolescent athletes. Am J Sports Med 25:682–686, 1997.
4. Chapman MW, Gordon JE, Zissimos AG: Compression plate fixation of acute fractures of the diaphyses of the radius and ulna. J Bone Joint Surg 71A:159–169, 1989.

5. Crenshaw AH Jr: Fractures of shoulder girdle, arm, and forearm. In Canale ST (ed): Campbell's Operative Orthopaedics, 9th ed. St. Louis, Mosby, 1998, pp 2309–2323.
6. Edwards GS Jr, Jupiter JB: Radial head fractures with acute distal radioulnar dislocation: Essex-Lopresti revisited. Clin Orthop 234:61–69, 1988.
7. Esser RD, Davis S, Taavo T: Fractures of the radial head treated by internal fixation: Late results in 26 cases. J Orthop Trauma 9:318–323, 1995.
8. Geel CW, Palmer AK, Ruedi T, et al: Internal fixation of proximal radial head fractures. J Orthop Trauma 4:270–274, 1990.
9. Henley MB, Bone LB, Parker B: Operative management of displaced intraarticular fractures of the distal humerus. J Orthop Trauma 1:24–35, 1987.
10. Kurer MH, Regan MW: Completely displaced supracondylar fracture of the humerus in children: A review of 1708 comparable cases. Clin Orthop 256:205–214, 1990.
11. Ring D, Jupiter JB: Current concepts review. Fracture dislocation of the elbow. J Bone Joint Surg 80:566–580, 1998.
12. Wolfgang G, Burke F, Bush D, et al: Surgical treatment of displaced olecranon fractures by tension band wiring technique. Clin Orthop 224:192–204, 1987.

V. Hand and Wrist

37. ANATOMY OF THE HAND

Vern J. Prochaska, M.D.

1. Name the bones of the proximal and distal carpal rows.
The bones of the proximal carpal row, from radial to ulnar, are the scaphoid, lunate, triquetrum, and pisiform. The distal row comprises the trapezium, trapezoid, capitate, and hamate.

2. How much of wrist flexion and extension occurs at the midcarpal joint?
Wrist kinematics are quite complex, and the exact amount of motion that occurs at the radiocarpal and midcarpal joints is debated. In the simplest terms, 50% of wrist motion occurs at the midcarpal level. A greater proportion of flexion occurs at the midcarpal joint, whereas most of wrist extension occurs at the radiocarpal joint.

3. List the contents of the carpal tunnel.
The normal carpal tunnel contains the median nerve and nine flexor tendons: the four sublimis tendons, the four profundus tendons, and the flexor pollicis longus.

4. What is Guyon's canal?
Guyon's canal is the triangular canal immediately ulnar to the carpal tunnel in the wrist. The ulnar nerve and ulnar artery traverse the canal, which may be a site of ulnar nerve entrapment.

5. List the contents of the six dorsal wrist compartments.
The dorsal wrist compartments are numbered from radial to ulnar and contain the extensor tendons. The contents of the compartments are listed in the table below. A helpful mnemonic to remember the number of tendons in each compartment is 2-2-1-2-2-1.

Dorsal Wrist Compartments

COMPARTMENT	CONTENTS
1	Abductor pollicis longus Extensor pollicis brevis
2	Extensor carpi radialis longus Extensor carpi radialis brevis
3	Extensor pollicis longus
4	Extensor digitorum communis Extensor indicis proprius
5	Extensor digiti minimi
6	Extensor carpi ulnaris

6. How much motion occurs at the fifth carpometacarpal joint?
The fifth carpometacarpal joint is a saddle joint and the most mobile of the carpometacarpals. Cadaveric studies demonstrate 15° of motion, but many authors give 20–30° as a functional range of motion for the ulnar side of the hand.

7. How much motion occurs at the third carpometacarpal joint?

No motion occurs at the third carpometacarpal joint. It acts as a central stable post for the hand, and its axis is used as the reference for adduction and abduction of the digits.

8. What muscles are innervated by the median nerve distal to the carpal tunnel?

The median nerve supplies motor branches to the lateral two lumbricals, abductor pollicis brevis, flexor pollicis brevis, and opponens pollicis. All but the opponens pollicis are difficult to isolate and test for evaluation of wrist lacerations or for carpal tunnel syndrome. Opposition of the thumb is easily and reliably tested by having the patient ouch the tips of the small finger and thumb.

9. Why is the recurrent motor branch of the median nerve at risk during carpal tunnel release?

The recurrent motor branch has a variable course across the wrist. It may leave the median nerve proximal (most common) or distal to the transverse carpal ligament, or it may pass through the ligament (up to 30% in some series).

10. What is the action of the interosseous muscles?

The dorsal interossei abduct the digits and assist in metacarpophalangeal (MCP) flexion. The palmar interossei adduct and assist in MCP flexion; they also play a role in extension of the interphalangeal (IP) joints through their attachment to the extensor hood.

11. What is unique about the lumbrical muscles?

The lumbrical muscles are unique in that they take their origin from a tendon. Arising from the tendons of the flexor digitorum profundus in the palm, these muscles join the extensor expansion and act as flexors of the MCP joints and extensors of the IP joints.

12. What are the borders of the anatomic "snuff box"?

The snuff box lies just distal to the radial styloid process. The radial border is composed of the abductor pollicis longus and extensor pollicis brevis. The ulnar border is the extensor pollicis longus. The floor of the snuff box is the scaphoid bone.

13. What is Allen's test?

Allen's test evaluates the circulation of the radial and ulnar arteries in the hand. The patient opens and closes the fist several times, then the examiner occludes the radial and ulnar arteries at the wrist with the fist closed. Next the patient opens the fist and the examiner releases one of the arteries. The hand should flush immediately. The procedure is repeated, with release of the other artery. Failure to flush or slow return of color to the hand suggests occlusion of one of the arteries.

14. Which artery is dominant?

Although the radial artery is more easily palpated, the ulnar artery is usually the dominant source of blood to the hand. Radial artery puncture for blood gases and blood pressure monitoring might not be done so liberally if the radial artery were the dominant source of blood.

15. Where is "no man's land" of the hand?

Bunnel first described no man's land, the area in which *both* the flexor tendons of the fingers pass through a tight fibrous tunnel. Designated as zone II, it is the area between the distal palmar crease and the insertion of the flexor superficialis at the midportion of the middle phalanx. Repair of tendon lacerations in this region requires meticulous technique and knowledgeable postoperative management.

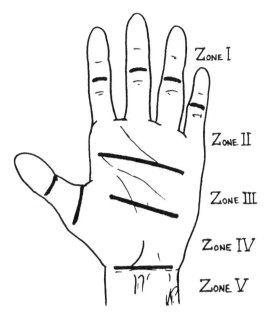

Zones of flexor tendon injury. Zone II: "no man's land."

16. What are the vincula tendinum?
The vincula are thin fibrous slips, covered by synovial membrane, that transmit blood vessels to the flexor tendons. Each tendon has a vinculum breve and a vinculum longum.

17. What structure is involved in Dupuytren's contracture?
Dupuytren's contracture is a progressive contracture of the fingers into the palm caused by cords of palmar fascia. It commonly begins with the fourth and fifth fingers and may involve the entire palm. Baron Dupuytren is given credit for identifying the cause of the contracture and for the first successful surgical release.

18. What deformity is caused by rupture of the central extensor tendon of the digit?
Rupture of the central slip allows the lateral bands to drop volar to the axis of the proximal interphalangeal (PIP) joint. the lateral bands then become flexors of the PIP as the joint "buttonholes" through the rupture. The distal interphalangeal (DIP) joint then undergoes a compensatory hyperextension. This loss of extension of the PIP and hyperextension of the DIP is called a boutonnière (buttonhole) deformity.

19. Where do most wrist ganglia originate?
The most common ganglion is the dorsal wrist ganglion, which originates from the scapholunate ligament and accounts for approximately 60–70% of all hand ganglia. The second most common is the volar ganglion (18–20%). Ganglia of the flexor tendon sheath at the A-1 pulley are the third most common (10–12%).

20. Which of the annular pulleys of the flexor tendon are the most important in preventing bowstringing?
Five annular fibrous tissue bands overlie the synovial sheath of the flexor tendons. They are numbered from proximal to distal. The A-2 and A-4 pulleys are the strongest and most important for preventing the tendons from bowstringing.

Retinacular pulley system. *A*, Annular pulley, with flexor digitorum superficialis omitted. *B* and *C*, Demonstration of function of annular pulleys and tendon bowstringing with absent A-2 and A-4.

BIBLIOGRAPHY

1. American Society for Surgery of the Hand: The Hand: Examination and Diagnosis, 3rd ed. New York, Churchill Livingstone, 1990.
2. Doyle JR: Anatomy of the flexor tendon sheath and pulley system: A current review. J Hand Surg 14A:349, 1989.
3. Kaplan EB: Functional and Surgical Anatomy of the Hand, 2nd ed. Philadelphia, J.B. Lippincott, 1965.
4. Kugzynski K: The proximal interphalangeal joint: Anatomy and causes of stiffness in the fingers. J Bone Joint Surg 50B:656, 1968.
5. Landsmeer JMF: Atlas of Anatomy of the Hand. Edinburgh, Churchill Livingstone, 1976.
6. Lichtman DM, Alexander AH (eds): The Wrist and Its Disorders. Philadelphia, W.B. Saunders, 1997.
7. Matloub HS, Yousef NJ: Peripheral nerve anatomy and innervation patterns. Hand Clin 8:201, 1992.
8. Netter FH: Atlas of Human Anatomy. New Jersey, Ciba-Geigy, 1989.
9. Palmer AK, Werner FW, Murphy D, Glisson R: Functional wrist anatomy: A biomechanical study. J Hand Surg 10A:39, 1985.
10. Romanes GJ: Cunningham's Manual of Practical Anatomy, vol 1: Upper and Lower Limbs, 15th ed. Oxford, Oxford University Press, 1986.
11. Tubiana R (ed): The Hand, vol v. Philadelphia, W.B. Saunders, 1999.

38. FRACTURES AND DISLOCATIONS OF THE HAND AND WRIST

Vern. J. Prochaska, M.D.

1. What is a mallet finger? How is it treated?

Mallet finger describes a flexion deformity of the distal interphalangeal (DIP) joint due to loss of continuity of the extensor tendon with the distal phalanx. It may be due to an avulsion of the tendon or avulsion fracture at the tendon insertion. Splinting of the DIP in extension is the preferred method of treating both types of injury. Many authors advocate surgical treatment if the fracture involves a significant portion of the articular surface and the joint is subluxed.

2. What structure is frequently injured in crush injuries of the distal phalanx?

The nailbed is frequently involved in crush injuries but often neglected. Care should be taken to repair the nailbed with a fine, absorbable suture. Fractures of the distal phalanx rarely require more than simple splinting for protection.

3. What are the indications for open reduction and internal fixation of proximal and middle phalangeal fractures?

Indications for surgery on proximal and middle phalangeal fractures, which do not differ significantly from indications for other fractures, include unstable fractures that cannot be reduced and maintained by closed means, most intraarticular fractures, multiple fractures in an extremity, and open fractures with associated soft-tissue injury.

4. What methods of fixation are available for fractures of the metacarpals and phalanges?

The most common method of fixation of small bones is by Kirschner wires, either with open or closed reduction. Intraosseous, tension-band, and cerclage-wiring techniques are also useful. Intermedullary fixation has been described but is less popular. Small-plate and screw fixation (as described by the AO group) is technically demanding and recommended only for those very familiar with the technique.

5. What structure is ruptured in dorsal dislocations of the proximal interphalangeal (PIP) joint?

The volar plate is always ruptured in dorsal dislocations (the most common dislocations of the PIP joint). To protect the volar plate injury, some authors recommend splinting the PIP in 20–30° of flexion for 2–3 weeks. Others advocate early mobilization and buddy taping.

6. What is a boxer's fracture?

A boxer's fracture is a fracture of the fifth metacarpal neck. It is one of the most common hand fractures and is usually seen in brawlers or persons who strike a wall or other unyielding object in anger.

7. How is a boxer's fracture treated?

Considerable variation exists in the literature regarding treatment of boxer's fractures. Recommendations range from minimal immobilization with no attempt at reduction to closed reduction and pin fixation; occasionally open reduction also is recommended. Because of the mobility of the carpometacarpal joint of the fifth finger, dorsal angulation of up to 40° appears to be well tolerated. Rotational malalignment, however, is not acceptable. Acute fractures are generally treated by closed manipulation and immobilization in a plaster splint for 3–4 weeks.

8. How can rotational malalignment be evaluated?

Even very small rotational discrepancies at the base of the finger can be magnified at the finger tips, causing overlap or divergence of the digits with flexion. To evaluate rotational alignment, have the patient flex the metacarpophalangeal (MCP) and PIP joints, and look at the alignment of the fingers. They should point toward the scaphoid bone. Subtle differences sometimes can be seen by looking at the semiflexed fingers end-on and comparing the planes of the fingernails with those of the unaffected.

9. What is a "fight bite"? Why is it significant?

The term fight bite refers to a laceration over the knuckles caused by a clenched fist striking a tooth. These initially innocuous-appearing wounds lead to serious and rapidly progressive infections from oral flora. All wounds on the dorsum of the fist sustained during a fight should be considered human bites, whether or not the patient admits to striking the teeth. Treatment includes prompt surgical debridement, irrigation, and initiation of appropriate antibiotics.

10. What is the safe position for hand immobilization?

The safe position, also called the intrinsic-plus position and the James position, can be used for many fractures of the metacarpals and phalanges as well as soft-tissue injuries. In this position, the MCPs are in 70° of flexion, the PIPs in 15–20° of flexion, and the DIPs in 5–10° of flexion. Due to the cam shape of the metacarpal head, the MCPs tend to become stiff when immobilized in extension. The interphalangeal (IP) joints are more likely to become stiff in flexion and, therefore, are placed in relative extension.

11. What is a complex dislocation of the MCP joint?

Dorsal dislocations of the MCP are divided into simple or complex dislocations. Both are caused by hyperextension injuries. Simple dislocations may be treated by closed reduction and splinting or buddy taping. Complex dislocations require open reduction because of the interposition of the volar plate between the metacarpal head and the proximal phalanx. Improper reduction of simple dislocations may convert them to complex dislocations.

12. How can I tell the difference between a simple and a complex dislocation?

Simple dislocations present with the proximal phalanx hyperextended (60–90°) on the dorsum of the metacarpal head. The joint surfaces are still partially in contact on a lateral radiograph. Complex dislocations present with the digit in a less dramatic position. The MCP is slightly hyperextended, and the IPs are slightly flexed. A hollow can be felt proximal to the dorsal base of the proximal phalanx, and the metacarpal head is prominent in the palm. Skin is often puckered in the palm. On radiographs the joint space is widened and the proximal phalanx is usually displaced toward the central digits. A pathognomonic finding is the presence of a sesamoid within the joint space on a radiograph. The sesamoid is in the volar plate, which is interposed between the phalanx and the metacarpal head.

13. What is a Bennett fracture?

A Bennett fracture is actually a fracture-dislocation of the base of the thumb metacarpal joint. Described by Edward Halloran Bennett in 1882, it consists of an intraarticular fracture separating a volar lip fragment from the metacarpal shaft. The shaft is displaced radially and dorsally at the base by the abductor pollicis longus. The pull of the adductor pollicis on the distal shaft increases the displacement of the base in abduction.

14. How is Bennett's fracture treated?

Multiple treatment methods have been reported to produce good results. The most common current recommendation is attempted closed reduction and percutaneous pinning of the metacarpal to the trapezium. If adequate reduction cannot be obtained, then open reduction and pin fixation are advised. A small AO cortical screw also can be used if the fragment is large enough.

15. Name the other fracture at the base of the thumb.

Rolando described an intraarticular fracture at the base of the first metacarpal in 1910. Rolando's fracture can be viewed as a Bennett's fracture with a second large dorsal fragment in creating a T- or Y-shaped pattern. True Rolando's fractures are less common than more severely comminuted intraarticular fractures. Such fractures are more difficult to treat and have a less favorable outcome.

16. What is gamekeeper's thumb?

The term *gamekeeper's thumb* has come to mean almost any injury of the ulnar collateral ligament of the thumb MCP. It was coined by Campbell in 1955 to describe a chronic stretching of the ulnar collateral ligament, causing instability. Specifically it refers to an occupational deformity of the hands of British gamekeepers due to their methods of killing rabbits. Skier's thumb is a more appropriate name for an acute injury. It is commonly seen in skiers because of forced abduction of the thumb against a planted ski pole. It is also frequently seen in ball-handling athletes.

17. What is a Stener lesion?

Stener reported a series of cases in which the adductor pollicis aponeurosis was interposed between the avulsed ligament and its site of insertion. He pointed out that healing of a ligament cannot be expected to occur under these circumstances. Repair of complete tears of the ulnar collateral ligament gives the most predictable results.

18. Which carpal bone is fractured most often?

The scaphoid (carpal navicular) is the most commonly fractured bone in the carpus. After distal radius fractures, it is the most common fracture of the wrist. Its function as a link between the proximal and distal carpal rows makes it vulnerable to injury. Approximately 80% of such fractures occur at the waist of the scaphoid.

19. Fractures at which location in the scaphoid have the lowest rate of healing? Why?

Fractures of the proximal third of the scaphoid have nonunion or avascular necrosis rates in the neighborhood of 30%. Fractures of the tuberosity or distal third have healing rates approaching 100% and waist fractures heal in 80–90% of cases. The major blood supply to the scaphoid is a branch of the radial artery that enters the dorsal ridge distally. The remaining 30% of the distal scaphoid is supplied by a second group entering the tuberosity.

20. What should be done if no fracture is seen on the radiograph but the snuff box area is tender?

It is best to assume that there is a fracture in the presence of significant tenderness. The wrist and thumb should be immobilized if a fracture is suspected. The radiographs should be repeated in 2–3 weeks. Normal resorption along the fracture site may make the fracture line evident at that time.

21. What is scapholunate dissociation? Why is it important?

Tears of the scapholunate interosseous ligament lead to separation of the scaphoid and lunate. A scapholunate interval ≥ 3 mm (Terry Thomas sign) is confirmatory. This lesion also presents with persistent snuff box tenderness and should be considered in all cases of suspected scaphoid fractures. It may lead to progressive carpal collapse and disability.

22. What should be done if no fracture is visible at 3 weeks but tenderness remains?

Special radiographic views, including the clenched-fist view, can help to delineate fractures from ligamentous injury. Tomography and bone scans are also useful. More recently, magnetic resonance imaging (MRI) has been shown to be a highly sensitive test for fractures of the scaphoid.

23. How is a scaphoid fracture treated?

Nondisplaced scaphoid fractures are generally treated in a thumb spica cast. Debate persists regarding the merits of immobilizing the elbow. Long arm casts appear to reduce the time to healing compared with short arm casts. A long arm cast for 6 weeks, followed by a short arm cast until radiographic evidence of healing is seen, is an acceptable method. Displaced or unstable fractures require percutaneous pin fixation or compression screw fixation.

24. What should be done if a scaphoid fracture does not heal?

The treatment of choice for nonunion of the scaphoid is bone grafting. Volar grafting, as popularized by Russe, is the most common procedure.

25. What is a chauffeur's fracture?

A fracture of the radial styloid is known as a chauffeur's fracture or back-fire fracture. It was commonly seen in the early 1900s when a car back-fired on starting, causing the crank to strike the distal radius or to wrench the hand back violently. A chauffeur's fracture is generally treated by closed reduction and percutaneous pin fixation.

26. What is a Colles' fracture?

A Colles' fracture is a metaphyseal fracture of the distal radius that is dorsally angulated. It may extend into either the radiocarpal and/or the radioulnar surface.

27. What is a Smith's fracture?

A Smith's fracture is a volar angulated fracture of the distal radius. It is also called a reverse Colles' fracture. A Type I Smith's fracture is extraarticular. A Type II fracture enters the dorsal rim of the articular surface. A Type III fracture enters the middle of the radiocarpal surface.

28. What is a Barton's fracture?

A Barton's fracture is actually a fracture-dislocation of the distal radius. It may be displaced either volarly or dorsally. A Type III Smith's fracture is equivalent to a volar Barton's fracture.

29. What is the Frykman classification of distal radius fractures?

The Frykman classification distinguishes between extraarticular and intraarticular fractures involving either the radiocarpal joint or the distal radionuclear joint. It is further modified by the presence of a distal ulnar fracture.

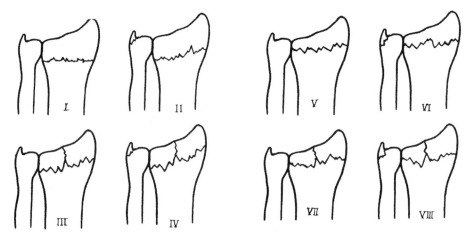

Frykman classification.

30. What is the universal classification of distal radius fractures?

The universal classification system can be used for all distal radius fractures. It is more useful in making treatment decisions than the Frykman classification.

Type I	Extraarticular, nondisplaced
Type II	Extraarticular, displaced
Type III	Intraarticular, undisplaced
Type IV–a	Intraarticular, reducible, stable
Type IV–b	Intraarticular, reducible, unstable
Type IV–c	Intraarticular, irreducible, unstable

31. How is a Colles' fracture treated?

Types I, II and III Colles' fractures are treated by closed reduction and application of a sugar-tong plaster splint, which is later converted to a standard plaster or fiberglass cast. The reduction maneuver usually requires a combination of pronation rotation with a volar and ulnar-directed force. If a satisfactory reduction cannot be achieved or maintained, then surgical methods should be employed.

Primary external fixation (possibly including percutaneous pin fixation) should be considered for Type IV–a and Type IV–b fractures.

Other treatment methods include percutaneous pin fixations (radius only, Kapandji intrafocal pinning or transulnar) and open reduction with internal fixation. Combinations of any of the above methods are common.

32. What is an acceptable reduction?

The goal is to restore the distal radius length, radial slope, and palmar tilt. Length should be compared with the contralateral side. Radial slope averages $22°$ and palmar tilt averages $11°$. Poor results are anticipated if length is not restored to at least the level of the ulna, if there is articular step-off of > 2 mm, or if there is dorsal tilt of $> 20°$.

33. How long should a Colles' fracture be immobilized if cast treatment is used?

The usual course of treatment consists of 1–2 weeks in a sugar-tong splint followed by another 3–5 weeks in a cast. It is imperative that radiographs of the fracture be obtained at 1–2 weeks, or fracture reduction may be lost in plaster. At 1–2 weeks a repeat reduction or conversion to another treatment method is still possible.

34. How should a Smith's fracture be treated?

Types I and II fractures follow the guidelines outlined in questions 30 and 31. Type III Smith's fractures usually require primary open reduction and volar buttress plate fixation.

35. What is Kapandji intrafocal fixation?

Intrafocal fixation involves percutaneous K-wire fixation in which at least one of the wires is inserted into the fracture, and is used to manipulate the displaced fragment as well as prevent later loss of reduction. Studies demonstrate that it is best used alone only in younger individuals with mild comminution.

36. What structure can be injured in fractures or dislocations of the distal radioulnar joint?

The triangular fibrocartilage complex may be damaged in injuries to the distal ulna. The complex consists of a triangular fibrocartilaginous structure and the ulnocarpal ligament. Its base is along the sigmoid notch of the radius, and its apex is attached to the ulnar styloid process.

BIBLIOGRAPHY

1. Ark J, Jupiter JB: The rationale for precise management of distal radius fractures. Orthop Clin North Am 24:205, 1993.
2. Ashkenaze DM, Ruby LK: Metacarpal fractures and dislocations. Orthop Clin North Am 23:19, 1992.
3. Barton N: Conservative treatment of articular fractures in the hand. J Hand Surg 14A:386, 1989.

4. Carter PR, Frederick HA, Laseter GF: Open reduction and internal fixation of unstable distal radius fractures with a low-profile plate: A multicenter study of 73 fractures. J Hand Surg 23A:300–307, 1998.
5. Cooney WP III, Dobyns JH, Linscheid RL: Non-union of the scaphoid: Analysis of the results from bone
   grafting. J Hand Surg 5:343, 1980.
6. Ford DJ, Ali MS, Steel WM: Fractures of the fifth metacarpal neck: Is reduction or immobilization necessary? J Hand Surg 14B:165, 1989.
7. Green DP (ed): Operative Hand Surgery, 4th ed. New York, Churchill Livingstone, 1998.
8. Hastings H II, Lebovic SJ: Indications and techniques of open reduction and internal fixation of distal
   radius fractures. Orthop Clin North Am 24:309, 1993.
9. Hubbard LF: Metacarpal phalangeal dislocations. Hand Clin 4:39, 1988.
10. Kaur JM: The distal radioulnar joint: Anatomic and functional considerations. Clin Orthop 275:37,
    1992.
11. Knirk JL, Jupiter JB: Intra-articular fractures of the distal end of the radius in young adults. J Bone Joint
    Surg 68A:657, 1986.
12. Livesley PJ: Conservative management of Bennett's fracture-dislocation: A 26 year follow-up. J Hand
    Surg 15B:291, 1990.
13. Lubahn JD: Mallet finger fractures: A comparison of open and closed technique. J Hand Surg 14A:394,
    1990.
14. Rikli DA, Kupfer K, Bodoky A: Long-term results of the external fixation of distal radius fractures. J
    Trauma 44:970–976, 1998.
15. Rockwood CA, Green DP, Bucholz RW, Heckman JD (eds): Rockwood and Green's Fractures in Adults,
    vols. 1 and 2, 4th ed. Philadelphia, J.B. Lippincott, 1996.
16. Royle SG: Rotational deformity following metacarpal fracture. J Hand Surg 15B:124, 1990.
17. Russe O: Fractures of the carpal navicular: Diagnosis, non-operative and operative treatment. J Bone
    Joint Surg 42A:759, 1960.
18. Trumble TE, Wagner W, Hanel DP, et al: Intrafocal (Kapandji) pinning of distal radius fractures with and
    without external fixation. J Hand Surg 23A:381–394, 1998.
19. Vaccaro AR, Kupcha PC, Salvo JP: Accurate reduction and splint of the common boxer's fracture.
    Orthop Rev 19:994, 1990.

39. CARPAL INSTABILITY

Jeffrey A. Rodgers, M.D.

1. Name the bones of the proximal and distal carpal rows.

The proximal row consists of the scaphoid, lunate, and triquetrum, whereas the distal row consists of the trapezium, trapezoid, capitate, and hamate. The pisiform is not considered a part of either row. It is of clinical importance to note that the scaphoid spans the midcarpal joint.

2. How many sets of joints compose the wrist joint?

The wrist joint is composed of four distinct joints: the distal radioulnar joint, radiocarpal joint, midcarpal joint, and carpometacarpal joint.

3. What are the anatomic links of the proximal and distal carpal rows?

There are none. The proximal and distal carpal rows are in fact intercalated segments with no muscle or tendon attachments. The scaphoid has been proposed to function as the slider-crank control that links motion at the radiocarpal and intercarpal joints.

4. How is relative carpal motion affected in radial and distal carpal rows?

With radial deviation, flexion occurs in the proximal carpal row through a mechanism that is not completely understood. However, it is thought that the flexion of the scaphoid is transmitted to the lunate by the scapholunate interosseous ligament. With ulnar deviation, the proximal row extends under the influence of the hamate-triquetral interaction.

5. Compare a normal versus functional range of motion of the wrist.

Normal range of motion of the wrist consists of 70° extension and 80° of flexion. Functionally, however, only 10° of flexion and 30° of extension are required for adequate hand function and grip strength.

6. What is the most common form of carpal instability?

The most common form of carpal instability is dorsiflexion-intercalary segment instability (DISI), which usually is associated with an injury to the scapholunate ligament that results in loss of the normally coordinated motion of the proximal carpal row. However, Dobyns described a series of patients who demonstrated the same pattern of instability without injury to the scapholunate ligament. The diagnosis of DISI deformity is based on a lateral radiograph. The normal scapholunate angle is 30–60°. With DISI, however, this angle has been defined to be > 70°. The capitolunate angle is usually < 20°. Characteristically, the lunate translates volarly and extends while the scaphoid flexes.

In dorsiflexion–intercalated segment instability (DISI), the lunate extends and the scaphoid flexes, resulting in a scapholunate angle > 70°. (From Cooney WP, Linscheid RL, Dobyns JH: Carpal instability: Treatment of ligament injuries of the wrist. AAOS Instructional Course Lectures 41:33–44, 1992, with permission.)

7. Who was Terry Thomas and what does he have to do with wrist instability?

Terry Thomas was a famous comedian with an all-star spitting gap between his incisors. The Terry Thomas sign is an eponym describing a scapholunate disassociation on the anteroposterior (AP) radiograph of the wrist. By definition, a diastasis > 3 mm is pathognomonic for scapholunate disassociation. Another sign of the DISI deformity on the AP radiograph is the double cortical ring of the scaphoid produced by the overlay of the distal pole on the palmar-flexed scaphoid when viewed end-on.

8. Describe Mayfield's classification of perilunate instability.

Mayfield described a sequential pattern of injury after a fall on the outstretched hand, using a cadaver model in which the wrists were loaded in extension, ulnar deviation, and intercarpal supination. He described progressive perilunate instability in four stages: stage 1, scapholunate diastasis; stage 2, dorsal dislocation of the capitate; stage 3, disruption of the lunotriquetral interosseous ligament; and stage 4, complete dislocation of the lunate. Such injuries represent "lesser arc" injuries. "Greater arc" injuries involve fracture of one or more of the carpal bones; i.e., transscaphoid perilunate dislocation.

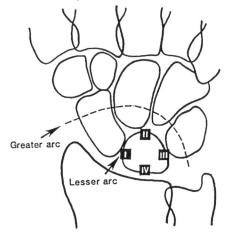

Greater and lesser arc injuries.

9. Describe further work-up of the painful wrist when plain radiographs are normal.

In the setting of an acute wrist injury with normal AP and lateral radiographs, stress radiographs should be obtained, including AP views in ulnar and radial deviation and a clenched fist-supination view to demonstrate dynamic instability of the scaphoid.

10. What is the scaphoid shift test?

1. The scaphoid shift test as described by Dr. Kirk Watson is a provocative maneuver in which the examiner may reproduce the patient's sensation of instability or even cause subluxation of the proximal pole of the scaphoid by stabilizing the scaphoid palmarly while bringing the wrist from ulnar to radial deviation. A palpable click and pain with this maneuver indicate dynamic rotatory subluxation of the scaphoid.

2. The exam should be considered abnormal only if different from the uninjured wrist.

11. What other special studies or procedures can be used to evaluate the painful wrist?

A three-phase bone scan is helpful to rule out occult carpal bone fracture or early avascular necrosis of the lunate. Arthrography, including injection of the radiocarpal, midcarpal joint, and distal radioulnar joints may reveal interosseous ligament tears or injury to the triangular fibrocartilage. The test has a high false-positive rate, and many hand surgeons recommend diagnostic wrist arthroscopy instead.

12. What pattern of instability is found with injury of the lunotriquetral ligament?

Volar flexion-intercalary segment instability (VISI) occurs with injury of the lunotriquetral ligament. Radiographs show a scapholunate angle < 30°, and volar flexion of the lunate results in a capitolunate angle > 20°. Diastasis is uncommon between the lunate and the triquetrum. Lunotriquetral ligament disruption only recently has been recognized as a distinct carpal injury by Reagan et al. Although much less common than DISI, VISI can occur with injury to the lunotriquetral (LT) ligament if injury to the extrinsic scaphotriquetral and radiotriquetral ligaments also has occurred. LT ligament injury alone usually does not result in static radiographic instability.

VISI

In volar flexion–intercalated segment instability (VISI), the lunate is flexed and the scaphoid remains in neutral to slight flexion, resulting in a scapholunate angle of 30° or less. (From Cooney WP, Linscheid RL, Dobyns JH: Carpal Instability: Treatment of ligament injuries of the wrist. AAOS Instructional Course Lectures 41:33–44, 1992, with permission.)

13. Can VISI or DISI deformities occur without injury to either the scapholunate or lunotriquetral intercarpal ligaments?

Yes. This pattern of injury has been described by Dobyns as carpal instability, nondisassociative (CIND). Patients have a normal arthrogram, because no interosseous ligament injury is present.

14. What is the natural history of untreated, chronic scapholunate disassociation?

Chronic scapholunate disassociation commonly results in osteoarthritis and subluxation in what has been termed *scapholunate advanced collapse* (SLAC). Degeneration typically occurs between the radial styloid process and the scaphoid and later in the unstable lunocapitate joint as the capitate subluxes dorsally in the lunate.

15. What treatment options are available for scapholunate disassociation?

Two schools of thought exist with regard to treatment of this difficult problem. The first classifies the injuries as acute (< 4 weeks from time of injury), subacute (> 4 weeks from time of injury), and chronic (> 12 months from time of injury). Treatment options include arthroscopic reduction and percutaneous pinning in the acute phase, open repair techniques in the subacute phase, and open repair or limited intercarpal fusion for chronic instability. The other school of thought, however, believes that the limited intercarpal fusion of the scaphotrapeziotrapezoid (STT) joint has the best chance of good results, especially in young athletes or manual laborers.

16. What is midcarpal instability?
Midcarpal instability consists of either congenital laxity or ligament attenuation between the scaphoid and capitate and/or the triquetrum and capitate. VISI deformity usually results, with a painful "clunk" during activities that involve ulnar deviation and pronation of the wrist.

17. How is the diagnosis of midcarpal instability confirmed?
Standard radiographs show a VISI deformity. During cineradiography, as the wrist is taken into ulnar deviation, the proximal carpal row snaps suddenly from a palmarflexed to a dorsiflexed position, reproducing the patient's symptoms.

BIBLIOGRAPHY

1. Cooney WP, Linscheid RL, Dobyns JH: Carpal instability: Ligament repair and reconstruction. In Nevaiser RJ (ed): Controversies in Hand Surgery. New York, Churchill Livingstone, 1990, pp 125–145.
2. Cooney WP, Linscheid RL, Dobyns JH: Carpal instability: Treatment of ligament injuries of the wrist. AAOS Instructional Course Lectures 41:33–44, 1992.
3. Cooney WP, Linscheid RL, Dobyns JH: Fractures and dislocations of the wrist. In Rockwood CA, Greene DP, Bucholz RW (eds): Rockwood and Greene's Fractures in Adults. New York, J.B. Lippincott, 1991, pp 563–678.
4. Kleinman WB: Long term study of chronic scapho-lunate instability treated by scapho-trapezio-trapezoid arthrodesis. J Hand Surg 14A:429–445, 1989.
5. Lichtman DM, Schneider JR, Swafford AR, et al: Ulnar midcarpal instability: Clinical and laboratory analysis. J Hand Surg 8:515–523, 1981.
6. Linscheid RL, Dobyns JH, Babout JW, Bryan RS: Traumatic instability of the wrist: Diagnosis classification in pathomechanics. J Bone Joint Surg 54A:1612–1632, 1972.
7. Reagan DS, Linscheid RL, Dobyns JH: Lunotriquetral sprains. J Hand Surg 9(A):502–514, 1984.
8. Ritt MJ, Linscheid RL, Cooney WP, Bergen RA, Kai-Nau A: The lunotriquetral joint: Kinematic effects of sequential ligament sectioning, ligament repair and arthrodesis. J Hand Surg 23(A):432–445, 1998.
9. Ruby LK: Wrist biomechanics. AAOS Instruction Course Lectures 41:25–32, 1992.
10. Taleisnik J: Current concepts review: Carpal instability. J Bone Joint Surg 70A:1262–1268, 1988.
11. Watson HK, Ballet FL: The SLAC wrist: Scapholunate advanced collapsed pattern of degenerative arthritis. J Hand Surg 9A:358–365, 1984.

40. TENDON INJURIES OF THE HAND AND WRIST

John A. Miyano, M.D.

1. How do you test the function of the flexor digitorum profundus (FDP) tendon?
The function of the FDP is assessed by active flexion of the distal interphalangeal (DIP) joint with the proximal interphalangeal (PIP) joint held in passive extension, which indicates an intact FDP tendon.

2. Does active flexion at the PIP joint rule out a flexor digitorum superficialis (FDS) laceration?
No. The PIP joint can be flexed using the pull of the FDP tendon. To isolate the FDS, the PIP joint must be actively flexed with the other fingers held in full extension to limit FDP activity.

3. **Define the zones of injury of the flexor tendons in the hand and wrist.**
   Zone I: Insertion of the FDP at the distal phalanx to the middle of the middle phalanx
   Zone II: Middle of the middle phalanx to the distal palmar crease
   Zone III: Distal palmar crease to the distal edge of the carpal tunnel
   Zone IV: Carpal tunnel
   Zone V: Proximal edge of the carpal tunnel to the musculotendinous junction

4. **Which zone is referred to as "no man's land" and why?**
   Historically, it has been most difficult to obtain successful repairs of flexor tendon lacerations in zone II, in which the FDP and FDS tendons run together in a tight, fibroosseous tunnel. Adhesions to the tunnel and between the tendons may develop, compromising tendon gliding.

5. **When repairing a flexor tendon in the finger, which portion(s) of the fibroosseous tunnel is/are the most critical to preserve?**
   The annular pulleys (A1–A5) keep the tendons from bowstringing during active flexion. A2 and A4 are over the shafts of the proximal and middle phalanges, respectively, and must be preserved for normal function.

6. **Define a jersey finger.**
   A jersey finger is an avulsion of the FDP tendon from its insertion on the distal phalanx. It is commonly a sports injury that occurs when a player tries to make a tackle by grabbing another player's jersey. The resisted, forceful flexion causes the tendon to avulse. Treatment is early surgical repair.

7. **Which nerve(s) is/are at risk of injury when the flexor carpi radialis (FCR) is lacerated at the wrist? When the flexor carpi ulnaris (FCU) is lacerated at the wrist?**
   The median nerve is just below the FCR and the palmaris longus at the level of the wrist and is vulnerable to injury. The ulnar nerve (and artery) is deep to the FCU at the level of the wrist.

8. **What is a Mannerfelt lesion?**
   A Mannerfelt lesion is an attritional rupture of the FPL over an osteophyte arising from the scaphoid within the carpal tunnel. It is most commonly seen in rheumatoid arthritis.

EXTENSOR TENDONS

9. **Describe mallet finger.**
   A mallet finger is a flexion deformity of the DIP joint caused by rupture or avulsion of the terminal extensor tendon from the distal phalanx.

10. **What is the treatment for mallet finger?**
    Full-time immobilization of the DIP joint only in extension for a minimum of 6 weeks is required, which may be accomplished with a molded plastic splint (Stack splint), aluminum and foam splint, or surgical pinning across the DIP joint.

11. **When evaluating a laceration to the dorsum of the hand, does active PIP extension rule out a complete tendon laceration? Why or why not?**
    It does not. Active PIP extension can be maintained by the intrinsic muscles (interossei and lumbricals) pulling through the lateral bands. This also may be demonstrated in individuals with radial nerve palsies in which active PIP extension may be preserved in spite of loss of wrist and metacarpophalangeal joint extension.

12. **What is the difference between a swan-neck deformity and a boutonnière deformity?**
    A swan-neck deformity is hyperextension of the PIP joint combined with flexion of the DIP joint (creating the appearance of the head and neck of a swan). A boutonnière deformity is flexion of the PIP joint combined with extension of the DIP joint.

13. What are the deforming forces in a boutonnière deformity?

The initial problem is disruption of the extensor tendon insertion into the middle phalanx, known as the central slip. Over time, the lateral bands migrate volar to the axis of rotation of the PIP joint, thereby becoming PIP flexors instead of extensors.

BIBLIOGRAPHY

1. Canale ST (ed): Campbell's Operative Orthopaedics, 9th ed. St. Louis, Mosby, 1998.
2. Doyle JR: Extensor tendons: Acute injuries. In Green DP (ed): Operative Hand Surgery, 3rd ed. New York, Churchill Livingstone, 1993, pp 1925–1954.
3. Geyman JP, Fink K, Sullivan SD: Conservative versus surgical treatment of mallet finger: A pooled quantitative literature evaluation. J Am Board Fam Pract 11:382–390, 1998.
4. Leddy JP: Flexor tendons: Acute injuries. In Green DP (ed): Operative Hand Surgery, 3rd ed. New York, Churchill Livingstone, 1993, pp 1823–1852.
5. Leddy JP, Packer JW: Avulsion of the profundus tendon insertion in athletes. J Hand Surg Am 2: 66–69, 1977.
6. Mannerfelt L, Norman O: Attrition ruptures of flexor tendons in rheumatoid arthritis caused by bony spurs in the carpal tunnel. J Bone Joint Surg Br 51:270–277, 1969.
7. Strickland JW: Flexor tendon injuries: Part I and part II. J Am Acad Orthop Surg 3:44–62, 1995.

41. SOFT-TISSUE INJURIES AND DISORDERS OF THE HAND

John A. Miyano, M.D.

FINGERTIP INJURIES

1. Discuss the treatment for a subungual hematoma.

Painful hematomas may be decompressed by perforating the nail with a heated paper clip, a battery-powered cautery, or a large needle (16-gauge) used like a drill. Some advocate nail plate removal and nail bed repair if the hematoma is larger than 25–50% of the nail surface.

2. What is the treatment for nail bed lacerations?

Nail bed lacerations should be repaired primarily with a fine (5-0 or 6-0) absorbable suture, such as plain gut. Part or all of the nail plate may have to be removed to allow for adequate visualization and access. After the repair is completed, the nail plate should be reinserted underneath the eponychial fold to prevent scarring of the eponychium to the nail bed.

3. What size fingertip avulsions or amputations will heal without skin grafting or flaps?

Defects up to 1 square cm will heal with dressing changes over a period of 3–6 weeks. Larger defects may require local skin flaps (e.g., V-Y advancement flaps, cross-finger flaps).

4. What is the treatment for a distal phalangeal tuft fracture?

Commonly the result of fingertip crush injuries, most tuft fractures can be treated symptomatically with a brief period (2–3 weeks) of protection. Aluminum and foam splints may be used to make a "bumper" over the tip of the finger.

5. Describe the difference between a paronychia and a felon.

A paronychia is an infection of the eponychial fold (around the edge of the nail plate). A felon is an infection of the fingertip pulp.

6. What is the treatment of a paronychia or felon?

Both require incision and drainage. A paronychia can be drained by incising and sometimes elevating the eponychial fold. A felon can be drained through an incision on the side of the fingertip that extends into the pulp, thereby opening the septal compartments.

7. What causes soft-tissue damage in frostbite?

The damage is caused by vascular compromise. The early response to extreme cold is vasoconstriction, followed by thrombosis of damaged vessels.

8. What is the initial treatment for frostbite?

Initial treatment is rapid rewarming in a water bath at approximately 40°C. Blisters should be left intact.

BURNS

9. Define the different degrees of burns.

A first-degree burn is superficial, characterized by pain and erythema; a second-degree burn is a partial-thickness burn characterized by pain and blistering; and a third-degree burn is a full-thickness burn characterized by painless, blanched skin secondary to nerve death and thrombosis.

10. What is the treatment for most small and medium-sized second-degree burns?

Most can be treated with local wound care, including topical antibiotics (e.g., silver sulphadiazine) and dressing changes. Tetanus status should be checked for all patients.

11. What is the best way to limit edema in burned extremities?

Elevation and early mobilization are important in the reduction of postburn swelling. Compression dressings are generally contraindicated, especially if the circulation is already compromised.

12. What is the clinical significance of a circumferential burn?

Circumferential burns often cause vascular compromise due to tissue edema and loss of skin elasticity (eschar). Even noncircumferential burns are at risk. Escharatomies and fasciotomies are performed if any compromise is detected.

13. What are the two most common mechanisms of injury in an electrical burn? Which is usually more serious?

Injury is usually caused by either surface burns from the initial flash and fire or deep burns from electrical current conducting through the tissues. Conduction burns occur when an individual is grounded (e.g., standing in a pool of water) and usually cause more severe damage to both superficial and deep tissues.

14. When evaluating patients with conduction electrical burns, what must be examined besides the point of contact?

An exit point also must be sought. Unless the area of exit is broad enough to dissipate the energy, a second burn results.

15. Why must urine output be measured in patients with conduction electrical burns?

Conduction burns are associated with significant muscle necrosis and secondary myoglobin release (rhabdomyolysis). If untreated, this may result in acute renal failure. Hydration to maintain a urine output of at least 75 ml/hr is recommended until the breakdown products have cleared.

16. What is the initial treatment for most chemical burns?

Unless a specific neutralizing agent is known, most chemical burns should be irrigated copiously with water.

17. What acid burn classically continues to damage tissue long after exposure?

Hydrofluoric acid, used in industry for such tasks as etching glass, continues to burn unless the tissues are infiltrated with calcium gluconate or calcium chloride.

DUPUYTREN'S CONTRACTURE

18. What is Dupuytren's contracture?

Dupuytren's contracture is a proliferative fibroplasia of the subcutaneous tissues of the palm and fingers, often leading to progressive flexion contractures.

19. What is the etiology of the fibroplasia?

It is believed that myofibroblasts are somehow stimulated, forming type III collagen. Why this occurs is not clear. A genetic predisposition may exist; the fibroplasia is more common in Caucasians of Northern European ancestry. Numerous associated risk factors include smoking, alcohol abuse, and epilepsy.

20. Which fingers are most commonly involved?

The ring and small fingers are most commonly involved. Occasionally, the long finger, thumb, and index finger also may be involved.

21. Who develops Dupuytren's disease more frequently, men or women?

Men develop the disease more frequently than women, at a ratio of 7:1.

22. Which tissues are primarily affected?

Dupuytren's disease is primarily a fibroplasia of palm and finger fascia (e.g., the pretendinous band, natatory ligament, spiral band, lateral digital sheet, Grayson's ligament). Secondary thinning of the subcutaneous fat, as well as thickening and dimpling of the overlying skin, may occur.

23. What other connective tissue disorders are associated with Dupuytren's?
- Plantar fibromatosis (Lederhose's disease)
- Knuckle pads (Garrod's nodes)
- Peyronie's disease

24. Involvement of which portion of the palmar fascia causes contracture of the metacarpophalangeal (MCP) joint?

The pretendinous band.

25. Name the three main cords that develop and cause contracture of the PIP joint.

The central, lateral, and spiral cords. The retrovascular cord is less often the primary lesion, but may be involved in recurrence or incomplete correction.

26. What is the indication for surgical intervention for involvement of the MCP joint?

Consideration for surgery is usually given for contracture > 30°. The MCP joint is tolerant of contracture, and even long-standing deformity > 30° can be reliably corrected. As a general rule, if the patient can place his or her palm flat on a table, operative intervention is not required.

27. How much angular deformity is acceptable in the PIP joint?

Unlike the MCP joint, the PIP joint is not tolerant of contracture. Some believe that any rigid contracture of the PIP joint is indication for surgery, because advanced contracture is very difficult to correct.

28. What is the recurrence rate after surgical intervention?

The recurrence rate may be > 50%, depending on the technique used. However, recurrence may not be rapid or require reoperation. Generally, correction of contracture at the MCP joint is more reliable.

BIBLIOGRAPHY

1. Benson LS, Williams CS, Kahle M: Dupuytren's contracture. J Am Acad Orthop Surg 6:24–35, 1998.
2. Green DP: Operative Hand Surgery, 3rd ed. New York, Churchill Livingstone, 1993.
3. Lister G: The Hand: Diagnosis and Indications, 3rd ed. New York, Churchill Livingstone, 1993.

42. ARTHRITIS AND ARTHROPLASTY OF THE HAND AND WRIST

Jeffrey J. Tiedeman, M.D.

1. Which joints are most commonly involved in a patient with osteoarthritis of the hand and wrist?

The joints most prone to osteoarthritis in the hand and wrist include the distal interphalangeal (DIP) joints and the carpometacarpal (CMC) joint of the thumb. The signs and symptoms are usually localized to the involved joints. Pain is common after joint use and is relieved by rest. In contrast to patients with rheumatoid arthritis, those with osteoarthritis usually have little problem in the morning on rising, but pain increases as the day progresses. Night pain is also common and may interfere with sleep. On physical examination pain with passive motion and crepitus in the joint are prominent findings. Joint enlargement from synovitis and ligamentous laxity are also common features.

2. What are Heberden's nodes?

Heberden's nodes are bone spurs that form on the dorsal aspect of the DIP joints of the fingers. Although typically small in size, such exostoses around the DIP are readily apparent and give the joint a knobby appearance. Similarly, Bouchard's nodes are osteophytes that develop at the proximal interphalangeal (PIP) joint, which is a much less frequent site of osteoarthritis.

3. Which patients are at risk of developing degenerative arthritis after a fracture of the distal radius?

Patients with intraarticular extension of the fracture either into the radiocarpal joint or the distal radioulnar joint are at greatest risk for developing degenerative arthritis. Specifically, fractures that extend into the radiocarpal joint and subsequently heal with > 2 mm of intraarticular incongruity have been shown to be at increased risk for developing degenerative arthritis. Consequently, the goal of treatment for this particular type of fracture is restoration of normal anatomy with reduction of the intraarticular component, particularly in young active individuals.

Knirk JL, Jupiter JB: Intra-articular fractures of the distal end of the radius in young adults. J Bone Joint Surg 68A:647–659, 1986.

4. What is a SLAC wrist?

SLAC wrist refers to scapholunate advanced collapse, which is the most common form of arthritis in the wrist. The degenerative change typically goes through a specific sequence and is caused by articular alignment problems among the scaphoid, the lunate, and the radius. The degenerative arthritis initially involves the radioscaphoid joint. The radiolunate joint is generally spared as the process progresses to the capitolunate joint.

5. Describe the treatment options for CMC arthritis of the thumb.

The CMC joint is the second most frequently involved joint in osteoarthritis of the hand after the DIP joint. The disease process, also known as basal joint arthritis, has a predilection for postmenopausal women and is 10 times more common in women, usually after the fifth decade of life. Conservative treatment includes oral antiinflammatory medication, splints, thenar strengthening exercises, and modification of activity. Pain unresponsive to conservative measures and subsequent loss of function or joint instability are the primary indications for operative intervention. Surgical options include CMC joint arthrodesis or trapezial excision, with either silicone implant arthroplasty or tendinous interpositional graft. An arthrodesis or fusion is a suitable option in a patient with arthritis confined to the CMC joint, particularly in a young person with a demanding occupation. With pantrapezial arthritis good results have been obtained by excising the trapezium and filling the space either with silicone arthroplasty or a tendon graft.

Lins RE, Gelberman RH, McKeown L, et al: Basal joint arthritis: Trapeziectomy with ligament reconstruction and tendon interposition arthroplasty. J Hand Surg 21A:202–209, 1996.

RHEUMATOID ARTHRITIS

6. What is caput ulna syndrome?

Caput ulna syndrome refers to the destructive process initiated by synovitis of the distal radioulnar joint. Characteristic findings include loss of wrist rotation (pronation/supination) and dorsiflexion, weakness, dorsal prominence and instability of the distal ulna, soft-tissue swelling over the distal ulna secondary to synovitis, loss of normal action of the extensor carpi ulnaris tendon, and occasionally loss of extension of the small, ring, and long fingers as a result of extensor tendon ruptures.

7. Name the indications and contraindications for total wrist arthroplasty.

The **major indication** for total wrist arthroplasty is rheumatoid arthritis with wrist pain secondary to advanced destructive changes in the radiocarpal joint. The operation is best suited for patients who also have involvement of several other joints in the upper extremities with resultant limitation of forearm rotation, elbow flexion, shoulder motion, and motion of the digits. Total wrist arthroplasty is desirable in such patients because the only surgical alternative is wrist arthrodesis, which unfortunately eliminates remaining wrist motion and typically diminishes rather than improves overall upper extremity function. Wrist arthrodesis, however, is the preferred procedure for the vast majority of patients with advanced radiocarpal arthritis not due to rheumatoid arthritis, because it generally provides predictable pain relief with a relatively low complication rate.

The **only true contraindication** for total wrist arthroplasty is active infection. In rare cases of juvenile rheumatoid arthritis the diameter of the medullary canal of the distal radius is too narrow to accommodate the stem of the prosthesis, thereby precluding total wrist arthroplasty.

Gelberman RH: The Wrist: Total Wrist Arthroplasty. New York, Raven Press, 1994, pp 253–278.

8. What are the most common complications of total wrist arthroplasty?

The most common complication of total wrist arthroplasty is loosening of the distal component, which has been found in approximately 20% of wrists over a 5-year period postoperatively. A second potential complication is dislocation of the prosthesis. Both complications may cause further problems, such as carpal tunnel syndrome. Failure of total wrist arthroplasty occasionally requires conversion to a wrist fusion.

Beer TA, Turner RH: Wrist arthrodesis for failed wrist implant arthroplasty. J Hand Surg 22A:685–693, 1997.
Gelberman RH: The Wrist: Total Wrist Arthroplasty. New York, Raven Press, 1994, pp 253–278.

9. Which flexor tendon most commonly ruptures in rheumatoid arthritis?

The flexor pollicis longus is the tendon that most commonly ruptures in rheumatoid arthritis (Mannerfelt syndrome). The rupture is usually due to attrition as the tendon passes over a bony spur or erosion in the carpal scaphoid. Treatment usually consists of surgical reconstruction with a tendon graft or a tendon transfer using a superficial digital flexor tendon.

10. What is a boutonnière deformity? Why does it occur?

A boutonnière deformity is a progressive condition that occurs frequently in patients with rheumatoid arthritis. The deformity has three components: (1) flexion of the PIP joint, (2) hyperextension of the DIP joint, and (3) hyperextension of the metaphalangeal (MP) joint. The primary inciting event is synovial proliferation within the PIP joint, which stretches the extensor mechanism. As a result, the patient is unable to maintain full extension of the PIP joint. The lateral tendinous bands subsequently displace volarward and become fixed in this position. Shortening of the oblique retinacular ligaments then results in hyperextension and limited active flexion of the DIP joint. Patients compensate for the flexion deformity of the PIP joint by hyperextending the MP joint. The deformity tends to progress from a supple and passively correctable condition to a fixed condition that may be functionally disabling.

11. What is swan-neck deformity?

Like the boutonnière deformity, swan-neck deformity is common in, but not unique to, rheumatoid arthritis. Swan-neck deformity is characterized by hyperextension of the PIP joint, flexion of the DIP joint, and weakening of the periarticular structures of the PIP joint due to synovitis. Tightness of the intrinsic musculature then creates an abnormal force across the joint, resulting in swan-neck deformity.

12. What is a Brewerton view?

A Brewerton view is a variant of an anteroposterior radiograph of the hand. It should be obtained in all patients evaluated for rheumatoid arthritis. The fingers are placed flat on the radiographic plate, and the metacarpals are inclined at a 65° degree. The radiographic tube is then inclined 15° toward the ulnar side of the hand. The Brewerton view may show bony erosive changes beneath the collateral ligaments of the MCP joints early in the course of rheumatoid arthritis, when standard anteroposterior radiographs of the hand show little change.

13. In advanced rheumatoid arthritis, what MCP joint deformity is typically seen? What are the underlying causes?

The classic deformity seen in rheumatoid arthritis is ulnar drift of the digits and volar dislocation of the proximal phalanges. Various factors are responsible for the pathophysiology, including MCP joint synovitis, articular cartilage erosion and bony destruction, extensor tendon subluxation or dislocation (secondary to selective stretching of the support structures on the radial side), ligamentous and volar plate disruption, intrinsic tightness, and finally the forces of gravity and pinch. The ulnar drift of the fingers is often accompanied by radial deviation of the wrist, creating the characteristic Z-plasty deformity of the hand and wrist often seen in patients with rheumatoid arthritis.

14. What potential complications are associated with silicone MCP joint arthroplasty?

The most common complications are infection, prosthetic breakage, prosthetic dislocation, recurrent deformity, limited motion, and pain. Silicone synovitis, a common problem after carpal bone silicone replacement, is relatively infrequent in MCP joint arthroplasty. Despite these complications, MCP arthroplasty has proved to be an effective, predictable, and long-lasting procedure with high patient satisfaction.

Swanson AB, de Groot Swanson G: Flexible implant resection arthroplasty. In Strickland JW (ed): Master Techniques in Orthopaedic Surgery: The Hand. Philadelphia, Lippincott-Raven, 1998.

UNUSUAL ARTHRITIS DISORDERS

15. What characteristic manifestations are found in the hands of patients with systemic lupus erythematosus (SLE)?

SLE is a connective tissue disorder that occurs primarily in young adult women. A common clinical feature of SLE is polyarthritis, usually in the small bones of the hands and feet. Ligamentous laxity with subsequent instability of the distal radioulnar joint, intercarpal joints, MCP joints, and all three thumbs is a distinctive feature of the disease. Raynaud's phenomena may also exist in up to 50% of patients.

16. What is Jaccoud's syndrome?

Jaccoud's syndrome, a classic condition associated with SLE, involves flexion deformities and ulnar deviation of the MCP joints and swan-neck deformities of the digits. As is typical of SLE, the major problem is soft-tissue attenuation with resultant ligamentous laxity. In this particular syndrome the involved tissue includes the radial portion of the dorsal capsular hood of the MCP joint with ulnar subluxation of the extensor digitorum communis tendons and hyperextension of the PIP joints. The resultant deformity may appear quite similar to that seen in rheumatoid arthritis; radiographs, however, usually reveal preservation of the joint space, which is consistent with the nonerosive synovitis of SLE.

17. What are the typical manifestations of psoriatic arthritis?

Approximately 5% of patients with psoriasis develop arthritis that involves mainly the small bones of the hand and feet. Patients classically present with diffuse swelling throughout an entire digit, which is termed a "sausage digit." Joint involvement is most frequent at the DIP and PIP levels. Erosive articular destruction is common and results in pencil and cup deformities of the joints, which may be seen radiographically. Progressive distal phalangeal osteolysis with tuft resorption is also highly suggestive of psoriatic arthropathy. Spontaneous fusion of the DIP joint and intercarpal joints is also common. The severity of joint destruction often parallels the degree of accompanying fingernail deformities, which include pitting, ridging, thickening, and detachment of the nail.

BIBLIOGRAPHY

1. Azar FM: Arthrodesis of shoulder, elbow, and wrist. In Canale ST (ed): Campbell's Operative Orthopaedics, 9th ed. St. Louis, Mosby, 1998, pp 203–206.
2. Beer TA, Turner RH: Wrist arthrodesis for failed wrist implant arthroplasty. J Hand Surg 22A:685–693, 1997.
3. Gelberman RH: The Wrist: Total Wrist Arthroplasty. New York, Raven Press, 1994, pp 253–278.
4. Green DP: Operative Hand Surgery, 2nd ed. New York, Churchill Livingstone, 1993.
5. Knirk JL, Jupiter JB: Intra-articular fractures of the distal end of the radius in young adults. J Bone Joint Surg 68A:647–658, 1986.
6. Lins RE, Gelberman RH, McKeown L, et al: Basal joint arthritis: Trapeziectomy with ligament reconstruction and tendon interposition arthroplasty. J Hand Surgery 21A:202–209, 1996.
7. Swanson AB, deGroot Swanson G: Flexible implant resection arthroplasty. In Strickland JW (ed): Master Techniques in Orthopaedic Surgery: The Hand. Philadelphia, Lippincott-Raven, 1998, pp 421–438.

43. ARTHRODESIS OF THE HAND AND WRIST

Ian D. Crabb, M.D.

1. What two main symptoms may lead a clinician to consider wrist arthrodesis?

Severe wrist pain or carpal instability/subluxation are the indications for wrist arthrodesis. Numerous etiologies may lead to such symptoms. The most common is a ligamentous or bony injury to the wrist that leads to subsequent degenerative arthritis. The arthritis often begins in the radioscaphoid articulation and ultimately progresses to carpal arthritis. Other etiologies of a painful, unstable wrist include infection, inflammatory arthritis (such as rheumatoid arthritis), or after tumor resection.

2. When is wrist fusion more appropriate than performing an arthroplasty?

The need for wrist stability and strength often outweighs the need for range of motion in the wrist. Complete wrist fusion is a reliable, durable, and functional solution to end-stage wrist arthritis. In contrast, wrist arthroplasties have many complications and are rarely recommended in a high-demand hand.

3. What is the optimal position for wrist fusion?

The optimal position for wrist fusion is continually debated. Clearly some tasks are better served with extension and some with flexion. Perineal care is aided by slight wrist flexion, whereas grip strength is better in extension. In practice, a neutral flexion extension and slight ulnar deviation is best.

4. Name the two main complications of wrist arthrodesis.

The main complications of wrist arthrodesis are nonunion and delayed union.

5. Can patients return to work after wrist arthrodesis?

Successful wrist arthrodesis yields a stable and pain-free arm. Most patients can return to even heavy work. The impairment rating for a wrist arthrodesis in $0°$ of flexion and $0°$ radioulnar deviation is 30% of the upper extremity or 18% of the whole person.

6. Define limited carpal arthrodesis.

The definition of a limited carpal arthrodesis is fusion between one or several carpal bones. Many combinations are used.

7. When should a limited wrist arthrodesis be considered?

Limited wrist arthrodesis is best used for localized carpal arthritis. Limited arthrodeses also may be used to treat instability patterns of the wrist that are not amenable to soft tissue reconstruction. By their nature, limited wrist arthrodeses shift stresses from one articulation to another. Load shifting may lead to accelerated degeneration of the more stressed joint.

8. Discuss the advantages and disadvantages of limited carpal arthrodesis.

The main advantage of a limited carpal arthrodesis is the ability to retain some wrist motion. The average postoperative range is approximately one-half of the normal range of motion. The ability to retain some motion is of significant psychological benefit to patients contemplating this type of surgery. The main disadvantage of limited carpal arthrodesis is that the full force of carpal loading is transmitted over a smaller surface area, which leads to increased pressure and the potential for cartilage wear and failure.

9. Describe the common sequence of radiocarpal degenerative arthritis.

The common sequence of arthritis at the radiocarpal joint begins with an instability pattern, which develops between the scaphoid and the lunate after disruption of the scapholunate ligament. Because of the abnormal rotation of the scaphoid, the radioscaphoid articulation will then develop into degenerative arthritis with wear of the articular cartilage, swelling, and pain. Mechanical instability and collapse may persist for years before painful arthritis ensues.

10. How is the common pattern described in question nine used in planning limited carpal arthrodesis?

The pattern of radiocarpal degeneration tends to exclude the radiolunate articulation until very late in the disease. The articulation can thus be used as a base for a limited carpal fusion. The most commonly used arthrodesis currently is the four-corner arthrodesis, in which the lunate capitellum triquetrum and hamate are fused and the scaphoid is excised.

11. What is a four-corner fusion?

A four-corner fusion involves the lunate, capitate, triquetrum, and hamate.

12. What is a triscaphe fusion?

Triscaphe fusion is the fusion of the scaphoid, trapezius, and trapezoid.

13. When is arthrodesis considered in the fingers?

The primary indication for arthrodesis in the finger joints is pain. As a practical matter, arthrodesis in any one of the finger joints causes significant functional morbidity and is a procedure of last resort.

14. Which finger joints are most amenable to fusion?

Fusion of the distal interphalangeal (DIP) joint causes the least functional disability. Fusion of the proximal interphalangeal (PIP) joints and the metacarpophalangeal (MCP) joints causes significant functional disability. The one exception is the thumb MCP joint, which in most people can be fused with very little residual morbidity.

15. How does one choose between arthroplasty or fusion in the hand?

As a general rule, you would fuse the DIP joints, fuse the index and middle PIP joints if absolutely necessary, and may consider arthroplasty for the small and ring finger PIP joints. Arthroplasty may be considered for the MCP joints, with the exception of the thumb.

16. What are the complications of finger arthrodesis?

• Nonunion
• Delayed union
• Malunion with a rotational or angular deformity

17. Which thumb joint can be fused with little consequence for overall function?

The MCP joint of the thumb can be fused with little affect on grip strength or mobility of the hand.

18. What are the indications for thumb carpometacarpal (CMC) joint fusions?

A thumb CMC joint fusion may be considered in a younger patient or one who is involved in heavy labor. The thumb CMC joint is a critical joint that allows the thumb to move from the plane of the palm to a position of opposition. Many arthritic conditions in the CMC joint are handled by a ligament reconstruction and arthroplasty of the basal joint. Young or very active patients are candidates for fusion. The advantage of fusion is that it is durable and gives reasonably good function. The limitation of the thumb CMC fusion is the inability to fully flatten the hand to reach into small spaces or pockets.

BIBLIOGRAPHY

1. American Medical Association: Guides to the Evaluation of Permanent Impairment, 4th ed. Chicago, June 1993.
2. Beer TA, Turner RH: Wrist arthrodesis for failed wrist implant arthroplasty. J Hand Surg (Am) 20:965–970, 1995.
3. Jones BF, Stern PF: Interphalangeal joint arthrodesis. Hand Clin 10:267–275, 1994.
4. Kuschner SH, Lane CS: Surgical treatment for osteoarthritis at the base of the thumb. Am J Orthop 25:91–100, 1996.
5. Larsen CF, Jacoby RA, McCabe SJ: Nonunion rates of limited carpal arthrodesis: A meta-analysis of the literature. J Hand Surg (Am) 22:66–73, 1997.
6. Leibovic SJ: Internal fixation for small joint arthrodesis in the hand. The interphalangeal joints. Hand Clin 13:601–613, 1997.
7. Lee DH, Carroll RE: Wrist arthrodesis: A combined intramedullary pin and autogenous iliac crest bone graft technique. J Hand Surg (Am) 19:733–740, 1994.
8. Mih AD: Limited wrist fusion. Hand Clin 13:615–625, 1997.
9. Pellegrini VD, Burton RI: Osteoarthritis of the proximal interphalangeal joint of the hand: Arthroplasty or fusion? J Hand Surg (Am) 15:194–209, 1990.
10. Weiss AP, Hastings H: Wrist arthrodesis for traumatic conditions: A study of plate and local bone graft application. J Hand Surg (Am) 20:50–56, 1995.
11. Wyrick JD, Stern PJ, Kiefhaber TR: Motion-preserving procedures in the treatment of scapholunate advanced collapse wrist: Proximal row carpectomy versus four-corner arthrodesis. J Hand Surg (Am) 20:965–970, 1995.
12. Zachary SV, Stern PJ: Complications following AO/ASIF wrist arthrodesis. J Hand Surg (Am) 20:339–344, 1995.

44. KIENBÖCK'S DISEASE

Gregory G. Degnan, M.D., Atul B. Joshi, M.D., and David M. Lichtman, M.D.

1. Describe the pathologic changes in Kienböck's disease.
The pathologic changes in the lunate are due to avascular necrosis. Decreased lunate vascularity, fragmentation, and osseous necrosis are consistent histologic findings.

2. What causes Kienböck's disease?
The exact cause is unknown. It is thought to be due to repeated stress or an acute fracture that leads to interruption of blood supply in a susceptible or "at-risk" lunate.

3. What is the role of trauma in the etiology of Kienböck's disease?
Numerous authors, including Kienböck himself, have implicated trauma or acute fracture as a cause of the avascular necrosis (AVN). Some series have reported an incidence of fracture lines in the lunate as high as 82%. It is not clear, however, whether the fractures are the cause or the result of AVN.

White and Omer pointed out that classic AVN of the lunate is rare after fracture/dislocation or dislocation of the carpus. Their series of cases demonstrated transient vascular ischemia of the lunate after such injuries, along with radiographic density of the lunate consistent with Kienböck's disease. The clinical course, however, was resolution rather than progression.

4. Discuss the three basic patterns of extraosseous blood supply to the lunate.
In his cadaver experiments Lee noted three predictable patterns of extraosseous blood supply:
1. A single volar or dorsal vessel supplying the entire bone;
2. Several vessels, volar and dorsal, without central anastomosis;
3. Several vessels, volar and dorsal, with central anastomosis.

Lee theorized that patients with patterns 1 and 2 are at greater risk for developing Kienböck's disease.

5. Discuss the three basic patterns of intraosseous blood supply to the lunate.
Gelberman found three basic patterns of intraosseous blood supply:
1. Y pattern in 59%;
2. I pattern in 31%;
3. X pattern in 10%.

His study revealed that the least vascular zone was in the proximal subchondral area adjacent to the radial articular surface, where subchondral fractures and early collapse are most commonly noted.

6. What is the incidence and effect of ulnar variance on predisposition for the development of Kienböck's disease?
Hulten reported a 78% incidence of short ulna (ulnar minus variant) in his patients with Kienböck's disease compared with an incidence of 23% in the normal population. Numerous authors subsequently confirmed the increased incidence of ulnar minor variance. In Japan, however, ulnar positive variance is equally common in the normal population. Recently in the Netherlands, D'Hoore showed an insignificant difference in ulnar variance between people with normal wrists and those with Kienböck's disease.

7. How does ulnar variance predispose to Kienböck's disease?
A short ulna causes increased shear forces on the lunate, predisposing it to injury with repetitive stress. Originally a theory, this has been confirmed by laboratory studies.

8. What radiographic view is required to define the true degree of ulnar variance? Describe how the patient is positioned.

The neutral position posteroanterior (PA) view is the standard view used to determine variance. The patient is positioned so that the shoulder is abducted 90°, the elbow is flexed 90°, and the palm of the hand is placed flat on the cassette.

9. Describe the lunate at risk for Kienböck's disease.
- Lunates with a single extraosseous nutrient vessel
- Lunates with poor intraosseous vascular anastomoses
- Lunates subject to increased shear stress (e.g., negative ulnar variance)

10. What are the criteria for diagnosing Kienböck's disease?

Kienböck's disease is a radiographic diagnosis based on characteristic radiographic density changes in the lunate. Increased density is later followed by fracture lines, fragmentation, and collapse. Kienböck's disease should be included in the differential diagnosis of any chronic wrist pain.

11. Describe the radiographic findings in stage I Kienböck's disease.

Radiographs are normal except for the possibility of a linear or compression fracture of the lunate. Bone scan shows increased uptake around the lunate; magnetic resonance imaging (MRI) shows loss of signal intensity on T1-weighted images.

Stage I Kienböck's disease.

12. Describe the radiographic findings in stage II Kienböck's disease.

Stage II is characterized by a definite increase in the density of the lunate relative to the other carpal bones (see figure, top left of next page). Late in stage II there may be some loss of height on the radial side of the lunate.

13. Describe the radiographic findings in stage III Kienböck's disease.

Stage III is a transitional stage in which the disease begins to affect the carpal structure. Radiographs show collapse of the lunate in the frontal plane and elongation in the sagittal plane. The capitate shows proximal migration. Scaphoid foreshortening and scapholunate dissociation may or may not be present. (See figure, top right of next page.)

14. Describe the radiographic findings in stage IV Kienböck's disease.

All of the radiographic findings of stage III are present along with generalized carpal degenerative arthritis.

Stage III Kienböck's disease.

Stage II Kienböck's disease.

15. What is the difference between stages IIIA and IIIB Kienböck's disease?

Stage IIIA is characterized by lunate collapse without fixed scaphoid rotation. In stage IIIB lunate collapse is accompanied by fixed scaphoid rotation and other secondary carpal derangements.

16. How is the carpal height ratio measured? What is its significance?

The carpal height ratio, as described by Youm, is a measure of the degree of collapse of the wrist related to lunate collapse and proximal migration of the capitate. Carpal height is the distance between the distal articular surface of the third metacarpal and the distal radial articular surface. The carpal height ratio is defined as the carpal height divided by the length of the third metacarpal. The normal value is 0.54 ± 0.03.

17. What is the treatment of stage I Kienböck's disease?

For newly diagnosed cases, immobilization is the treatment of choice. Some authors apply an external fixator to relieve compression across the lunate. If symptoms persist after 2–3 months of immobilization, it is probably best to proceed with treatment as in stage II or IIIa.

18. Discuss the treatment options for stage II Kienböck's disease.

For stage II with ulnar minus variance, an equalization procedure decreases shear and compressive forces across the lunate and allows possible revascularization. Radial shortening is currently the most popular method, but excellent results also have been reported with ulnar shortening. **For stage II with ulnar positive or neutral variance,** a lunate revascularization procedure is indicated. Popular methods of revascularization include vascular pedicle bone graft and direct implantation of a dorsal metacarpal vessel.

19. Discuss the treatment options for stage IIIA Kienböck's disease.

For **stage IIIA with ulnar minus variance,** an equalization procedure is still acceptable, although some authors recommend limited intercarpal fusion across the midcarpal row. For **stage**

IIIA with an ulnar positive or neutral variance, revascularization of the lunate is indicated, although some authors again recommend limited intercarpal arthrodesis.

20. Discuss the treatment options for stage IIIB Kienböck's disease.

For stage IIIB disease, limited intercarpal arthrodesis is indicated to restore carpal stability and to prevent further degeneration. Triscaphe fusion is preferred, although scaphocapitate and scaphocapitolunate fusion accomplishes the same objectives. In addition, if significant synovitis and local fragmentation is present, excision of the lunate is recommended.

21. Discuss the treatment options for stage IV Kienböck's disease.

For stage IV disease salvage operations are indicated. Good results have been reported with both proximal row carpectomy and wrist arthrodesis. The choice of procedure depends on the needs of the patient and the integrity of the articular surfaces of the lunate fossa and the capitate.

22. What is the role of silicone replacement arthroplasty in the treatment of Kienböck's disease?

Once a widely used procedure, silicone lunate replacement arthroplasty has been abandoned; particulate synovitis has been described in many recipients because of stress erosion of the implant.

CONTROVERSIES

23. Should Kienböck's disease be treated conservatively or aggressively?

The precise pathogenesis and natural history of Kienböck's disease are still undetermined. It is possible for progression of the disease to arrest at any stage and for revascularization to occur spontaneously. Some authors, therefore, recommend a nonoperative approach, using cast immobilization to treat symptomatic stages. Most cases, however, continue to progress over time and result in carpal instability and arthritis. We recommend a more aggressive approach, basing our treatment plan on the stage of the disease and ulnar variance.

24. What is the role of venous congestion in the etiology of Kienböck's disease?

In a recent study, the intraosseous venous pressure in Kienböck's disease was significantly higher than in the normal lunate. If venous pressure is higher than the arterial inflow pressure, ischemia will result. Therefore, venous anomalies may represent another form of an at-risk lunate.

25. What is the role of wrist arthroscopy in the management of Kienböck's disease?

The exact role of arthroscopy in Kienböck's disease is still not defined. However, it does provide direct visualization of the lunate surface and surrounding ligaments. A yellowish discoloration as well as detachment of the cartilaginous surface has been identified. Such findings may aid in diagnosis and surgical decision-making.

26. What is the appropriate role of revascularization procedures?

The positive results following most types of revascularization procedures are based on empirical observation rather than laboratory evidence. Clinical studies have not been well controlled. Some authors, therefore, prefer equalization or intercarpal arthrodesis for stage II or III disease, regardless of the ulnar variance.

27. What is the appropriate role of external fixation?

Some authors believe that the application of an external fixator decompresses the lunate and enhances revascularization, especially when combined with a revascularization procedure. This concept must be tested by long-term follow-up of a sufficient number of cases before it can be universally recommended.

28. What are the surgical treatment options for Kienböck's disease in a patient with ulnar neutral or positive variance?

In Japan, where many cases of Kienböck's disease have ulnar positive variance, opening- or closing-wedge osteotomies have become popular. Recent evidence has shown that capitate shortening (Almquist procedure) can also effectively decrease shear stress across the lunate.

BIBLIOGRAPHY

1. Almquist EE: Capitate shortening in the treatment of Kienböck's disease. Hand Clin 9:505–512, 1983.
2. Armistead RB, Linscheid RL, Dobyns JH, et al: Ulnar lengthening in the treatment of Kienböck's disease. J Bone Joint Surg 64A:170–178, 1982.
3. Beckenbough RD, Shives TC, Dobyns JH, et al: Kienböck's disease: The natural history of Kienböck's disease and consideration of lunate fractures. Clin Orthop 149:98–106, 1980.
4. D'Hoore K, De smet L, Verellen K, et al: Negative ulnar variance is not a risk for Kienböck's disease. J Hand Surg (Am) 19:229–231, 1994.
5. Gelberman RH, Bauman TD, Menon J, et al: The vascularity of the lunate bone and Kienböck's disease. J Hand Surg 5A:272–278, 1980.
6. Gelberman RH, Salamon PB, Jurist JM, et al: Ulnar variance in Kienböck's disease. J Bone Joint Surg 57A:674–676, 1975.
7. Gelberman RH, Szabo RM: Kienböck's disease. Orthop Clin North Am 15:355–367, 1984.
8. Hori Y, Tomai S, Okuda H, et al: Blood vessel transplantation to bone. J Hand Surg 4A:23–33, 1979.
9. Lichtman DM, Alexander AH: The Wrist and its Disorders, 2nd ed. Philadelphia, W.B. Saunders, 1997.
10. Lichtman DM, Alexander AH, Mack GR, et al: Kienböck's disease: Update on silicone replacement arthroplasty. J Hand Surg 7A:343–347, 1982.
11. Lichtman DM, Degnan GG: Staging and its use in the determination of treatment modalities for arthroplasty. Hand Clin 9:409–416, 1993.
12. Lichtman DM, Mack GR, MacDonald RT, et al: Kienböck's disease: The role of silicone replacement arthroplasty. J Bone Joint Surg 59A:899–908, 1977.
13. Miura H, Sugioka Y: Radial closing osteotomy for Kienböck's disease. J Hand Surg (Br) 21:1029–1034, 1996.
14. Palmer AK, Glisson RR, Werner FW: Ulnar variance determination. J Hand Surg 7A:376–379, 1982.
15. Schiltenwolf M, Martini AK, Mau HC, et al: Further investigation of the intraosseous pressure characteristics in necrotic lunates (Kienböck's disease). J Hand Surg (Am) 21:754–758, 1996.
16. Sheetz KK, Bishop AT, Berger RA: The arterial blood supply of the distal radius and ulna and its potential use in vascularized pedicle bone graft. J Hand Surg (Am) 20:902–914, 1995.
17. Sundberg SB, Linscheid RL: Kienböck's disease—Results of treatment with ulnar lengthening. Clin Orthop 187:43–51, 1984.
18. Trail IA, Linschid RL, Quenzer DE, Scherer PA: Ulnar lengthening and radial recession procedures for Kienböck's disease. Long term clinical and radiographic follow-up. J Hand Surg (Br) 21:169–176, 1996.
19. Viola RW, Kiser PK, Bach AW, et al: Biomechanical analysis of capitate hamate fusion in the treatment of Kienböck's disease. J Hand Surg (Am) 23:395–401, 1998.
20. Watson HK, Ryu J, DiBella A: An approach to Kienböck's disease: Triscaphe arthrodesis. J Hand Surg 10A:179–187, 1985.
21. Weiss AC, Weiland A, Moore JR, et al: Radial shortening for Kienböck's disease. J Bone Joint Surg 73A:384–391, 1991.

45. NERVE ENTRAPMENTS OF HAND AND WRIST

Jeffrey J. Tiedeman, M.D.

1. What is the most commonly encountered compressive neuropathy of the upper extremity? In whom does it occur?

The most common compressive neuropathy of the upper extremity is carpal tunnel syndrome (CTS) or median nerve compression at the wrist. The carpal tunnel is a narrow, fibroosseous canal rigidly bound by the carpal bones and roofed by the transverse carpal ligament, containing the median nerve and the nine extrinsic flexors of the fingers and thumb with their synovial sheath. CTS is most commonly encountered during middle or advanced age; > 80% of patients are more than 40 years of age at the time of diagnosis. It is twice as frequent in women.

2. What are the most common causes of CTS?

Median nerve compression may occur with decreased canal size or increased volume of the contents in the canal. Consequently, a multitude of clinical entities can give rise to the condition. Nonspecific tenosynovial proliferation in otherwise healthy individuals is the most common cause of increased canal contents. The mnemonic **PRAGMATIC** can be used to remember the other common causes of CTS:

P = **P**regnancy
R = **R**heumatoid arthritis
A = **A**rthritis (degenerative)
G = **G**rowth hormone abnormalities (acromegaly)
M = **M**etabolic (hypothyroidism, gout, diabetes mellitus)
A = **A**lcoholism
T = **T**umors
I = **I**diopathic
C = **C**onnective tissue disorders (amyloidosis, hemochromatosis)

3. What are the most common symptoms associated with CTS?

The median nerve is responsible for sensory innervation of the thumb and index and long fingers as well as the radial border of the ring finger. It also supplies the thenar musculature at the base of the thumb and the two radial lumbrical muscles. The most frequent complaint is numbness, which typically involves the fingers innervated by the median nerve. Patients also may complain of numbness and tingling in the entire hand. Pain also may occur over the same distribution or more proximally in the forearm as the result of median nerve compression in the carpal tunnel. Nocturnal symptoms are common and frequently awaken patients from sleep. Clumsiness or lack of dexterity with the hand is a frequent complaint because of sensory loss or weakness of the thenar musculature.

4. Name the provocative tests used to substantiate the diagnosis of CTS.

A median nerve percussion test is performed by percussion with a finger or reflex hammer over the median nerve in the wrist or palm. A positive test produces paresthesias in the median nerve distribution (Tinel's sign). Phalen's test is performed with the wrist in full, unforced flexion, which is achieved by putting the dorsum of one hand against the dorsum of the other while the fingers are held dependent. This position increases carpal canal pressures and decreases local median nerve blood flow. A positive test produces paresthesias or sensory disturbances mimicking the patient's symptoms within 60 seconds.

5. What other diagnostic studies should be performed when evaluating a patient for CTS?

Laboratory studies should be obtained to screen for diabetes mellitus, gout, and renal, thyroid, and collagen vascular diseases. Radiographs of the wrist should be obtained to document a fracture, tumor, or arthritis as a possible cause of median nerve compression. Finally, electrodiagnostic studies are the most sensitive and objective tests for the diagnosis of CTS. They always should be obtained before surgical treatment of CTS to corroborate the diagnosis, to rule out other disorders, and to provide baseline nerve function data. Up to 10% of patients with clinically evident CTS, however, produce normal electrodiagnostic studies.

6. Describe the most common complications resulting from carpal tunnel release.

The results from surgical decompression of the median nerve at the carpal tunnel are reliably good. The complication rate is low, ranging from 2–15%. Complications include incomplete release of the transverse carpal ligament, injury to the palmar cutaneous branch or recurrent motor branch of the median nerve, reflex sympathetic dystrophy, finger stiffness, decreased strength, and persistent tenderness in the palmar scar.

7. What is Guyon's canal?

Guyon's canal is a fibroosseous tunnel bound by the hamate and pisiform. The roof is the transverse carpal ligament. The ulnar artery and nerve pass through Guyon's canal. Unlike the carpal tunnel, no tendons pass through Guyon's canal.

8. What causes compressive neuropathies in Guyon's canal?

(1) Trauma, (2) ganglia, (3) lipomas, and (4) fractures of the hamate or pisiform. The most common traumatic mechanism is pressure from bicycling. Sensory neuropathy is usually from a distal canal lesion, whereas motor weakness is from a lesion proximal to or within the canal.

9. What is bowler's thumb?

Bowler's thumb is a traumatic neuropathy of the ulnar digital nerve to the thumb. It is due to repeated friction or compression of the nerve by the edge of the thumb hole at the bowling ball. Early ball adjustment is necessary. The size, fit, spacing, and angulation of the holes should be altered. On rare occasions, transposition or neurolysis is required for relief of severe symptoms.

Digital compression neuropathy also may occur in racquet sports (pressure on the thumb ulnar digital nerve from the grip) or handball (direct compression from the ball strike). Digital nerve compressions will usually occur where the nerve passes near a sesamoid bone.

10. Can posterior interosseous nerve (PIN) compression occur at the wrist?

Yes. Repeated forceful wrist dorsiflexion (such as in gymnastics) may irritate the PIN. The diagnosis is one of exclusion. Carpal instability, ganglia, and dorsal osteophytes must be excluded. Rest, splinting, and NSAIDs should alleviate the symptoms.

11. How does palmar cutaneous nerve compression occur?

Blunt trauma results in transient neurapraxia. Patients have pain over the thenar eminence and may have a Tinel's sign at the proximal edge of the transverse carpal ligament. Conservative treatment usually suffices.

12. What is double crush syndrome?

Simultaneous compression of a peripheral nerve at more than one location is referred to as double crush syndrome. In fact, a compressive lesion at one point on a peripheral nerve will lower the threshold for occurrence of compression neuropathy at another location (distal or proximal) on the same nerve. For instance, less compression of the median nerve is necessary at the carpal tunnel level to produce symptoms when coexistent cervical nerve root compression is present.

BIBLIOGRAPHY

1. Carr D, Davis P: Distal posterior interosseous nerve syndrome. J Hand Surg 10A:873, 1985.
2. Dobyns JH, O'Brien ET, Linscheid RC, et al: Bowler's thumb: Diagnosis and treatment. A review of seventeen cases. J Bone Joint Surg 54A:751, 1972.
3. Eversman WW: Compression and entrapment neuropathies of the upper extremity. J Hand Surg 8:759, 1983.
4. Glowacki KA, Breen CJ, Sachar K, et al: Electrodiagnostic testing and carpal tunnel release outcome. J Hand Surg 21A:117–122, 1996.
5. Gonzalez del Pino J, Delgado-Martinez AD, Gonzalez Gonzalez I, et al: Value of the carpal compression test in the diagnosis of carpal tunnel syndrome. J Hand Surg [Br] 22:38–41, 1997.
6. Szabo RM, Steinberg DR: Nerve entrapment syndromes in the wrist. J Am Acad Orthop Surg 2:115–123, 1994.
7. Watchmaker GP, Weber D, Mackinnon SE: Avoidance of transection of the palmar cutaneous branch of the median nerve in carpal tunnel release. J Hand Surg 21A:644–650, 1996.

46. TENOSYNOVITIS OF THE HAND, WRIST, AND FOREARM

Julian S. Arroyo, M.D.

1. How many dorsal compartments are found at the wrist? What do they contain?

The six dorsal compartments at the wrist contain the extensor tendons to the wrist and fingers and the abductors to the thumb.

2. Name the tendons in each dorsal compartment.

1st: Abductor pollicis longus	4th: Extensor digitorum
Extensor pollicis brevis	Extensor indicis
2nd: Extensor carpi radialis longus and brevis	5th: Extensor digiti minimi
3rd: Extensor pollicis longus	6th: Extensor carpi ulnaris

One way to remember the number of tendons in each compartment is to remember the sequence 2-2-1-2-1-1.

3. What is de Quervain's disease?

De Quervain's disease is stenosing tenosynovitis of the first dorsal compartment at the wrist. It is most commonly seen in women between 30 and 50 years of age.

4. What are the chief complaints in de Quervain's disease?

Most patients complain of pain and tenderness localized to the radial aspect of the wrist. The pain is worsened with thumb movement because the thumb extensor and abductor travel in this compartment.

5. What is the differential diagnosis for de Quervain's disease?

Arthritis of the first carpometacarpal joint may mimic de Quervain's disease. It can be differentiated by radiographs and physical exam, with a positive grind test. The two lesions, however, commonly coexist. Another possibility is a **scaphoid fracture or arthrosis** involving the radiocarpal or intercarpal joints. Finally, **intersection syndrome** may resemble de Quervain's disease.

6. What are the causes of de Quervain's disease?

The most common cause is an overuse injury of the wrist and hand. The disorder is also seen in patients with inflammatory arthritis.

In some patients the first dorsal compartment is subdivided by a septum, with the extensor pollicis brevis on the ulnar side. This phenomenon has been seen in 20–30% of reported cases. Some patients also have an anomalous tendon in a third tunnel. These septi cause stenosis and are thought to be a cause of de Quervain's disease.

7. What is the treatment of de Quervain's disease?

Nonoperative therapy consists of rest, thumb and wrist immobilization, local steroid injections, and systemic antiinflammatories. If this regimen fails, surgical release of the compartment is recommended.

8. Which nerve and artery are at risk during surgical release of the first dorsal compartment?

The superficial sensory branch of the radial nerve has two or three terminal divisions that are located directly over the first dorsal compartment. Transection of these nerves may lead to a painful neuroma. The radial artery is also at risk, because it passes through the anatomic snuff box.

9. What is intersection syndrome?

Tenosynovitis of the second dorsal compartment.

10. What are the symptoms of intersection syndrome?

The most common symptoms are pain and swelling approximately 4 cm above the wrist as the extensor pollicis brevis and abductor pollicis longus cross or intersect the extensor carpi radialis longus and brevis. In severe cases, there may be audible crepitus.

11. What is the cause of intersection syndrome?

Intersection syndrome is frequently associated with repetitive use of the wrist.

12. What is the treatment of intersection syndrome?

Nonoperative therapy consists of rest, work modification, and local steroid injections. The vast majority of cases respond to nonoperative treatment, but occasionally the second dorsal compartment requires surgical release.

13. What are the symptoms of stenosing tenosynovitis of the flexor tendons (trigger finger)?

Patients complain of catching or triggering of the finger with locking in flexion. They often complain of pain at the proximal interphalangeal (PIP) joint, but the lesion occurs at the metacarpophalangeal (MCP) joint. Often there is a palpable nodule on the flexor tendon proximal to the MCP joint. Most commonly the ring and middle fingers are affected, but any digit may be involved.

14. Where is the anatomic lesion that causes trigger finger?

The fingers have four annular (A-1–A-4) and three cruciform (C-1–C-3) pulleys in the fingers that prevent the flexors from bowstringing. The A-1 pulley becomes thickened and narrowed from chronic inflammation and entraps the flexor tendon. A reactive nodular fusiform enlargement of the tendon sheath may compound the entrapment.

15. What other problems caused by stenosing tenosynovitis of the hand are commonly seen with trigger finger?

De Quervain's disease and carpal tunnel syndrome are two other hand problems that are caused by stenosing tenosynovitis and that frequently coexist with trigger finger.

16. In what age group is trigger finger most common?

Two age groups are commonly affected: middle-aged women and neonates. Of congenital trigger fingers, 25% are noted at birth. The condition may present as late as 2 years of age. Unlike the adult type, congenital trigger finger presents with a persistent flexion deformity without triggering. Spontaneous resolution occurs in approximately 30% of cases that present in the first year of life.

17. What is the treatment for trigger finger?

Nonoperative treatment consists of splinting and local injection of steroids into the flexor sheath. Surgical treatment simply involves incising the A-1 pulley. Care must be taken to avoid cutting the A-2 pulley. Studies have shown that the A-2 pulley, attached to the proximal phalanx, and the A-4 pulley, attached to the middle phalanx, are the most important pulleys for prevention of bowstringing.

18. How does the treatment of stenosing tenosynovitis differ in rheumatoid patients?

In rheumatoid patients the surgeon should preserve the A-1 pulley to prevent bowstringing and ulnar drift. Therefore, the tendon sheath is explored with removal of any nodules within the flexor tendons. A complete tenosynovectomy is performed. Some authors suggest removing one arm of the sublimis tendon to create room for the flexor as they pass through the pulleys. This method is not universally accepted.

BIBLIOGRAPHY

1. Canale ST (ed): Campbell's Operative Orthopaedics, 9th ed. St. Louis, Mosby, 1998.
2. Green DP (ed): Operative Hand Surgery, 3rd ed. New York, Churchill Livingstone, 1993, pp 2217–2134.

47. PEDIATRIC HAND AND WRIST

Keith R. Gabriel, M.D.

1. Define polydactyly, macrodactyly, and syndactyly.

Polydactyly is duplication of one or more digits. Macrodactyly is an enlarged digit. Syndactyly is fusion of digits.

2. Is there a racial predilection for postaxial (ulnar-side) polydactyly?

Yes. Duplication of the small finger is 10 times more common in African-Americans than in Caucasians. Postaxial polydactyly in Caucasians may indicate serious associated abnormalities.

3. Is there a similar racial predilection for preaxial (thumb) polydactyly?

The incidence is similar in African-Americans and Caucasians but slightly higher in Asians and Native Americans.

4. Does a significant association between preaxial polydactyly and other congenital disorders exist?

Although syndactyly may occur, most duplicated thumbs present as an isolated anomaly and do not demonstrate the same frequency of serious associated abnormalities as postaxial polydactyly in whites.

5. In central polydactyly, which finger is most commonly duplicated?

The ring finger is commonly duplicated. Duplication of the index finger is rare.

6. When a duplicate digit is represented only by a skin tag, simple ligation in the nursery is sometimes advocated. What are the possible serious sequelae?

There are reports of infants who have bled to death.

7. How common is macrodactyly?

Macrodactyly is one of the rarest congenital malformations of the upper extremity. It is usually caused by conditions such as neurofibromatosis, Proteus syndrome, lymphangioma, or arteriovenous malformation.

8. An infant presents with absence of one thumb. The index finger is short, and the entire hand deviates toward the radial side of the forearm. The distal end of the ulna is quite prominent. What is the likely diagnosis?

The likely diagnosis is radial club hand. The degree of radial deficiency and the resulting appearance and function are quite variable.

9. How is the stethoscope helpful in evaluating the patient with a radial deficiency?

Radial defects are frequently associated with cardiovascular defects. Gastrointestinal (GI) and genitourinary systems must be carefully evaluated. Aplastic (Fanconi) anemia and platelet defects also should be considered.

10. What interventions are usually recommended for the initial treatment of radial club hand?

Initial treatment usually consists of passive stretching and splinting of the wrist and hand toward a central or even ulnarly deviated position.

11. An infant presents with absence of the small finger, ulnar deviation of the hand and wrists, and a shortened forearm that is bowed toward the ulnar side. What are the major differences between this entity and radial club hand?

Ulnar club hand is less common (reported ratios range form 1:4 to 1:10) than radial club hand. The expression in the limb is even more variable and may include absence of radial rays, limitation of elbow motion, and humeral shortening. Associated anomalies are usually restricted to the musculoskeletal system.

12. Central deficiency of the hand (cleft hand) may be associated with what other cleft deficiencies?

Cleft hand is usually bilateral. Frequent associations are cleft foot, cleft lip, and cleft palate. Noncleft anomalies often are seen in the cardiac and GI systems.

13. How does a trigger digit in the infant differ from a trigger digit in the adult?

In the infant the thumb is more commonly involved, the condition is frequently bilateral, and the presentation is likely to be fixed-flexion posture rather than clicking or "triggering."

14. What is the management of trigger thumb in the infant (> 1 year of age)?

Initial treatment consists of splinting in extension. Perhaps 30% of cases resolve without surgery. After 1 year of age, most thumbs require surgical release.

15. What is the difference between camptodactyly and clinodactyly?

Strictly speaking, both terms mean "bent finger." Both conditions usually occur in the small finger. Camptodactyly is angulation in the anteroposterior plane; that is, a flexion contracture. Clinodactyly is angulation in a radioulnar direction.

16. In what age groups does camptodactyly usually present?

Camptodactyly usually presents in infancy or adolescence.

17. Mild clinodactyly is common in normal children. Marked clinodactyly is associated with what condition?

Mental retardation.

18. The nursery discharge note says the infant has a simple, incomplete syndactyly between the ring and long fingers. Describe the deformity.

A web of skin joins the fingers (simple), extending from the commissure but not reaching the fingertips (incomplete). In most cases the web extends to the middle of the proximal phalanx.

19. Describe a complex, complete syndactyly.

"Complex" indicates that the bones of the adjacent fingers are fused together. "Complete" means that the syndactyly extends to the fingertips.

20. What factors influence the timing of surgery to separate syndactyly.

Expected differential growth of the involved digits is a key factor. For instance, the thumb and index must be separated early, whereas syndactyly of the ring and long fingers may be delayed for 2 or 3 years. In practice, most separations are done between 6 months and 1 year of age.

21. When should a surgical procedure to alter prehensile patterns be performed?

Prehensile patterns begin to develop at about 1 year of age and are well established by the age of 3 years. Therefore, a surgical procedure to alter prehensile patterns should be done before the age of 3 years.

22. What is Streeter's dysplasia?

Streeter's dysplasia is a syndrome of congenital constriction bands that may affect any part of the body. In the fingers the constriction may range from simple indentation to congenital amputation. In many cases, surgical release by Z-plasty is necessary to relieve distal circulatory embarrassment.

23. What is Madelung's deformity? Where is the growth disturbance?

The articular surface of the distal radius becomes progressively tilted in an ulnar and palmar direction because of growth disturbances at the ulnar-palmar aspect of the distal radial physis.

24. A young female gymnast presents with bilateral wrist pain. Radiographs show widening and irregularity of the physis of the distal radius. What is the likely diagnosis?

The likely diagnosis is epiphysiolysis of the distal radius. This condition, which is seen almost exclusively in young gymnasts, is analogous to a stress fracture. It is treated symptomatically, with restriction of activity or splinting. In severe cases, premature closure of the physis of the distal radius has been reported.

25. Hyperflexion injury to the distal interphalangeal joint in the adult may cause disruption of the extensor tendon ("mallet finger"). What is the analogous injury in the preadolescent?

The analogous injury in the preadolescent is a displaced Salter-Harris type I or II separation of the physis of the distal phalanx. The nailbed remains firmly affixed to the distal fragment; thus any bleeding around the nail indicates an open injury.

26. The term *extra-octave fracture* refers to which injury?

An extra-octave fracture is a Salter-Harris type I or II fracture at the base of the proximal phalanx of the small finger, angulated so that the small finger points toward the ulna, as if the patient had been trying to span a few too many piano keys. This injury is also called a "pencil fracture," because physicians place a small pencil or pen between the small and ring fingers to assist with the reduction maneuver.

27. Are fractures of the carpal bones in the preadolescent as common as they are in the adult?

No. Such fractures are uncommon in preadolescents. Apparently the thick cartilaginous construction of the growing carpals gives them sufficient resilience to avoid most fractures.

28. Dislocations of the proximal interphalangeal (PIP) joint usually occur in what direction?

Such dislocations usually occur dorsally, in response to a hyperextension force. Specifically, the base of the middle phalanx dislocates dorsal to the tip of the proximal phalanx. Lateral dislocations also occur. In the child, a volar dislocation is rare.

29. How long do you expect to see soreness and swelling after a jammed finger or after reduction of a simple PIP dislocation?

Soreness and swelling persist for 3–6 months. It is imperative that the patient and the parents be properly informed when such injuries are first diagnosed.

30. What is the characteristic hand position in spastic cerebral palsy?

The thumb is clasped into the palm, the fingers flexed at the metacarpophalangeal joints, the wrist flexed, and the forearm pronated.

31. Surgery of the upper extremity (hand) is most often indicated in what general category of patients with cerebral palsy?

Surgery is most often indicated in patients with spastic hemiplegia.

32. What congenital bony connection between the radius and ulna, usually located proximally, prevents forearm rotation?

Radioulnar synostosis.

BIBLIOGRAPHY

1. Albanese SA, Palmer AK, Kerr DR, et al: Wrist pain and distal growth plate closure of the radius in gymnasts. J Pediatr Orthop 9:23–28, 1989.
2. Askins G, Ger E: Congenital constriction band syndrome. J Pediatr Orthop 8:461–466, 1988.
3. Bayne LG, Costas BL, Lourie GM: The upper limb. In Morrissy RT, Weinstein SL (eds): Lovell and Winter's Pediatric Orthopaedics, 4th ed. Philadelphia, Lippincott-Raven, 1996, pp 781–848.
4. Busch MT: Sports medicine. In Morrissy R, Weinstein SL (eds): Lovell and Winter's Pediatric Orthopaedics, 4th ed. Philadelphia, Lippincott-Raven, 1996, pp 1181–1228.
5. Graham TJ, O'Brien ET: Fractures of the hand and wrist region. In Rockwood CA JR, Wilkins KE, Beaty JH (eds): Fractures in Children, 4th ed. Philadelphia, Lippincott-Raven, 1996, pp 323–448.
6. Koman LA, Gelberman RH, Toby EB, Poehling GG: Cerebral palsy. Management of the upper extremity. Clin Orthop 253:62–74, 1990.
7. Ogden JA: Skeletal Injury in the Child, 2nd ed. Philadelphia, W.B. Saunders Company, 1990.
8. Rao SB, Esposito PW, Crawford AH: Congenital and developmental wrist disorders in children. In Lichtman DM, Alexander AH (eds): The Wrist and its Disorders. Philadelphia, W.B. Saunders, 1997, pp 509–539.
9. Slakey JB, Hennrikus WL: Acquired thumb flexion contracture in children: Congenital trigger thumb. J Bone Joint Surg Br 78:481–483, 1996.
10. Tachdjian MO: Pediatric Orthopedics, 2nd ed. Philadelphia, W.B. Saunders, 1990.

VI. The Spine

48. CERVICAL SPINE DISEASE

Stephen R. Pledger, M.D.

1. In what phase of embryo life do the somites develop into cervical vertebrae?
At 5–6 weeks the embryo begins to resegment, and the somites become vertebrae. Resegmentation occurs when the right and left somites at each level fuse across the midline, incorporating the notch cord.

2. In the third week of embryonic life the embryonic spinal cord is developed. What mesenchymal tissues form the notch cord?
In the third life of embryonic life, ectodermal cells sink into the dorsal surface of the caudal end of the embryo and push forward between the ectoderm and endoderm to form mesoderm. In the middle the mesoderm coalesces into an axial segmental rod called the natal cord.

3. How many vertebrae make up the cervical spine?
The cervical spine consists of the first seven vertebrae of the spinal column.

4. Do any of the cervical vertebrae have bifid spinous processes?
The spinous processes at the third, fourth, and fifth cervical vertebrae are bifid.

5. The articulations between the vertebral arches of the cervical spine are maintained by what anatomic structures?
The articulations between the vertebral arches are maintained by (1) the supraspinous ligaments, which in the cervical spine have evolved into the ligamentum nuchae; (2) the interspinous ligaments; (3) the ligamentum flavum at each level; and (4) the synovial facet joints.

6. What artery has an intimate relationship with the cervical spine and serves as the major source of blood to the cervical cord and cervical spine?
The vertebral artery is the major source of blood for the cervical cord and cervical spine. The vertebral arches originate from the subclavian artery on each side and are usually the first and largest branches of the subclavian artery.

7. Which elements of the cervical spine are responsible for its mobility?
The elements primarily responsible for the mobility of the spine are the discs in the apophyseal joints. Each of these elements provides a relative contribution to degree and pattern of motion, such as flexion/extension and rotation.

8. Which vertebrae are responsible primarily for the rotation of the cervical spine?
The atlantoaxial joints (C1 and C2) are responsible for right and left lateral rotation.

9. Which vertebrae are responsible for flexion/extension?
Primary flexion of the cervical spine is determined from C3 to C7 with the primary movement coming from the C2–C3, C3–C4, and C4–C5 vertebral spaces.

10. Is the atlantoaxial joint (C1, C2) a stable or unstable joint?
The atlantoaxial joints are unstable because of their opposed convexity with a small contact area between the joint surfaces. This configuration is necessary for the joint to perform movements in all directions; flexion/extension, lateral flexion, and rotation. Stability between the atlas and axis depends on the transverse ligament.

11. Which type of injuries are responsible for the majority of cervical spine fractures from C2 to C7: flexion, extension, or axial compression?
Extreme cervical compression is the major cause of cervical spine fractures from C2 to C7. Such compression may occur from diving, American football, and trampoline injuries; automobile accidents; and emergency aircraft egress (ejection-seat injuries). Compression forces are responsible for the majority of nonfatal cervical fractures.

12. The teardrop fracture of the cervical spine is caused by what type of injury: hyperflexion, hyperextension, or compression?
The mechanism of injury is hyperflexion. The term teardrop reflects the sadness often associated with a neurologic sequela.

13. The unilateral facet dislocations are caused by what external forces?
The unilateral facet dislocation is assumed to occur from axial rotation movements as well as flexion movements and distraction. Tearing of the interspinous ligaments and variable amounts of ligamentum flavum and capsule in one of the facet joints leads to facet dislocation.

14. Which cervical arthrosis is the most effective in controlling flexion/extension, rotation, and lateral bending?
The halo vest or cast is the most effective in controlling rotation, flexion/extension, and lateral bending. The second most effective device is a rigid cervicothoracic brace, followed by a four-poster brace. The least effective is a soft cervical collar.

15. What is the recommended cervical orthotic device for cervical strain?
Philadelphia collar.

16. What is the most commonly recommended orthotic for most cervical spine fractures?
The halo vest or cast is recognized for most cervical spine fractures. The cervicothoracic brace is used for less unstable fractures.

17. In cervical trauma, which radiograph should be obtained, before anything else is done, to evaluate the stability of the cervical spine?
The initial radiograph is a lateral radiograph of the cervical spine, preferably made with the patient still on the transportation stretcher. All handling should be postponed until the results of the radiographic examination are known. If handling is necessary, the patient should be lifted "as one piece" by at least four persons to avoid cervical cord injury, especially in the unconscious patient.

18. When the fracture is not obvious on a lateral radiograph of the cervical spine, what is initially evaluated to help determine whether fracture has occurred?
Because swelling is noted in the prevertebral soft tissue after cervical spine fractures, the midposition of C3–C7, where most fractures occur, should be evaluated. At C3, 3.5 mm is standard; at C4, 5.0 mm; and at C5, C6, and C7, approximately 15 mm, with up to 20 mm at the distal portion. If abnormal widening is noted at any area along the anterior cervical spine, fracture should be suspected.

19. What other radiographs are helpful in determining cervical fractures or dislocations?
The oblique views are essential in evaluation of the apophyseal joints, which indicate either unilateral or bilateral facet dislocation. Tomograms are also helpful in determining odontoid fractures.

20. Is there a normal subluxation (spondylolisthesis) or stepped-off formation in the cervical spine of children?

Yes. Normal variants of a type of subluxation that occurs in the posterior borders of vertebral bodies at C2, C3 and C3, C4 often have led to the diagnosis of subluxation in children. Understanding that this phenomenon is a normal variation or pseudosubluxation is important. Evaluation of vertebral swelling helps to determine whether or not an acute injury is involved.

21. What type of spinal instability is commonly found in children with Down syndrome?

The incidence of C1, C2 subluxation is 20%. This lesion is found in all age groups, with no preponderance at any age.

22. Which radiographic imaging study is the most helpful in determining herniated discs of the cervical spine?

The gold standard is the myelogram with subsequent computed tomographic (CT) scan. However, magnetic resonance imaging (MRI) is quickly becoming the gold standard. The CT scan alone, without contrast or myelogram, is contraindicated.

23. Is the CT scan contraindicated for any cervical spine abnormalities?

No. The CT scan is indispensable in determining bony problems of the cervical spine, whether tumors or fractures are involved. CT is the imaging study of choice for all victims of trauma.

24. In evaluating a cervical spine problem, what abnormal findings are expected with a C5, C6 nerve abnormality (e.g., herniated disc, trauma)?

Expected findings include decreased sensation in the thumb and index finger, with weakness of the deltoid and biceps muscles, absence of the biceps reflex, and weakness of the extensor carpi radialis longus.

25. What abnormalities are expected with a C7 abnormality (e.g., herniated disc at C6, C7)?

Expected findings include numbness in the long finger and potentially in the index finger, slight weakness of the triceps, and absence of the brachioradialis reflex.

26. What abnormality is expected with a C8 nerve abnormality (e.g., herniated disc at the C7, T1 area)?

Expected findings include numbness in the ulnar nerve distribution of the little finger and ring finger, a claw-hand deformity, weakness of the triceps muscle, and absence of the triceps reflex.

27. What is os odontoideum?

Os odontoideum is a congenital anomaly of the odontoid. Patients may present clinically with no symptoms, local neck symptoms and transitory episodes of paresthesia after trauma, or frank myelopathy. Clinical manifestations are limited to neck pain and torticollis; depending on the severity, frank brainstem abnormalities may be present.

28. How is os odontoideum treated when patients present with transitory myelopathy?

Nonoperative treatment is sufficient for the patient presenting with a relatively stable os odontoideum and little compromise of the spinal cord. For marked instabilities, however, a cervical fusion of C1 and C2 is the procedure of choice.

29. What are the most common clinical findings in Klippel-Feil syndrome?

The classic clinical findings are a short neck, a low posterior headline, and a limited range of neck motion. However, fewer than 50% of patients have all three elements of the triad.

30. What are the most common radiographic findings of Klippel-Feil syndrome?

The most common findings are congenitally fused vertebrae from C2 to C7. The fusions may be multiple-level or single-level.

31. Do patients with Klippel-Feil syndrome have any auditory abnormalities?

Yes. Deafness was first associated with Klippel-Feil syndrome by Jalladeau in 1936. The incidence in Klippel-Feil syndrome is approximately 30%.

32. What other spine abnormality is most commonly associated with Klippel-Feil syndrome?

Scoliosis is the most commonly associated spinal abnormality in Klippel-Feil syndrome. Approximately 50% of patients report cases of scoliosis, either alone or in combination with kyphosis.

33. What is the most common congenital abnormality found in patients with quadriplegia due to football injury?

Torg reported that the most common congenital abnormallity is stenosis of the cervical spine canal, with the quadriplegia occurring at the stenotic level. Any football player with transient neurologic abnormalities should be evaluated; if cervical stenosis is found, it is recommended that the patient quit playing football.

34. The Jefferson fracture involves what type of injury to the cervical spine?

The Jefferson fracture is a unique fracture of the first cervical vertebra. Axial loading directly downward on the ring of C1 causes multiple fractures of the ring and usually a spreading of the fragments.

35. The hangman's fracture involves what lesion of the cervical spine?

The hangman's fracture is scientifically termed a traumatic spondylolisthesis of the axis or C2. The weakest length of the vertebrae is the pars interarticularis of C2, a narrow isthmus located between the superior and inferior facets. This injury usually occurs during rapid deceleration in a motor vehicle accident, when the victim is thrown forward with the head striking the windshield. The accident usually involves head-on collision with another vehicle or with a fixed object.

36. Give the most common signs and symptoms of hangman's fracture.

The most common symptoms are not highly specific. The patient often feels marked apprehension and fear with a sense of subjective instability. Pain radiating along the course of the greater occipital nerve (C2), so-called occipital neuralgia, is frequent and leads to marked guarding of neck motion. Another common finding is direct trauma to the top of the forehead of the skull.

37. In an unconscious patient with obvious blunt trauma to the forehead, what type of injuries must be ruled out immediately?

With obvious head trauma and unconsciousness, one needs to rule out a cervical spine fracture. This is best done with a scout lateral radiograph of the cervical spine.

38. Where is the most common injury to the cervical spine in children?

Injuries to the cervical spine are rare in children. The most common, however, occur from the occiput to C3. Lesions at the atlantoaxial joint are noted in 70% of children < 15 years of age but in only 16% of adults.

39. Athletic injuries to the cervical spine associated with quadriplegia are the result of what mechanism?

Athletic injuries to the cervical spine associated with quadriplegia most commonly occur as a result of axial loading. Examples include spearing in football (when a player strikes an opponent with the crown of his helmet); a poorly executed dive into a shallow body of water; with the head striking the bottom; or pushing a hockey player into the boards headfirst. The fragile cervical spine is compressed between the rapidly decelerated head and the continued momentum of the body.

40. In C4 quadriplegia, with lesion between C4 and C5 vertebrae, what changes in motor function, sensory function, or reflexes are expected?

In C4 quadriplegia, you expect the patient to breathe spontaneously because C4 innervates the diaphragm. The patient is able to shrug the shoulders independently but lacks functional abdominal muscles. Sensation is present in the upper anterior chest wall but not in the upper extremities. All reflexes are absent.

41. In C5 quadriplegia, what motor, sensation, and reflex changes are expected?

In C5 quadriplegia, the deltoid muscle and a portion of the biceps muscle are functioning. The patient is able to perform shoulder abduction and flexion/extension as well as some elbow flexion. However, all these functions are weak. Sensation is normal over the upper portion of the anterior chest wall and the lateral aspect of the arm from the shoulder to the elbow crease. The biceps reflex may be normal or slightly decreased.

42. In C6 quadriplegia, what motor functions, sensations, and reflexes remain intact?

Both the biceps and rotator cuff muscles continue to function.

Motor: The most distal functional muscle group is the wrist extensor group. The extensor carpi radialis longus and brevis and extensor carpi ulnaris may not be functioning. The patient has almost full function of the shoulder, full flexion of the elbow, full supination and partial pronation of the forearm, and partial extension of the wrist. The strength of wrist extension is normal, because some power for the extension is supplied predominantly by the extensor carpi radialis longus and brevis.

Sensation: The lateral side of the entire upper extremity as well as the thumb, index, and half of the middle finger have normal sensory power.

Reflexes: Both the biceps and the brachioradialis reflexes are normal.

43. In C7 quadriplegia, what motor functions, sensations, and reflexes remain intact?

C7 quadriplegia involves the vertebral level of C7, T1.

Motor: With the C7 nerve root intact, the triceps, wrist flexors, and long-finger extensors are functional. The patient can hold objects, but the grasp is extremely weak. Although still confined to a wheelchair, the patient may be able to attempt parallel bar and brace function for general exercise.

Sensation: C7 has little pure sensory representation in the upper extremity. No precise zone for C7 sensation may be mapped.

Reflexes: The biceps, brachioradialis, and triceps reflexes are normal.

44. What is a central cord injury?

A central cord injury is an incomplete spinal cord lesion that most commonly occurs in the elderly and results from an extension injury. This type of quadriplegia involves the upper extremities more than the lower extremities. Seventy-five percent recover and are ambulatory.

45. What is Brown-Séquard syndrome?

The syndrome results from an incomplete spinal cord injury in which ipsilateral motor loss, contralateral pain, and temperature loss are found. The recovery rate is 90%.

46. What is anterior cord syndrome?

Characterized by complete motor deficit with preservation of deep pressure and proprioception resulting from an incomplete spinal cord injury. Fifty percent of patients recover weak motor skills, but only 10% ambulate.

47. What role (if any) do steroids have in the treatment of acute spinal cord injuries?

Bracken et al. (1990) reported significant improvement in motor and sensory deficits in incomplete motor lesions with methylprednisone administered within 8 hours (30 mg/kg then 5.4 mg/kg for 23 hrs). After 8 hours, only sensory deficits improved.

48. Define spinal cord shock.
Spinal cord shock is a temporary physiologic loss of spinal cord activity that results in areflexia.

49. What physical finding signals the end of spinal shock?
The bulbocavernous reflex signals the end of spinal shock.

50. What is the most common pain pattern of herniated cervical disc?
The most common pain pattern for the cervical disc is radiation into the scapular area and down the lateral aspect of the arm in to the forearm and hand.

51. Name the most common methods of conservative treatment of herniated cervical disc.
The most common methods of treating a herniated cervical disc include a cervical collar, physical therapy with cervical traction, epidural steroid blocks, nonsteroidal antiinflammatory drugs (NSAIDs), and tincture of time.

52. What is the most common surgical treatment for a herniated cervical disc?
The most common surgical treatment is anterior cervical discectomy and fusion (ACDF) with an iliac crest allograft or autogenous graft. The second most common is cervical laminectomy with removal of the herniated fragment.

53. What is the rate of success for conservative treatment of herniated cervical discs?
Conservative treatment of herniated cervical discs is highly successful in 50–60% of cases. A minimum of 3 months of conservative care should be given before considering surgical intervention.

BIBLIOGRAPHY

1. Chewning S: Comprehensive Review Course—Cervical Spine Trauma. American Academy of Orthopedic Surgeons, 1998.
2. Clark CR, Ducker T, Dvorak J, et al (eds): The Cervical Spine, 3rd ed. Philadelphia, Lippincott-Raven, 1997.
3. Hoppenfeld S: Orthopaedic Neurology: A Diagnostic Guide to Neurological Levels. Philadelphia, J.B. Lippincott, 1977.
4. Walt RT: Comprehensive Review Course—Rehabilitation of Spinal Cord Injuries. American Academy of Orthopedic Surgeons, 1998.

49. LOW BACK PAIN, LUMBAR DISC DISEASE, SPINAL STENOSIS, AND LUMBAR FUSION

Stephen E. Doran, M.D., and Randall D. Neumann, M.D.

LOW BACK PAIN

1. What is the lifetime incidence of low back pain?
The lifetime incidence of low back pain ranges from 50–70%, whereas the incidence of sciatica ranges from 13–40%.

2. What risk factors are associated with the development of back pain?
Risk factors include jobs that require heavy and repetitive lifting, use of jackhammers and machine tools, and operation of motor vehicles. Smokers are at greater risk for low back pain, which may be severe. Individuals slightly above normal body weight are more likely to report back pain than those below or at normal weight.

3. Where does acute low back pain originate?

All structures of the lumbar spine can contribute to significant back pain, including the paraspinous muscles, ligaments, facet joints, annulus fibrosus, disc, and nerve roots.

4. What is the differential diagnosis of low back pain?

Multiple entities may produce back pain, ranging from spinal diseases to vascular diseases.

Common Conditions That Cause Low Back Pain

Spinal disorders	Herniated disc Spondylolisthesis Spinal stenosis Osteoarthritis	Metabolic disorders	Osteoporosis Osteomalacia Paget's disease
		Trauma	Fracture
Rheumatologic conditions	Rheumatoid arthritis Reiter's syndrome Psoriatic arthritis Ankylosing spondylitis	Hemoglobinopathies	Sickle-cell disease
		Renal disorders	Stones Tumors Infection
Tumor	Benign Malignant Metastatic	Female genital disorders	Ovarian cysts Ovarian tumors
Infections	Bacterial Tuberculosis	Vascular disease	Aortic aneurysm
		Gastrointestinal disease	Peptic ulcer Pancreatic disease Gall bladder

5. What is the treatment for acute low back pain?

The vast majority of patients with low back pain improve within 2 months. Patients should be treated symptomatically with aspirin and nonsteroidal antiinflammatory drugs (NSAIDs). No drug treatment has proved superior to aspirin alone, although some medications may have fewer side effects. Bedrest should be limited to 1–2 days while spasms subside. No evidence shows that prolonged bed rest is of benefit in patients with acute low back pain. The use of corsets, transcutaneous nerve stimulation (TENS), or conventional traction for the treatment of back pain remains controversial; no studies have proved the efficacy of these treatments. Some evidence suggests that exercise provides some benefit, and patients should begin with general stretching and range-of-motion activities.

6. List the other symptoms that should be evaluated in patients with acute low back pain and their possible etiologies.

Evaluation of Symptoms in Patients with Low Back Pain

SYMPTOM	LABORATORY	DIAGNOSTIC	PROCEDURE	POSSIBLE ETIOLOGY
Fever or weight loss	Culture	Radiograph Bone scan CT scan MRI	Biopsy Surgery	Infection Tumor
Night pain	Complete blood count Sedimentation rate Chemical profile	Radiograph Bone scan CT scan MRI	Biopsy Surgery	Tumor Spinal cord tumor

Table continued on following page.

Evaluation of Symptoms in Patients with Low Back Pain (Continued)

SYMPTOM	LABORATORY	DIAGNOSTIC	PROCEDURE	POSSIBLE ETIOLOGY
Morning stiffness	RA factor ANA Sedimentation rate	Radiographs		RA Ankylosing spondylitis Psoriatic arthritis
Colicky pain	Urinalysis Urine C&S Amylase	IVP Gallbladder scan CT Aortogram Ultrasound	GI workup Surgery Biopsy	Kidney Gallbladder Aneurysm Peptic ulcer Pancreas

7. What is the treatment for chronic low back pain?

Chronic low back pain is defined as pain that persists for more than 6 months. Less than 5% of patients with low back pain develop chronic back pain syndrome; these patients, however, account for approximately 85% of the total cost of back pain care. Because chronic back pain is often due to multiple factors, such as pathology of the intervertebral disc, facet joints, and soft tissues, amelioration of symptoms is difficult. Anatomic and psychological factors both contribute to the development and persistence of chronic low back pain. Psychosocial factors such as narcotic dependency, depression, and litigation/compensation issues may perpetuate or intensify the anatomic factors that cause back pain. Successful treatment of chronic low back pain addresses both the anatomic and psychosocial factors. Physical therapy is beneficial for improving flexibility, strength, and endurance. TENS units decrease pain for some patients. Antidepressants and counseling may benefit patients experiencing depression. Some patients successfully return to their occupations via work-hardening/conditioning programs. Injections of local anesthetics or epidural/caudal corticosteroids may reduce pain for a small number of patients with chronic symptoms, but are much more effective in relieving acute symptoms of back and radicular pain. Lumbar fusion may be helpful for a selected group of patients whose symptoms are primarily due to intervertebral disc degeneration.

LUMBAR DISC DISEASE

8. Describe the usual history of patients with lumbar disc herniation.

Most people relate back and leg pain to a traumatic event, but close questioning sometimes reveals that patients have had intermittent episodes of back pain for months or years. The pain may be brought on by heavy exertion, repetitive bending, twisting, or heavy lifting. Pain usually begins in the low back and radiates to the sacroiliac region and buttocks. Radicular pain usually extends below the knee and follows the dermatome of the involved nerve root. When patients have sustained a disc herniation, the pain is generally worse in the leg than in the back. Pain may be intermittent in nature and usually increases with activities, especially sitting in a car for a long period of time. The pain may be relieved by standing or by bed rest. The hallmark is exacerbation of leg pain by straining, sneezing, or coughing. Patients may complain of weakness. The weakness is usually localized to the neurologic level of involvement. Paresthesias are common and follow the nerve root distribution for the sensory areas.

9. What is cauda equina syndrome?

Cauda equina syndrome is a large midline disc herniation that may compress several roots of the cauda equina; it occurs in only 2% of patients with a herniated disc. The L4–L5 disc is the most commonly offending herniation. The mode of onset may be rapid or slowly progressing. Often back pain or perianal pain predominates, and disc symptoms are minimal. Patients complain of difficulty with urination, increased frequency, or overflow incontinence. In men, a recent history of impotence may be elicited. Patients may have leg pain that progresses to severe numbness of the feet and difficulty with walking. Myelography shows a complete block with large disc herniations. Prompt surgical intervention is the treatment of choice.

10. Describe the physical examination for patients with lumbar disc disease.

Patients should be examined in the standing, sitting, and lying positions. A list or limp can be seen with the patient walking. Range of motion of the spine should be examined. Patients with disc herniation frequently complain of leg pain on forward flexion, whereas patients with spinal stenosis often have leg pain on back extension. Muscular atrophy or muscle spasm should be identified with range-of-motion evaluation. Weakness is also determined. A complete neurologic examination is necessary, including testing of motor strengths, reflexes, and sensory deficits. The presence or absence of tension sign is the most important finding in patients suspected of having disc herniation. Evaluation should include examination for hip and knee pathology.

11. What are the physical findings in patients with unilateral disc herniation at the L3–L4 disc?

Unilateral herniation at the L3–L4 disc generally involves compression of the L4 nerve root, with possible sensory deficits in the posterolateral thigh, anterior knee, and medial leg. Motor weakness is variable in the quadriceps and hip adductors. Changes also are apparent in the patellar reflex.

12. What are the physical findings in patients with unilateral disc herniation at the L4–L5 disc?

The L5 nerve root is compressed with disc herniation at L4–L5. Sensory deficit occurs in the anterolateral leg, dorsum of the foot, and great toe. Motor weakness includes the extensor hallucis longus, gluteus medius, and extensor digitorum longus and brevis. Usually no reflex changes are present.

13. What are the physical findings in patients with unilateral disc herniation at the L5–S1 disc?

Disc herniation at L5–S1 signifies compression of the S1 nerve root. Sensory deficits occur in the lateral malleolus, lateral foot, heel, and web of the fourth and fifth toes. Motor weakness involves the peroneus longus and brevis, gastrocnemius-soleus complex, and gluteus maximus. The Achilles reflex is usually diminished.

14. What is a far lateral disc herniation?

A far lateral disc herniation occurs when the disc herniation occurs lateral to the spinal canal and neural foramen, producing pressure on the nerve root cephalad to the disc of origin. For example, a far lateral L4/5 disc herniation produces a L4 radiculopathy as opposed to the expected L5 radiculopathy. Conservative treatment is identical to other disc herniations. Surgical management requires an approach lateral to the spinal canal and facet joints.

15. What are the "tension" signs in lumbar disc herniation?

Tension signs are maneuvers that tighten the sciatic nerve and in doing so further compress an inflamed nerve root against a herniated lumbar disc. Variations of the test include the following:

1. **Lasegue's test.** This classic straight-leg raising test is performed with the patient in the supine position and the head flat or on a low pillow. One of the patient's hands is placed on the ilium to stabilize the pelvis. The other hand slowly elevates the leg by the heel, with the knee straight. The patient should be questioned as to whether the maneuver produces leg pain. Only when leg pain or radicular symptoms are produced is the test considered positive; back pain alone is not a positive finding.

2. **The bowstring sign.** This variation of the straight-leg raising test is performed as usual until pain is elicited. At this point, the knee is flexed, usually with significant reduction of symptoms. Finger pressure applied to the popliteal space over the terminal aspect of the sciatic nerve reestablishes the painful radicular symptoms.

3. **The sitting root test.** With the patient sitting and the cervical spine flexed, the knee is extended while the hip remains flexed to 90°. The patient may complain of leg pain or may attempt to extend the hip, again indicating nerve root compression.

4. **Contralateral straight-leg raising test.** This test is performed in the same manner as the straight-leg raising test, except that the nonpainful leg is raised. If this maneuver produces the patient's sciatica in the opposite extremity, the test is considered positive. A positive test is highly suggestive of a herniated disc and usually indicates the location of the extrusion. This test is commonly positive in patients who have disc herniations medial to the nerve root in the axilla.

5. **Reverse straight-leg raising test.** This test may be done with the patient in a prone position or in a lateral position with the unaffected side down. The test involves hip extension and knee flexion, exactly opposite to the standard straight-leg raising test. A positive result signifies irritation in the roots of the femoral nerve, commonly the L4 nerve root.

16. What is a list?

A list is produced when patients have herniation of a lumbar disc. Herniation that is lateral to the nerve root produces what is called a list away from the side of the irritated nerve root. Herniation of the disc that is medial to the nerve root, however, in what is called the axillary position, usually produces a list toward the side of the irritated nerve root. When the disc herniation is lateral, patients feel that they must move from the side of the irritated nerve in an attempt to draw the nerve root away from the disc fragment. When the herniation is in the axillary position medial to the nerve root, the patient lists toward the side of the nerve root in an attempt at decompression.

17. What other tests should be done in evaluation for lumbar disc disease?

No back examination is complete without evaluation of the peripheral circulation. The posterior tibial and dorsal pedis artery should be examined. Vascular claudication is an important cause of leg pain and may mimic lumbar disc disease. The hip and knee also should be evaluated. Limitations in range of motion of the hip, particularly in rotation, along with groin discomfort, is indicative of hip disease. Tenderness over the piriformis muscle in external rotation may implicate piriformis syndrome. Rectal tone should be evaluated in patients suspected of having cauda equina syndrome.

18. Are routine radiographs helpful in evaluation of lumbar spine disease?

Only 1–2% of the spine radiographs in patients with back pain between 20 and 50 years of age have unsuspected findings. Most studies have found some disc space narrowing or osteophyte formation in this age group. Spondylolisthesis and spondylolysis may be seen on radiographs, along with some disc space narrowing at the affected level. Such findings, however, are also present in patients with no back pain and no clinically significant pathology.

19. What imaging techniques are used in evaluation of lumbar disc disease?

1. **Myelography.** Indications include suspicion of an intraspinal lesion or questionable diagnosis resulting from conflicting clinical findings in other studies. Myelography has value in previously operated spines and in spinal stenosis, especially in conjunction with CT. Water-soluble contrasts are the most popular contrast agents. Because myelography is an invasive study, reactions may occur, including headache, pain, nausea, vomiting, meningitis, and localized infection.

2. **Computed axial tomography.** The advantages of CT over myelography include better visualization of lateral lesions, such as foraminal stenosis and lateral disc herniations, lower radiation dose, and absence of adverse reactions. CT generally allows discrimination between neural compression caused by soft tissue and that caused by bone. CT is extremely useful in the diagnosis of lateral or foraminal herniations of the lumbar disc. The disadvantages are that more radiology centers scan the third lumbar through the sacral disc. Higher lesions may be missed if scanning is limited to the levels.

3. **Magnetic resonance imaging.** The advantage of MRI over a CT scan includes the ability to demonstrate intraspinal tumors, to examine the entire spine, and to identify degenerative discs.

Anatomic detail of neural elements is much better than CT, but MRI does not demonstrate bone anatomy as well as CT.

   4. **Bone scan.** Bone scans can be used when physicians suspect diseases other than lumbar disc disease or spinal stenosis. Bone scan confirms neoplastic, infectious, traumatic, or arthritic problems of the spine.

20. Is electromyography useful in patients with lumbar disc disease?

Electromyography is commonly used to help in differentiating radicular symptoms from peripheral neuropathy or upper motor neuron lesions and in determining the presence or absence of generalized myopathy.

21. Compare the natural history of conservative and surgical treatment in patients with lumbar disc herniation.

In a controlled prospective study of 280 patients with lumbar disc herniation, treatment included conservative or surgical treatment. The surgically treated group was doing better at 1-year follow-up. However, comparison of the results at 4 and 10 years revealed no statistically significant difference in outcome. Surgery, therefore, provides more rapid relief of pain, but the ultimate endpoint is approximately the same, regardless of treatment.

22. What conservative treatment modalities can be used for patients with acute lumbar disc herniations?

Nonsurgical treatments include bed rest, oral medication, epidural steroids, physical therapy, bracing, traction, manipulation, and techniques such as TENS. A brief period of bed rest for 48–72 hours, along with nonopioid analgesics, should be used to control pain. Epidural steroids may be beneficial in eliminating acute pain but have not been shown to have long-term benefit. Only approximately 10% of patients with symptoms and signs ultimately require surgery. Therefore, physicians may expect a 90% relief rate with conservative treatment for patients with lumbar disc disease.

23. What surgical procedure is used for the treatment of lumbar disc disease?

The traditional surgery is laminectomy and lumbar disc excision by means of a midline incision. The paraspinous muscles are stripped from the lamina of the vertebra on each side of the lesion. The lamina is identified, and the ligamentum flavum is excised. Portions of the superior and inferior lamina may be removed. After the nerve root is retracted, the disc herniation identified and then removed, the disc is dissected free of loose fragments. Closure is routine. Patients are allowed to turn in bed, to walk, and to stand. General exercise is begun within the first 48 hours after surgery. Sitting is generally minimized, whereas lying and walking are progressively increased. Patients should refrain from long trips in a car for approximately 3 months. Exercises for lower extremity strength and rehabilitation are begun 6–8 weeks postoperatively. Patients are returned to sitting jobs within 4–6 weeks. The success rate for relief of leg pain is 93%; for relief of low back pain, 80%.

24. Describe microlumbar disc excision.

Microlumbar discectomy requires an operating microscope. The procedure is performed much like an open disc excision and laminectomy, except the laminae are not removed. Microlumbar discectomy requires less dissection and has the potential of less reactive scar tissue. Surgical results are approximately the same as with open disc surgery.

25. What are the complications of lumbar disc surgery?

Cauda equina syndrome	Dural tears
Thrombophlebitis	Nerve root injury
Pulmonary embolism	Cerebral spinal fluid fistula
Wound infection	Laceration of abdominal vessels
Pyogenic spondylitis	Injury to abdominal viscera
Postoperative discitis	

26. What minimally invasive techniques are available to treat lumbar disc herniations?

Most minimally invasive techniques attempt to treat disc herniations contained by the posterior longitudinal ligament (i.e., subligamentous disc herniations) and are ineffective in treating herniations in which a fragment of disc material has migrated cephalad or caudal to the disc space. Percutaneous injection of **chymopapain** into the intervertebral disc has been used in the past to partially dissolve the disc, reducing pressure on the nerve root. Most spine surgeons no longer use chymopapain because it is not very effective, has a small but significant risk of serious allergic reaction, and accelerates the degeneration of the disc, increasing the risk of chronic back pain. **Percutaneous automated discectomy** involves placing a cannula into the disc and aspirating disc material until the patient reports relief of radicular symptoms. This technique is not used widely because of a relatively high failure rate in relieving symptoms and the need to proceed with open techniques. **Endoscopic techniques** have been developed to treat lumbar disc herniations. An intradiscal approach involves placing a cannula within the disc and then removing disc material using an endoscope. A foraminal approach involves placing a cannula into the foramen of the nerve root and then removing disc material using an endoscope. This technique is most useful for far-lateral disc herniations. The most recently developed minimally invasive technique is **microendoscopic discectomy (MED™ Sofamor Danek).** Microendoscopic discectomy uses a posterior approach identical to standard lumbar discectomy or microdiscectomy. A cannula is docked onto the lamina under fluoroscopic guidance and a laminotomy; ligament removal and discectomy are then performed using an endoscope. Migrated disc fragments are accessible using this technique.

SPINAL STENOSIS

27. What is lumbar spinal stenosis?

Lumbar spinal stenosis is an abnormal narrowing of the osteoligamentous vertebral canal and/or vertebral foramina; the result is compression of the dural sac and/or the nerve roots. Lumbar spinal stenosis specifically excludes disc herniation as a causative agent.

28. What is the most common cause for neurologic leg pain in the older population?

Spinal stenosis.

29. What pathology is involved with spinal stenosis?

Spinal stenosis involves the three-joint complex of the disc facet joint and intervertebral disc. The intervertebral disc usually undergoes significant degenerative changes. Subsequent degeneration leads to collapse of the disc and facet arthritis, which tend to narrow the neural foramina progressively. Soft-tissue impression may result anteriorly from the disc or posteriorly from ligamentum flavum. On a mechanical basis, the neural foramina are then more narrowed with lumbar extension than with lumbar flexion. The site of such compression may either be centrally within the canal or more laterally within the lateral recess or neural foramina. Canal narrowing may be congenital, involving genetic conditions such as achondroplasia, or due to degenerative scoliosis or spondylolisthesis.

30. What is the classification of spinal stenosis?

Congenital
  Idiopathic
  Achondroplastic
Acquired
  Degenerative
    Central canal
    Peripheral canal, lateral recesses,
      nerve root canals
    Degenerative spondylolisthesis

Acquired *(cont.)*
  Iatrogenic
    Postlaminectomy
    Postfusion
    Postchemonucleolysis
  Posttraumatic
  Miscellaneous
    Paget's disease
    Diffuse interstitial skeletal hypertrophy

31. What is the most common cause of spinal stenosis?
Acquired degenerative spinal stenosis.

32. What is the differential diagnosis of spinal stenosis?
- Herniated disc
- Cauda equina syndrome
- Spinal cord tumor
- Primary or metastatic vertebral body tumors
- Infections
- Fractures
- Vascular insufficiency
- Peripheral neuropathy

33. Describe the epidemiology of spinal stenosis.
The age at onset of symptoms is variable, but the fifth and sixth decades are common. Achondroplasia usually presents in the fourth decade. Degenerative spondylolisthesis is infrequent in patients younger than 50 years. Distribution between men and women is equal. Degenerative spinal stenosis occurs more frequently in workers who have done heavy manual labor.

34. Describe the common history in patients with spinal stenosis.
Low back pain is a common finding but usually is not the reason for referral to an orthopedic surgeon. Patients describe feelings of aching and stiffness that often worsen with weather changes. The back pain is usually insidious rather than acute in onset. Pain is relieved with rest and generally aggravated by overactivity. Patients also describe buttock discomfort, tightness, or burning, induced by walking or standing. Patients complain of limited spine movement and increased amount of pain with extension of the spine. Urinary dysfunction is uncommon but occurs in approximately 3–4% of cases.

35. What presenting symptom is the hallmark of spinal stenosis?
Patients complain of pain that increases with walking or standing, whereas sitting and leaning forward or lying down alleviates the discomfort.

36. Distinguish neurogenic claudication from vascular claudication.
With vascular claudication, the claudication distance is usually fixed. Patients may stand in an erect position for relief of pain, which is brought on by walking uphill or bicycle riding. Pain is described as a cramp or a tightness in the calf. With neurogenic claudication, the claudication distance is generally variable. Patients must sit or get in a flexed position for relief of pain; walking uphill and bicycle riding usually do not induce pain. Patients describe neurogenic claudication as numbness, ache, or sharp pain; cramping is usually not included.

37. What radiographic examinations are important in the diagnosis of spinal stenosis?
Both CT scan and MRI provide excellent delineation of the stenotic areas. True stenosis is considered absolute with a 10–12 mm sagittal diameter. Both studies show the neural foramina, facet joints, ligamentum flavum, and any compression on the spinal canal. Other abnormalities, including posttraumatic deformities, overgrowth of spinal fusions, Paget's disease, vertebral ligament hypertrophy, and intraspinal masses also can be identified.

38. What is the treatment for spinal stenosis?
Nonoperative treatment involves a vigorous physical therapy program emphasizing postural changes, stretching, and strengthening of the tightened lumbar and lower extremity musculature. Biofeedback may be helpful. Transcutaneous electrical nerve stimulator units occasionally have been successful in relieving acute pain. Epidural steroids remain controversial. NSAIDs, particularly aspirin, may reduce leg and back pain. Braces may be used to decrease lumbar lordosis.

39. What are the indications for surgery with spinal stenosis?
Surgery is indicated in patients with severe spinal stenosis and intractable pain and in patients who fail an appropriate nonoperative course. Other causes of pain should be ruled out. Surgery is elective, except in the presence of bowel or bladder dysfunction.

40. What is the surgical treatment for spinal stenosis?

Surgical treatment involves removal of the lamina, ligamentum flava, spinous process, medial facets, and arthritis spurs in the lateral recesses. Attempts should be made to leave portions of the facet joints intact.

41. What complications are seen after decompression for spinal stenosis?

Instability	Arachnoiditis	Nerve root injury
Dural tears	Infection	Epidural scarring

LUMBAR FUSION

42. What are the indications for lumbar fusion?

Lumbar fusion is indicated for unstable fractures, symptomatic spondylolysis and spondylolisthesis, recurrent disc herniations, and disc degeneration (a.k.a. segmental instability). Examples of unstable lumbar fractures include burst fractures with greater than 50% canal compromise, compression fractures with significant angulation (> 35%), or chance fractures.

43. When is fusion indicated for spondylolysis and spondylolisthesis?

Patients who have significant back and/or radicular pain are candidates for decompression and possibly fusion if their symptoms do not respond to appropriate conservative care. Patients with spondylolysis without spondylolisthesis have been treated with decompression alone or with simultaneous fusion. Patients with spondylolysis and spondylolisthesis are usually treated with decompression and fusion. The treatment of patients with spinal stenosis and degenerative spondylolisthesis is controversial. Although some studies have shown improved outcome in patients treated with decompression and fusion, other studies have shown similar results with decompression alone.

44. When is fusion indicated for recurrent lumbar disc herniations?

Recurrent lumbar disc herniations may occur in up to 10–15% of patients. Fusion is usually not indicated for the first recurrent disc herniation. However, after the second recurrent disc herniation, fusion is often recommended, especially if the two recurrences occur soon after the original disc herniation.

45. When is fusion recommended for lumbar disc degeneration?

Fusion for lumbar disc degeneration is indicated for the treatment of low back pain of discogenic origin refractory to extensive conservative care (usually at least 6 months). Determining who may benefit from lumbar fusion for disc degeneration is a difficult decision. The primary challenge is determining whether the back pain originates from the disc or from other sources. Some surgeons rely on the appearance of the disc on MRI and x-ray to determine whether the back pain originates from the disc. A flattened disc with low signal characteristics on T2-weighted images is an indication of disc degeneration. Other surgeons rely on discography to determine whether a disc is the source of back pain. Discography involves the injection of contrast material into the disc space under fluoroscopic guidance. A discogram is considered positive if it provokes the patient's typical back pain or if an anatomic defect such as an annular tear is noted.

46. What are the surgical options available for lumbar fusion?

Lumbar fusion can be performed from a posterior approach with or without the simultaneous use of instrumentation. During a posterolateral fusion, bone graft is placed over the decorticated transverse processes, lateral facet joints, and sacral ala. During a posterior lumbar interbody fusion (PLIF), bone graft is placed into the disc space from a posterior approach. Spinal instrumentation increases fusion rates, especially if instability or spondylolisthesis is present. Posterior instrumentation usually involves placement of pedicle screws connected together with rods.

Lumbar fusion can also be performed from an anterior (either trans- or retroperitoneal) approach. During an anterior lumbar interbody fusion (ALIF), bone graft is placed into the disc space anteriorly and is often accompanied by posterior instrumentation.

More recently, threaded titanium cages have been developed that are placed into the disc space from either an anterior or posterior approach (ALIF or PLIF). Simultaneous pedicle screw instrumentation is usually not necessary because the cages provide adequate stability. Endoscopic techniques have been developed for the anterior placement of cages.

BIBLIOGRAPHY

1. Bridwell KH, DeWald RL, et al (eds): The Textbook of Spinal Surgery, 2nd ed. Philadelphia, Lippincott-Raven, 1997.
2. Frymoyer JW: Back pain and sciatica. N Engl J Med 318:291–300, 1988.
3. Lonstein JE, Winter RB, Bradford DS, Ogilvie JW (eds): Moe's Textbook of Scoliosis and Other Spinal Deformities, 3rd ed. Philadelphia, W.B. Saunders, 1995.
4. Herkowitz HN: Spinal stenosis: Clinical evaluation. In Instructional Course Lectures, vol XLI. Rosemont, IL, American Academy of Orthopedic Surgeons, 1992, pp 183–185.
5. McCowin PR, Borenstein D, Wiesel SW: The current approach to the medical diagnosis of low back pain. Orthop Clin North Am 22:315–325, 1991.
6. Menezes AH, Sonntag VK (eds): Principles of Spinal Surgery. New York, McGraw-Hill, 1996.
7. Tuite GF, et al: Outcome after laminectomy for lumbar spinal stenosis. Part I: Clinical correlations. J Neurosurg 81:699–706, 1994.

50. SCOLIOSIS AND KYPHOSIS

Glen M. Ginsburg, M.D.

1. What two deviations of the spine must be present in order to classify a curvature as scoliosis?

In order for a spinal deformity to be classified as scoliosis, both lateral (coronal plane) curvature and rotation (transverse plane) must be present.

2. What types of scoliosis are most commonly seen?

- Idiopathic (infantile, juvenile and adolescent)
- Neuromuscular
- Nonstructural
- Congenital

Scoliosis and kyphosis are also seen in other disease processes:

- Neurofibromatosis
- Traumatic (spinal cord) injuries
- Mesenchymal (Marfan syndrome, Ehlers-Danlos syndrome)
- Infections
- Metabolic disorders
- Tumors
- Spondylolisthesis
- Osteochondrodystrophy (dwarfism)
- Degenerative

3. What is the incidence of idiopathic scoliosis?

The incidence of scoliosis has been reported to be anywhere from 3–5%, with a slightly higher female predominance.

4. What are the three types of idiopathic scoliosis and their respective age groups?

The three types of congenital scoliosis are infantile (birth to 3 years), juvenile (3 years to puberty), and adolescent (at or just after puberty).

5. What is the most common curve pattern seen in infantile idiopathic scoliosis?

The most common curve pattern seen in infantile idiopathic scoliosis is a convex left thoracic curve, unlike adolescent idiopathic scoliosis, in which a left thoracic curve is rare and often is associated with intraspinal pathology.

6. Which radiographic measurement techniques are currently used to determine the prognosis of infantile idiopathic scoliosis?

The rib-vertebral angle difference of Mehta (RVAD) measures the intersection of a line perpendicular to the apical vertebral end plate and a line drawn for the midneck to the midhead of the right and left corresponding ribs A difference > 20° means that curve progression is likely. The rib phase describes the amount of overlap between the rib head and the vertebral body. A phase one rib does not overlap the body, and progression is unlikely. A phase two rib overlaps the vertebral body and means that progression is likely.

7. What two developmental anomalies of the vertebral anlage are responsible for the deformities seen in congenital scoliosis?

Congenital scoliosis results from either a failure of formation or a failure of segmentation of the vertebral anlage. Examples of failure of formation include hemivertebrae and butterfly vertebrae. Examples of failure of segmentation include unilateral bars and block vertebrae.

8. What other congenital anomalies (nonmusculoskeletal) are seen in association with congenital scoliosis?

Genitourinary anomalies are seen in 33% of children with congenital scoliosis. Klippel-Feil syndrome is seen in 25%. Fifteen percent will have intraspinal anomalies, and 10% will have congenital heart defects.

9. What does the term *segmentation* mean in reference to hemivertebra?

Segmentation of a hemivertebra means that it is separated from the adjacent vertebral body by a disc (and growth plate). A hemivertebra may be fully segmented (separated by a disc on both sides), semisegmented (a disc on one side only), or nonsegmented (no discs on either side). Obviously, a fully segmented hemivertebra has the greatest potential for growth.

10. What does the term *hemimetameric shift* mean?

Hemimetameric shift is the presence of hemivertebra on opposite sides of the spine that often will balance one another. This combination of deformities is often benign.

11. Which of the vertebral anomalies seen in congenital scoliosis causes the most rapid progression of deformity?

The most rapid progression of deformity seen in congenital scoliosis is a fully segmented hemivertebra with a contralateral unsegmented bar (up to 10°/year).

12. What is the treatment of choice for the anomalies described in questions 8–11?

The treatment of choice for a hemivertebra and a contralateral unsegmented bar is an in situ fusion as soon as the diagnosis is made. The fusion should include a mobile segment above and below the bar.

13. According to the Scoliosis Research Society, what is the minimal amount of lateral (coronal) curvature necessary to qualify as scoliosis?

Lateral (coronal) curvatures < 10° are generally not referred to as scoliosis.

14. Name three conditions that may cause lateral (coronal) curvature of the spine not associated with rotation (i.e., not true scoliosis).

Lateral (coronal) curvature of the spine without rotation can be seen with leg length discrepancy, posterior element tumors such as osteoid osteoma and osteoblastomas, and psychiatric conditions such as hysterical scoliosis.

15. What is the most frequently used clinical tool to measure spinal rotation?

The most commonly used clinical tool to measure spinal rotation is the scoliometer, which is drawn over the spinous processes of the patient while he or she bends at the waist with straight knees and dangling arms. The rotations in degrees are recorded at each spinal level.

16. How much spinal rotation should be present in order for a patient to be referred to an orthopaedic surgeon from a school nurse or primary care physician?

Under the guidelines of the Scoliosis Research Society, spinal rotations of greater than 7–8° are appropriate for referral to an orthopaedic surgeon. This amount of rotation corresponds to approximately 20° of coronal curvature on radiographs. At 5° of rotation, the false-positive rate for scoliosis referral (curves < 10°) was 36%.

17. What spinal radiograph measurement system is currently the most widely used, and how are radiographs measured with this system?

The Cobb method of radiographic measurement is currently the most widely used measurement system. A posteroanterior 3-ft standing radiograph is taken of the entire spine, including the iliac crests from a 6-ft distance. The superior and inferior vertebra of each curve is located. The superior and inferior surfaces of the vertebrae tilt maximally into the concavity of the curve. The superior and inferior surfaces of these vertebrae tilt maximally into the concavity of the curve. Perpendicular lines are then constructed from the superior end plate of the superior end vertebra and the inferior end plate of the inferior end vertebra. The angle subtended by the intersection of these two lines is the magnitude of the curve.

18. How are the apical and end vertebrae determined?

The vertebra that is maximally rotated and/or the most deviated from the vertical axis of the patient. More than one apical vertebra in a curve may be present if the apex is at a disc space. The superior end vertebra is the most cephalad vertebra of a curve whose superior surface tilts maximally into the concavity of the curve. The inferior end vertebra is the most caudad vertebra of a curve whose inferior surface tilts maximally into the concavity of the curve.

19. What are the neutral and stable vertebrae?

The neutral vertebrae are the first nonrotated vertebrae at the caudal and cranial ends of a curve. The stable vertebra is the vertebra that is bisected by the midsacral line (a vertical line erected from the S1 spinous process).

20. Describe the King classification of adolescent idiopathic scoliosis.

The King classification of thoracic idiopathic curves describes five patterns.

King I: a double thoracic and lumbar curve in which the lumbar curve is larger than the thoracic curve

King II: a structural thoracic curve and a compensatory lumbar curve

King III: a single thoracic curve with either no lumbar curve or a small lumbar curve that does not cross the midline

King IV: a long thoracolumbar curve in which L4 tilts into the curve

King V: represents a double thoracic curve in which T1 tilts into the structural upper curve that is structural on side bending.

21. Describe the Nash-Moe classification of vertebral rotation.

The Nash-Moe classification of vertebral rotation is based on the radiographic appearance of the apical vertebral pedicle shadows in reference to the sides of the vertebra. In grade 0 rotation, the pedicles of the apical vertebra are equidistant from the sides of the vertebra. In grade IV rotation, one pedicle has crossed the midline.

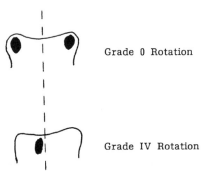

22. Describe the Risser radiographic classification of skeletal maturity.

The Risser classification of skeletal maturity is based on the ossification pattern of the iliac crest epiphysis. Ossification occurs from the anterior superior iliac spine to the posterior superior iliac spine. Excursion of ossification is divided into four grades:

Risser 1: 25% excursion   **Risser 4:** 100% (complete) excursion
Risser 2: 50% excursion   **Risser 5:** fusion of the epiphysis to the ilium,
Risser 3: 75% excursion   representing the end of spinal growth

23. What are the risk factors for progression of curvature in adolescent idiopathic scoliosis?

The risk factors for progression of idiopathic scoliosis are curve magnitude (the larger the curve, the greater the risk), growth potential of the patient (the more growth remaining, the greater the risk), and the curve type (double curves have a greater risk of progression). Female sex has not been statistically proven to increase the risk of progression because of the small numbers of males in the large reported series.

24. When is nonsurgical treatment of adolescent idiopathic scoliosis appropriate?

No treatment is generally required for patients with curves measuring < 20°. Nonsurgical treatment is indicated for curves measuring between 20° and 40–45° in skeletally immature patients.

25. What nonsurgical treatment of adolescent idiopathic scoliosis has been shown to alter the natural history of the disease?

The only nonsurgical treatment of adolescent idiopathic scoliosis that has been shown to alter the natural history is the use of a spinal orthotic (brace). Bracing is indicated in the child who presents with a curve of 30–40°, or who presents with a curve < 29° with a history of documented progression. Also, curves of 25–29° in the very young (Risser 0, Tanner 1) should be braced. Electrical stimulation, exercises, manipulation, and biofeedback have not been shown to alter the natural history.

26. What are the three most common types of braces used for adolescent idiopathic scoliosis, and how are they most effectively used?

The three most common types of spinal braces are the Milwaukee (apex T8 and above), TLSO or Boston (apex below T8), and the Charleston bending brace (nighttime use only).

27. What are the indications for operative treatment of adolescent idiopathic scoliosis?
Operative treatment of adolescent idiopathic scoliosis is recommended for curves > 40–45° in the skeletally immature patient, curves that progress despite bracing, or curves > 50–60° in the mature adolescent.

28. Describe the crankshaft phenomenon. How is this complication avoided?
The crankshaft phenomenon is the progression of spinal curvature despite solid posterior arthrodesis. It was described by Dubousset in 1973 and is thought to be related to continued anterior spinal growth against a posterior tether. This complication can be avoided by combining the posterior fusion with an anterior arthrodesis and is recommended in premenarchal patients, in patients who are Risser 1 or less, or in patients < 10 years of age with open triradiate cartilage.

29. What is kyphosis?
Kyphosis is a spinal deformity characterized by an increase in the posterior convex angulation in the sagittal plane. The normal posterior convex angulation of the thoracic spine is 20–40° measured by the Cobb method.

30. What types of kyphosis are normally seen?
- Scheuermann's
- Postlaminectomy
- Postural congenital
- Myelomeningocele
- Developmental (achondroplasia)
- Posttraumatic

31. Describe the two congenital defects that are most commonly seen in congenital kyphosis.
The two congenital defects commonly associated with congenital kyphosis are failure of formation (hemivertebra) and failure of segmentation (anterior unsegmented bar).

32. Which type of congenital kyphosis carries the greatest risk for neurologic impairment?
Failure of anterior formation of the vertebral body carries a high risk for paraplegia due to tethering of the cord over the sharp kyphus. Early (between 1 and 3 years of age) posterior fusion is the treatment of choice for this type of congenital kyphosis.

33. What is Scheuermann's kyphosis?
Scheuermann's kyphosis is a disorder of endochondral ossification that affects the vertebral endplates and ring apophyses, resulting in intravertebral disc herniation, anterior wedging of consecutive vertebra (≥ 5° in three adjacent thoracic vertebrae), and a fixed thoracolumbar kyphosis.

34. What is the prevalence of Scheuermann's kyphosis?
The prevalence of Scheuermann's kyphosis has been estimated to be between 0.4% and 8% of the general population, mainly affecting adolescents at puberty. The male:female ratio is about equal.

35. What is the etiology of Scheuermann's kyphosis?
The exact etiology of Scheuermann's kyphosis is unknown. A familial predilection has been theorized. Increased height and repetitive loading may be inciting factors.

36. What are the most common presenting symptoms of Scheuermann's kyphosis?
The most common presenting symptoms of Scheuermann's kyphosis are spinal deformity and pain at the apex, which is aggravated by prolonged sitting, standing, and activity. This disorder may account for as much at one-third of back pain complaints in pediatric patients.

37. What is the initial treatment of Scheuermann's kyphosis?
The initial treatment of Scheuermann's kyphosis is nonsurgical, consisting of thoracic extension, abdominal strengthening exercises, and avoidance of heavy lifting. Symptoms usually resolve by the end of growth.

38. When is bracing recommended for Schuermann's kyphosis?

Bracing is recommended in Scheuermann's kyphosis when the curve exceeds 70° in the skeletally immature patient. A Milwaukee brace is recommended for the thoracic form of the disease and a TLSO can be used for the atypical lumbar form. According to a recent natural history study, patients treated conservatively may have more pain at the apex of the curve as adults, but their overall quality of life should not be affected.

39. When is surgery recommended for Scheuermann's kyphosis?

Surgery is recommended for Scheuermann's kyphosis if the curve exceeds 75° and the patient is symptomatic or if neurologic signs appear. Restrictive lung disease may be seen if the kyphosis exceeds 100°.

40. What is the surgical treatment of choice for Scheuermann's kyphosis?

The surgical treatment of choice for symptomatic Scheuermann's kyphosis is anterior release and fusion (preferably with anterior column support), followed by a posterior arthrodesis with instrumentation of the entire kyphotic segment.

BIBLIOGRAPHY

1. Bodner RJ, Heyman S, Drummond DS, Gregg JR: The use of single-photon emission computed tomography (SPECT) in the diagnosis of low-back pain in young patients. Spine 13:1155–1160, 1988.
2. Freeman BL: Scoliosis and kyphosis. In Canale ST (ed): Campbell's Operative Orthopaedics, 9th ed. St. Louis, Mosby, 1998, pp 2849–2969.
3. Ginsburg GM, Bassett GS: Back pain in children and adolescents: Evaluation and differential diagnosis. J Am Acad Orthop 5:67–78, 1997.
4. Lonstein JE: Idiopathic scoliosis. In Lonstein JE, Winter RB, Bradford DS, Ogilvie TW (eds): Moe's Textbook of Scoliosis and Other Spinal Deformities, 2nd ed. Philadelphia, W.B. Saunders, 1995.
5. Lowe TG: Current concepts review: Scheuermann's disease. J Bone Joint Surg 72A:940–945, 1990.
6. McMaster MJ, Ohtsuka K: The natural history of congenital scoliosis. J Bone Joint Surg 64A:1128–1147, 1982.
7. Murray PM, Weinstein SL, Spratt KF: The natural history and long-term follow-up of Scheuermann's kyphosis. J Bone Joint Surg 75A:236–247, 1993.

51. SPONDYLOLYSIS AND SPONDYLOLISTHESIS

Glen M. Ginsburg, M.D.

1. Define spondylolysis.

Spondylolysis is the term used to describe a defect in the pars interarticularis, usually affecting the lumbar spine.

2. Define spondylolisthesis.

Spondylolisthesis is the term used to describe the slipping forward of an upper vertebral segment on the lower segment, usually occurring after a bilateral pars defect (spondylolysis) occurs at the same level.

3. What is the incidence of spondylolisthesis?

The incidence of spondylolisthesis is 5% for the general population. The incidence in adult Caucasian males is 5–6% and in females is 2–3%. In Eskimos, the incidence has been reported to be 50% and is < 3% in African-Americans. The incidence increases up to the age of 20 years and then remains constant. This lesion is rarely seen in children < 5 years of age.

4. Spondylolysis is strongly associated with what other adolescent spinal condition?

Spondylolysis is seen frequently in association with Scheuermann's kyphosis, in which the excessive lumbar lordosis places the L5–S1 articulation under shear. A study published in 1987 demonstrated a 50% incidence of spondylolysis in 18 patients with Scheuermann's kyphosis. The authors recommend obtaining oblique lumbar spine radiographs in patients with Scheuermann's kyphosis who develop low back pain.

5. Name the five common types of spondylolisthesis.

The five common types of spondylolisthesis are dysplastic, isthmic, degenerative, traumatic, and pathologic.

6. Describe the congenital defect associated with dysplastic spondylolisthesis.

The congenital defect associated with dysplastic spondylolisthesis is a deficiency in the inferior facets of L5 and/or the superior facets of S1, along with the elongation of the pars interarticularis. The pars have been likened to "pulled taffy."

7. What is the most common presenting symptom of spondylolysis or spondylolisthesis?

In both children and adults the most common presenting symptom of spondylolysis and spondylolisthesis is pain. In one study, spondylolisthesis was found in 47% of adolescent athletes complaining of back pain. The pain is usually lumbar in location and mild, but may radiate to the posterior thighs with increasing degrees of slip.

8. What repetitive motion has been postulated as the inciting factor in the development of isthmic spondylolisthesis?

The defect in isthmic spondylolisthesis has been attributed to repetitive hyperextension, which causes shear of the posterior elements.

9. Which sports have been linked to the development of isthmic spondylolisthesis?

Sports with cyclic flexion-extension activity have been positively associated with isthmic spondylolisthesis. An increased incidence has been reported in gymnasts, football lineman, new Army recruits, and weightlifters.

10. What physical findings have been associated with spondylolisthesis?

Several physical findings are commonly associated with spondylolisthesis. Hamstring tightness is very common, causing a stiff-legged gait with a short stride length ("pelvic waddle"). Forward bending is limited. Pain may be found on palpation of the paraspinal muscles. If the slip is severe, a step-off may be seen at the L5–S1 level. The buttocks may appear heart-shaped due to the verticality of the sacrum. The abdomen will protrude, causing the appearance of a transverse abdominal crease.

11. Describe the difference between the Scotty dog sign and the Greyhound sign.

The **Scotty dog sign** is the radiographic appearance of the pars interarticularis defect seen on oblique films in isthmic spondylolisthesis. The actual defect resembles a collar around the Scotty dog's neck. The **greyhound sign** is the radiographic appearance of the elongated pars interarticularis of L5 seen in chronic progressive slips.

12. Define stress reaction.

Stress reaction is the term used to describe the phase of spondylolysis before the appearance of the actual bony defect. Radiographically, a stress reaction can be associated with sclerosis or elongation of the pars. It is often seen with on the contralateral side of a unilateral spondylolysis.

13. How long after symptoms of back pain start before a technetium bone scan will show increased uptake at the level of the pars interarticularis?

A technetium bone scan will delineate an acute lesion within 5–7 days of the onset of symptoms.

14. What is the best study to diagnose spondylolysis in the symptomatic patient with normal radiographs and bone scan?

Single photon emission computed tomography (SPECT) has proven effective in cases in which positive symptoms exist in the presence of normal radiographs and bone scans. This test has been shown to be the most sensitive method of diagnosing stress reactions, making early diagnosis possible and treatment possible before the development of an established lysis.

15. How is the slip percentage and slip angle determined?

Slip percentage is measured by representing the distance between the posterior border of the body of L5 and the posterior border of the body of S1 as a percentage of the anteroposterior diameter of S1. The slip angle is measured by drawing a perpendicular to a line drawn along the posterior border of the sacrum, and another parallel to the inferior endplate of L5. The angle subtended by the intersection of these two lines is the slip angle.

16. How is spondylolisthesis classified?

The commonly accepted classification system for spondylolisthesis is Meyerding's, in which no anterior slip of the upper vertebral body on the lower is grade 0; 1–25% slippage is grade I; 26–50% slippage is grade II; 51–75% is grade III; and 76–100% is grade IV.

Complete anterior dislocation of the upper on lower vertebral body is referred to as spondyloptosis.

17. What percentage of spondylolisthesis will have occurred at the time of the first radiograph in the symptomatic patient?

According to a study of 272 patients by Seitsalo et al, 90% of the slip had occurred by the time the patient was first seen.

18. Which spinal segments are most commonly affected by spondylolysis/-listhesis?

The most common spondylolisthetic level is L5/S1, followed by L4/L5, and then L3/L4. Slips higher than L5 are usually seen in young adults and not in children or adolescents.

19. What is the treatment of choice for spondylolysis and grade I spondylolisthesis?

The treatment of choice for spondylolysis and grade I spondylolisthesis associated with a history of recent injury and short duration of symptoms involves restriction of any aggravating activities and a regimen of muscle strengthening for the back and abdomen. Healing may be monitored by the resolution of back pain and hamstring tightness. If symptoms do not resolve and a bone scan shows increased uptake in the area of the pars, a program of rest, NSAIDs, and the application of a TLSO or cast with a pantaloon extension down one thigh usually will alleviate symptoms. The pantaloon portion of the brace may be removed after pain resolves. If symptoms persist despite immobilization and the bone scan becomes "cold," primary repair of small defects (≤ 7 mm) with internal fixation and bone grafting has been successful.

A, L4/L5 spondylolysis. *B,* Anteroposterior (AP) radiograph after fusion with bone graft and fixation. *C,* Lateral radiograph after fusion with bone graft and fixation.

20. What is the Gill procedure and what role does it play in the treatment of spondylolysis-listhesis?

The Gill procedure involves complete removal of the loose laminar fragment posterior to the lysis, and has no role in the treatment of spondylolisthesis because it further destabilizes the spine.

21. What is the treatment of choice for spondylolisthesis of 25–50%?

Grade II slips in asymptomatic patients should be followed every 4–6 months with spot lateral radiographs of the lumbosacral junction until the end of growth. In situ posterior fusion without instrumentation of L5–S1 is recommended for patients with progressive slips, persistent back pain, or neurologic deficits.

22. What is the treatment of choice for spondylolisthesis of 50–75%?

In grade III slips, the procedure of choice is in situ posterior fusion, including L4 in the arthrodesis. Intertransverse fusion may be performed by either a midline incision with two paraspinal fascial incisions or by two paraspinal skin incisions. Anterior fusion has been reported with good results in adolescents, but carries greater potential morbidity than the posterior fusion.

23. What are the current indications for reduction of spondylolisthesis?

Reduction of spondylolisthesis is currently reserved for high-grade slips (grade III and IV) with a sagittal imbalance that is functionally debilitating, cosmetically unacceptable, or in the presence of a neurologic deficit in which a decompressive laminectomy would jeopardize the fusion.

24. What methods are currently used for slip reduction?

Current methods for slip reduction include closed reduction by gradual pelvic extension +/-, halo-femoral or halo-pelvic traction followed by pantaloon casting after in situ fusion, closed reduction and anterior fusion with pantaloon casting, or posterior transpedicular reduction and fusion with instrumentation.

BIBLIOGRAPHY

1. Bradford DS: Spondylolysis and spondylolisthesis. In Lonstein JE, Winter RB, Bradford DS, Ogilvie JW (eds): Moe's Textbook of Scoliosis and Other Spinal Deformities, 2nd ed. Philadelphia, W.B. Saunders, 1995.

2. Bradford DS, Hu SS: Spondylolysis and spondylolisthesis. In Weinstein SL (ed): The Pediatric Spine. New York, Raven Press, 1994.
3. Freeman BL: Scoliosis and kyphosis. In Canale ST (ed): Campbell's Operative Orthopaedics, 9th ed. St. Louis, Mosby, 1998, pp 2952–2961.
4. Ginsburg GM, Bassett GS: Back pain in children and adolescents: Evaluation and differential diagnosis. J Am Acad Orthop 5:67–78, 1997.
5. Hensinger RN: Current concepts review: Spondylolysis and spondylolisthesis in children and adolescents. J Bone Joint Surg 71A: 1098–1107, 1989.
6. Jackson DW, Wiltse LL, Cirincione RJ: Spondylolysis in the female gymnast. Clin Orthop 117:68–72, 1976.
7. Ogilvie JW, Sherman J: Spondylolysis in Scheuermann's disease. Spine 12:251–253, 1987.
8. Seitsalo S, Osterman K, Hyvarinen H, et al: Progression of spondylolisthesis in children and adolescents: A long-term follow-up of 272 patients. Spine 16:417–421, 1991.
9. Wiltse LL, Winter RB: Terminology and measurement of spondylolisthesis. J Bone Joint Surg 65A: 768–772, 1983.

52. SPINAL TRAUMA

Randall D. Neumann, M.D.

1. Discuss the mechanism of spinal injury.

It is helpful to think of the spine as divided into three columns. The anterior column includes the anterior longitudinal ligament, the anterior portion of the annulus, and the anterior half of the vertebral body. The middle column consists of the posterior longitudinal ligament, the posterior portion of the annulus, and the posterior portion of the vertebral body. The posterior column is made up of the pedicles, facets, lamina, and posterior ligamentous complex, including the interspinal ligaments, ligamentum flavum, and facet joint capsule. These columns may fail individually or in combination as a result of four basic mechanisms of injury: (1) compression, (2) distraction, (3) rotation, and (4) sheer forces. These forces result in the most common major types of spinal fractures.

2. What is the conus medullaris?

The conus medullaris is the end of the spinal cord and is usually found at the level of the first or second lumbar vertebra in a vertebral disc.

3. What is the cauda equina?

Below the level of the conus medullaris, the spinal canal is filled with the cauda equina, which consists of the motor and sensory nerve roots. These roots are less likely to be injured because they have more room in the canal and are not tethered to the same degree as the spinal cord.

4. Describe the sensory levels in the lower extremity.

Sensory Levels in the Lower Extremity

SENSORY LEVEL	AREA OF INNERVATION
L2	Anterior thigh
L3	Anterior knee
L4	Anterior lateral ankle
L5	Dorsum of the great and second toe
S1	Lateral side of the foot
S2	Posterior calf
S2–S5	Perianal sensation

5. Describe the muscle groups and their respective nerve root innervations in lower extremity examination.

Muscle Groups and Nerve Root Innervations

NERVE ROOT	MUSCLE GROUP
L1–L2	Hip adductors
L3–L4	Knee extension
L5–S1	Knee flexion
L5	Great toe extension
S1	Great toe flexion

6. What is neurogenic shock?
Neurogenic shock is defined as vascular hypotension with bradycardia as a result of spinal injury. Neurogenic shock is attributed to the traumatic disruption of the sympathetic outflow and unopposed vagal tone.

7. What is spinal shock?
Spinal shock is defined as a dysfunction of the nervous tissue of the spinal cord based on physiologic rather than structural disruption; it occurs after spinal cord injury. Shock is resolved when reflex arcs, including the bulbocavernosus reflex, resume function.

8. What is the bulbocavernosus reflex?
The bulbocavernosus reflex involves the S1, S2, and S3 nerve roots and a spinal cord-mediated reflex arch. Bulbocavernosus reflexes are tested by compressing the glans penis and observing contraction of the anal sphincter. When this reflex returns, spinal shock is resolved.

9. What is sacral sparing?
Sacral sparing means that an incomplete spinal cord lesion is present, with at least partial structural continuity of the white-matter long tracts. Sacral sparing is evidenced by perianal sensation, rectal motor function, and great toe flexor activity.

10. What is complete spinal cord injury?
A complete spinal cord injury is manifested by total motor and sensory loss distal to the injury level. When the bulbocavernosus reflex is positive but no sacral sensation or motor function has returned, the paralysis is permanent and complete in most patients.

11. What is an incomplete spinal cord injury?
In an incomplete spinal cord injury some motor or sensory function is spared distal to the cord injury. Several types of incomplete spinal cord syndromes have been identified:
1. **Brown-Séquard syndrome**, an injury to either half of the spinal cord, results either from lamina or pedicle fracture or from penetrating injury. Symptoms include motor weakness on the side of the lesion and contralateral loss of pain and temperature sensation. Prognosis for recovery is good; neurologic improvement often is significant.
2. **Anterior cord syndrome** is usually caused by a hyperflexion injury in which bone compresses the anterior spinal artery and cord. Patients have complete motor loss and loss of pain and temperature discrimination below the level of injury. Posterior columns, including deep-touch position sense and vibratory sensation, are spared. Prognosis for recovery is poor.
3. **Posterior cord syndrome**, which involves the dorsal columns of the spinal cord, is characterized by loss of proprioceptive vibratory sense with sparing of sensory and motor function. This syndrome is rare.
4. **Central cord syndrome**, which is the most common type of incomplete spinal cord injury, involves destruction of the central area of spinal cord. Centrally located arm tracts are most severely affected, whereas the leg tracts are affected to a lesser extent. Sensation is variably

spared. Central cord syndromes usually result from hyperextension injury in an older person with preexisting osteoarthritis of the spine or from flexion injuries in younger patients.

12. List the classification of thoracolumbar spine fractures.
   1. Compression
   2. Burst fracture
   3. Flexion–distraction injuries
   4. Extension injuries
   5. Dislocations

13. Describe a compression fracture.
   A compression fracture results in a typical anterior wedging of the vertebral body in the anterior column. The middle and posterior columns generally are not involved. Compression fractures are usually stable and rarely involve a neurologic deficit.

Compression fracture.

14. What is a burst fracture?
   A burst fracture is a fracture of the anterior and middle columns; varying degrees of the fracture fragments are displaced into the neural canal. Other common findings include spreading of the posterior elements and an increase in interpedicular distance.

Burst fracture.

15. What is a flexion–distraction injury?

A flexion–distraction injury, also known as a Chance fracture, is common in motor vehicle accidents when the victim is wearing only a lap seatbelt. The fracture involves the anterior, middle, and posterior columns or the posterior ligaments. With a true flexion–distraction injury, neurologic compromise occurs only with dislocation.

Chance fracture.

26. Describe a fracture–dislocation.

A fracture–dislocation involves disruption of all three columns by a combination of anterior compression with distraction and rotation. On the anteroposterior radiograph, significant translation is seen. This fracture is highly unstable and associated with significant neurologic deficit, dural tears, and infraabdominal injuries.

Fracture–dislocation.

17. Describe dislocations.

Dislocations are considered to be unstable because all three columns have failed. Usually multiple forces are involved, including rotation, distraction, compression, and sheer forces. Dislocations are highly unstable and are often associated with a neurologic deficit.

18. Describe an extension injury to the thoracolumbar spine.

When the lumbar spine is hyperextended, the usual result is an anterior vertebral body avulsion fracture accompanied by fractures of the posterior columns, including the spinous process, lamina, and occasionally pedicles. These fractures are generally stable.

19. What other fractures occur?

• **Transverse process fractures** result from blunt trauma, particularly at L5.
• **Spinous process avulsions** are stable injuries related to distraction.
• **Facet fractures** are uncommon but may occur in patients with prior laminectomies or stress fractures.

20. What radiographic examinations are necessary for patients with spinal cord injury?

Initial assessment consists of anterior and posterior lateral and oblique radiographs of the spine. Computed tomography (CT) demonstrates bony impingement on the neural canal and assesses stability. Conventional tomography is advantageous in the evaluation of transverse or axially oriented injuries, horizontal lamina fractures, and some facet injuries. Magnetic resonance imaging (MRI) may demonstrate more precisely the status of the intervertebral disc, potential sites of ligamentous injury, epidural hematoma, and extent of spinal cord injury.

21. Describe some of the various MRI findings that may be found with patients with spinal cord injuries.

1. Edema is seen as fusiform enlargement of the cord with increased signal intensity on T2-weighted images.
2. Hematoma is characterized by decreased signal intensity on T2 images acutely and is often surrounded by a halo of T2 enhancement from adjacent edema.
3. Extrinsic cord compression by osseous elements, soft tissue, or fluid.
4. Disk herniation
5. Transection

22. How often does noncontiguous, multilevel spinal injury occur?

Multilevel spinal cord injury is now more readily recognized with MRI. Various studies show an incidence between 4.5 and 16% of noncontiguous, multilevel spinal cord injury.

23. Describe the management of compression fractures.

Compression fractures generally are stable and rarely involve neurologic compromise. The patient may be treated effectively by hyperextension brace or casting. If the compression is minimal, the patient may be treated by hyperextension exercises and the avoidance of compression loads for approximately 3 months. Compression > 50% of the vertebral body height or multiple adjacent compression fractures are considered potentially unstable. Some authors recommend open reduction and internal fixation with posterior instrumentation and arthrodesis.

24. Describe the treatments for unstable thoracic fractures.

A posterior approach is commonly used. Reduction and fixation are performed with distraction and posterior instrumentation. Posterior instrumentation options include rods, sleeves, sublaminar wires, screws, and hooks. Iliac bone graft is used for fusion.

25. Describe the treatment for unstable thoracolumbar and lumbar fractures.

An anterior, posterior, or combined approach may be used. Various plates and screw devices are available anteriorly or posteriorly. Pedicle screws with rods or plates are placed posteriorly. For significant anterior decompression with removal of the vertebral body, an iliac strut graft is used.

26. What surgical approaches may be used for spinal fractures and dislocations?

1. **Anterior:** commonly used for anterior decompression of the cord by removing portions of the retropulsed vertebral body. Iliac strut grafts and plates are used for stabilization. Used mostly in the thoracolumbar junction and lumbar spine.

2. **Posterior:** used in thoracic spine in conjunction with posterior instrumentation and fusion. Laminectomy alone should never be the sole treatment with unstable spine injuries.

3. **Posterior lateral:** usually used in the thoracolumbar spine, removing portions of the transverse process and pedicle. Instrumentation and fusion may be difficult through this approach.

27. Discuss the common posterior instrumentation options for spinal stabilization.

1. Harrington rods: rod and hook device for distraction of the fracture.

2. Multiple hooks and rod: variation of the Harrington rod using hooks, rods, sleeves, and wire to increase translational and rotational stability.

3. Luque: rod with sublaminar wires.

4. Plate and screw constructs: wires or plates with pedicle screws.

BIBLIOGRAPHY

1. Bohlman HH, Ducker TB, Levine MD: Spine trauma in adults. In Herkowitz HN, Garfin SR, Balderston RA, et al (eds): Rothman-Simeone The Spine, 4th ed. Philadelphia, W.B. Saunders, 1999, pp 889–1070.
2. Bucholz RW, Gill K: Classification of injuries to the thoracolumbar spine. Orthop Clin North Am 17:67–73, 1986.
3. Frymoyer JW (ed): Orthopedic Knowledge Update Four. Rosemont, IL, American Academy of Orthopaedic Surgeons, 1993, pp 461–473.
4. Haher TR: Thoracic and lumbar fractures: Diagnosis and management. In Bridwell KH, DeWald RL (eds): The Textbook of Spinal Surgery. Philadelphia, J.B. Lippincott, 1991, pp 857–910.
5. Leventhal MR: Fractures, dislocations, and fracture dislocations of the spine. In Canale ST (ed): Campbell's Operative Orthopedics, 9th ed. St. Louis, Mosby, 1998, pp 2704–2790.
6. Spivak JM, Vaccaro AR, Cotler JM: Thoracolumbar Spine Trauma: I. Evaluation and classification. J Am Acad Orthop Surg 3:345–352, 1995.
7. Spivak JM, Vaccaro AR, Cotler JM: Thoracolumbar Spine Trauma: II. Principles of management. J Am Acad Orthop Surg 3:353–360, 1995.
8. Stauffer ES: Fractures and dislocations of the spine. In Rockwood CA, Green DP, Bucholz RW (eds): Rockwood and Green's Fractures in Adults, 3rd ed. Philadelphia, J.B. Lippincott, 1991, pp 1309–1395.
9. Vaccaro AR, An HS, Betz RR, et al: The management of acute spinal trauma: Pre-hospital and in-hospital emergency care. AAOS Instr Course Lect 46:113–125, 1997.

VII. Hip and Pelvis

53. EVALUATION OF HIP DISEASE

Randall D. Neumann, M.D.

1. What is the normal range of motion for the hip?

Extension	0°
Flexion	120°
Abduction	45°
Adduction	30°
External rotation	45°
Internal rotation	45°

2. What is pelvic obliquity?

Normally the iliac crests are at the same relative level on physical examination. When they are at different levels, the descriptive term is pelvic obliquity. This condition may be due to scoliosis or contractures about the hip. The most common contractures are adduction and flexion contractures.

3. In degenerative arthritis of the hip, where do most patients complain of pain?

Most patients describe pain in the groin area, with possible radiation into the anterior portion of the thigh. Patients rarely describe buttock or posterior pain, and the pain rarely radiates below the knee.

4. Differentiate referred pain from the spine and hip pain.

Most patients with hip pathology describe pain anterior to the hip or along the greater trochanteric region. Spinal pain usually involves the buttocks and posterior thigh.

5. What is the Thomas test?

The Thomas test assesses flexion contracture of the hip. Normal flexion allows the anterior portion of the thigh to rest against the abdomen, almost touching the chest. The patient holds one leg to the abdomen and lowers the other leg until it is flat on the examination table. If the hip does not extend fully, the patient has a fixed flexion contracture or a positive Thomas test.

6. What is a Trendelenburg test?

The Trendelenburg test assesses the gluteus medius muscle and the hip joint. The examiner stands behind the patient and observes the dimples overlying the posterior-superior iliac spine. The patients is asked to stand on one leg. As the patient stands erect, the gluteus medius muscle on the supported side should contract to keep the pelvis level. If the pelvis remains unsupported and the opposite side drops, the gluteus medius muscle is either weak or nonfunctioning, and the test is positive.

7. Describe a patient with a "hip limp."

During midstance the hip is displaced laterally by approximately one inch to the weight-bearing side. With a hip limp, lateral displacement is accentuated and results in an exaggerated limp.

8. What is the most common abnormality of patients with a congenitally dislocated hip?

Patients present with adduction contracture of the hip at 90° of flexion. Unilateral dislocation generally results in shortening of the involved leg.

9. What physical abnormality is seen in patients with slipped capital femoral epiphysis?

Because the femoral head is displaced in a posterior-inferior direction, patients generally have increased external rotation and diminished internal rotation of the leg. As the hip is flexed, it drifts into external rotation with more acute flexion.

10. Which motion is usually the last to be affected in patients with degenerative arthritis of the hip?

Most patients lose internal and external rotation before abduction and adduction. Flexion is usually maintained until severe changes occur.

11. What is the most common contracture in patients with cerebral palsy?

Patients with cerebral palsy generally have an adduction and flexion contracture of the hip. This contracture, along with scoliosis, may lead to the progressive development of dislocation.

12. What is the Ortolani maneuver?

The hip is gently abducted and the thigh is raised with the fingers to reduce the hip. When performing this test, the examiner should use one hand to stabilize the pelvis. The Ortolani maneuver is used to assess dislocation in a congenitally dislocated hip.

13. What is the Barlow test?

With the thumb placed on the inner aspect of the thigh and the hip adducted, longitudinal pressure is exerted on the thigh, pushing it toward the examination table. A dislocatable hip then becomes completely displaced, and when the leg is allowed to abduct, the hip reduces. The Barlow test establishes the diagnosis of a dislocatable hip.

14. What test is used to differentiate hip pathology from spine pathology?

The patient is placed on the examination table in a supine position and asked to perform a straight-leg raise with the heel approximately 12 inches off the table. Patients with hip pathology, such as fracture and degenerative arthritis, are unable to maintain the leg in the straight position. Reproduction of groin pain is common. Patients with spine pathology rarely have difficulty with this maneuver.

15. What physical abnormality is seen in patients with femoral neck or intertrochanteric fractures?

Patients who present with an intertrochanteric or femoral neck fracture have a shortening of the involved leg in external rotation. Generally the patient is unable to move the leg and finds it quite painful to place the hip through a passive range of motion.

16. List areas of tenderness about the hip and possible diagnoses.

Area of Tenderness	Diagnoses
Femoral triangle	Hernia
Trochanter	Trochanteric bursitis
	Snapping hip
Sciatic notch	Sciatic disorder
	Radiculopathy
Posterior trochanter	Pyriformis syndrome
Posterior iliac spine	Sacroiliac joint pathology
Sacrum	Insufficiency fracture
Coccyx	Coccydynia
Iliac crest	Iliac apophysitis
Anterior-superior iliac spine	Avulsion fracture

Area of Tenderness	Diagnoses
Iliac wing	Pelvic fracture
	Metastatic disease
	Primary tumors
Pubic rami	Stress fracture
	Metastatic disease
Proximal femur	Stress fracture
	Tumor

17. What is the differential diagnosis of patients who have catching in the hip?
- Arthritic conditions, including osteoarthritis and rheumatoid arthritis
- Loose bodies from chondral lesions or osteochondral lesions
- Pigmented villonodular synovitis
- Snapping hip syndrome

18. What range of motion test is a quick test for hip pathology?
The figure-four test is a quick test for hip pathology. The patient is in a supine position. The examiner flexes, externally rotates, and abducts the hip to place the heel across the uninvolved knee. Patients with hip pathology generally have diminished range of motion and are unable to perform the maneuver or do so without significant pain.

19. What radiographs are used to assess patients with hip pathology?
The standard radiographs are anteroposterior views of the pelvis, including the iliac crest, inferior portion of the spine, and hip joints. Cross-table lateral radiographs evaluate the lateral aspect of the hip and can be taken without moving the affected hip. In patients who have sustained trauma, inlet and outlet views of the pelvis, as described by Tile, are also recommended. If fractures involving the acetabulum are suspected, obturator and iliac oblique views of the acetabulum are taken.

20. When is hip aspiration useful?
Hip aspiration is extremely helpful in differentiating septic arthritis and transient synovitis of the hip in children. It may also be used to assess infectious processes after surgery, including hemiarthroplasty and total hip replacement. Hip aspiration for synovial fluid analysis and subsequent injection of steroids may be useful in differentiating hip pathology from spinal pathology.

21. What are the indications for tomography?
Tomography is normally used in victims of trauma. Its use has become limited, however, with the advent of computed tomography (CT). Plain tomography is still indicated in patients with nonunion of femoral neck fractures and internal fixation devices. It also may be helpful after reduction of a hip dislocation to look for loose bony fragments. The configuration of an acetabular fracture may be viewed on tomograms if a CT scan is not available. Tomograms also are helpful in evaluating the extent of stress fractures or femoral neck fractures.

22. Which hip disease processes are evaluated with magnetic resonance imaging (MRI)?
MRI has proved quite successful in evaluating transient osteoporosis of the hip, avascular necrosis, and both benign and malignant processes.

23. What are the indications for bone scan?
Bone scans are indicated for patients with hip disease that is not clearly defined by physical examination or plain radiographs. Examples include questionable infections; stress fractures; benign tumors, such as osteoid osteomas; and nondisplaced femoral neck fractures in the elderly. Bone scans are highly sensitive but generally nonspecific for differentiating disease processes.

24. Which areas are commonly affected with stress fractures about the hip?
Athletes may have stress fractures in the femoral neck and pubic rami, which usually are seen on plain radiographs. Patients with osteomalacia may develop bilateral stress fractures in the subtrochanteric region.

25. Which patients benefit from CT scans of the hip and pelvis?
CT scans are indicated for patients with traumatic conditions; they are highly effective in delineating the extent of fractures involving the acetabulum, iliac crest, and sacrum. Bony fragments in the acetabulum after hip dislocation are readily identified. Three-dimensional reconstructions of computed tomography are indicated preoperatively for difficult revisions of total hip arthroplasties and reconstruction procedures with ill-defined anatomy.

26. What are the indications for arthroscopy of the hip?
The following diagnostic and therapeutic objectives are indications for arthroscopic surgery of the hip:
1. Evaluation of a painful hip in which the diagnosis remains in question after other diagnostic techniques have failed
2. Exploration and debridement of interarticular debris after fracture dislocation of the hip
3. Exploration and removal of foreign bodies
4. Synovial loose body debridement
5. Synovectomy for pigmented villonodular synovitis
6. Synovial biopsy
7. Evaluation of osteochondritis dissecans
Arthroscopic surgery of the hip is quite demanding and should be done only by the most experienced arthroscopists.

BIBLIOGRAPHY

1. Glick JM: Hip arthroscopy. In McGinty JB, Casper RB, Jackson RW, Poehling GG (eds): Operative Arthroscopy. New York, Raven Press, 1991, pp 663–676.
2. Rockwood CA, Green DP, Bucholz RW, et al (eds): Fractures, 4th ed. Philadelphia, Lippincott-Raven, 1996.

54. PEDIATRIC HIP DISEASE

Walter W. Huurman, M.D.

1. What is developmental dysplasia of the hip?
Developmental dysplasia of the hip is a progressive condition in which the hip structures do not develop adequately. The condition has three characteristic components: (1) varying degrees of abnormality in the slope of the acetabulum; (2) excessive laxity of the hip joint that over time permits the femoral head to slide gradually upward and laterally out of its normal relationship with the acetabulum; and (3) abnormal torsion (rotation) of the upper end of the femoral shaft, which creates an abnormal relationship between the femoral head and the acetabulum. As a consequence, three stages may be identified: (1) the head of the femur is retained within an inadequate acetabulum, with minimal physical findings; (2) the head of the femur has moved slightly away from the acetabular medial wall; and (3) the head of the femur has slipped out of the acetabulum. The first two stages probably should be considered precursors to dislocation. Unfortunately, the examination may be normal in an infant or child at risk for developing a true dislocation.

2. How does developmental dysplasia differ from congenital dislocation of the hip?

The term *congenital* implies a condition present at birth. It has been recognized recently that hip dislocation may develop during the first year of life due to dysplasia of the hip's anatomic components; dysplasia without dislocation is often clinically undetectable at birth. The term *developmental dysplasia* encompasses hip dislocation developing in utero as well as that occurring postnatally.

3. What is subluxation of the hip?

By definition subluxation is a partial dislocation. The head of the femur has not completely lost contact with the articular surface of the acetabulum; therefore, physical findings may be entirely normal or reveal some degree of laxity on physical exam when the examiner attempts to passively dislocate the hip (Barlow test).

4. Describe the dislocated hip.

In a true dislocation of the hip, the head of the femur has completely lost contact with the articular surface of the acetabulum and is most commonly displaced posteriorly and upward out of the acetabulum. Various external factors may produce dislocation in the presence of a hypoplastic acetabulum. Efforts to bring the hip into extension tend to displace the hip laterally and superiorly due to tightness in the psoas muscle-tendon and ultimately may lead to dislocation. Use of confining swaddling clothes that bring the hip downward into premature extension may explain the high incidence of developmental dislocation in northern Italy around the turn of the century. Risk factors that point to the possibility of developmental dysplasia are now fairly well documented: (1) first child, (2) female sex, (3) breech delivery, and (4) family history. Family history of infantile hip disease in an infant, whether it be dysplasia or dislocation, should raise a red flag. Other coexisting contributory factors include teratologic and neurologic deficits, particularly meningoceles and cerebral palsy. In addition, the physician should be wary when abnormalities are noted in the physical examination of the lower extremity of a newborn infant, particularly the Galeazzi sign, Barlow test, and the Ortolani maneuver (see question 5).

5. Discuss the physical examination of a newborn infant, particularly with reference to the hip.

The examination must be carried out with all clothing removed and the infant placed in a warm, comfortable setting on a flat examining table—**not** in a bassinet or crib. The infant should be checked visually, particularly for neck motion and any abnormalities of the low back, such as dimpling over the distal sacrum or at the sacrococcygeal joint. There are three specific tests for hip abnormality, all of which may be normal in an infant who has only dysplasia when instability has not yet developed.

1. The **Galeazzi sign** is an evaluation of apparent thigh length. The child lies on his or her back, the thighs are held together and raised to a 90° hip and knee flexion position, and the level of the knees evaluated. Any difference in height between the knees should precipitate concern and further examination. Because a positive Galeazzi sign relies upon apparent shortening of one femur in comparison with a normal contralateral femur, it is negative in the presence of bilateral dislocation.

2. **Barlow's test**, which assesses the potential for passive dislocation of a located hip, also is done with the infant supine on an examining table. The hip and knee are flexed 90° and the thigh is held at right angles to the trunk in a slightly adducted position; gentle pressure is applied downward on the knee in an effort to slide the head of the femur out of a normal relationship to the acetabulum. The examiner looks for a piston-type motion, which may or may not be accompanied by a palpable clunk or jerking sensation as the femoral head slides out of the acetabulum.

3. The **Ortolani maneuver** usually is combined with Barlow's test. When the hip is gently abducted from 90° of flexion and adduction, a resistance may be felt. The examiner holds the knee flexed and the fingers gently hold the proximal femur between the thumb on the medial side and the index and long finger laterally at the greater trochanter, pressing upward on the greater trochanter. If abducting the hip with a little pressure over the trochanter produces a clunk that is

felt (rather than heard), the Ortolani test is positive. The "clicks" that are frequently felt in a new-born infant when the hips are passively moved are simply the iliopsoas tendon sliding over the crest of the ilium or the iliotibial band sliding across the greater trochanter. Ortolani's test may be negative with a completely dislocated hip; a negative test is simply a sign that the hip is firmly dislocated and cannot be reduced with manipulation in the nonanesthetized child.

If any physical findings are at all suspicious, further evaluation is necessary.

6. Describe the physical findings in a newborn infant with a developmentally dislocated hip.

If unilateral, Galeazzi's sign should be positive; Barlow's test is negative, and Ortolani's test may be positive or negative. Abduction limitation, the classic sign for dislocation, is not reliably present in a newborn infant.

7. Describe the physical findings in a 6-month-old infant with a developmentally dislocated hip.

The findings are usually fairly clear: short thigh and multiple folds in the medial skin on the dislocated side are evidence of proximal migration of the skeletal structures in the thigh. The trochanter is displaced upward in comparison with the normal side. The perineum on the side of the dislocation is broadened, indicating that the femoral head is displaced laterally. Hip abduction may be limited, but relying on this finding alone is dangerous.

8. Describe the physical findings in a 2-year-old child with a developmentally dislocated hip.

The usual presenting complaint is a limp; the limp of a unilateral hip dislocation is classic. The lurching gait has a tendency toward a Trendelenburg sway. This type of sway is not as clear in a young child as in a teenager or an adult, but it is still present in an effort to swing the center of gravity over the unstable hip joint. Parents often complain of unilateral toe walking. This is due to extremity shortening; they also may complain of intoeing or outtoeing. Bilateral hip dislocation often leads to a waddling gait that is frequently overlooked. A detailed examination (similar to that of a 6-month-old infant) of the lower extremity reveals shortening of the thigh, multiple skin folds, broad perineum, prominence of the trochanter, and shortening of the distance between the crest of the ilium and the tip of the trochanter. One of the best ways of measuring this distance is simply to use one's fingertips as a guide and compare the two sides.

9. What is the best radiographic evaluation?

Radiographic evaluation depends entirely on the age at first presentation. Ultrasound studies have changed the imaging evaluation of the hip joint in **newborn** infants. Such studies should be done as a dynamic test by an experienced ultrasonographer. The experienced examiner first visualizes the bony elements of the acetabulum and then identifies the elements that are inadequate. Laxity in the capsule may be noted when an effort is made to displace the femoral head out of the acetabulum or away from the medial wall of the acetabulum. Femoral head subluxation visible during real-time ultrasound scanning is evidence of hip joint laxity, which poses an immediate risk. In its more severe form, the femoral head displaces out of the acetabulum. If any of the findings are positive, anteroposterior radiographs of the pelvis (note: **pelvis**, not hip) should be done for confirmation. Infants older than 3–4 months are best diagnosed using anteroposterior and frog x-rays of the pelvis.

10. Describe the complete diagnosis in a newborn infant with hip abnormalities.

The best approach is to say simply that the hip is dysplastic and then describe the type: shallow acetabulum, hip joint laxity, subluxable hip, or dislocatable hip. A dislocatable hip should be additionally described as either reducible or not reducible.

11. What is the treatment for a newborn with developmental dysplasia of the hip?

At present the treatment of choice is a Pavlik harness, applied by an individual who is knowledgeable in harness fit, desired position, and potential complications. The principal effect of the

Pavlik harness is to hold the hips in flexion while permitting a moderate degree of abduction in the horizontal plane. This effect allows both maintenance of a stable position of the hip and a reasonable degree of motion, which is necessary for development of normal joint anatomy. More rigid braces and splints are also used but lack the freedom of motion that a Pavlik harness allows. If the hip is dislocated and not simply dysplastic or subluxable at birth, it is necessary to check the harness fairly frequently; if hip reduction has not been obtained by the time the harness has been worn for 3–4 weeks, additional treatment is necessary.

12. Describe the Pavlik harness.

The Pavlik harness was described first in 1958 by Arnold Pavlik in Czechoslovakia and was introduced into the United States several years later. The harness incorporates a chest component similar to ordinary suspenders with a cerclage strap around the thorax, forming a suspending medium for two stirrup-type boots. The boots are connected to the cerclage component by straps that hold the hips in flexion and control the degree of abduction. The anterior strap acts to flex, whereas the posterior strap maintains abduction. The harness should be worn continuously for the first weeks, depending on the developmental status of the hip. As the hip stabilizes, ultrasound examinations should be repeated at 1, 4, and 8 weeks, and a pelvic x-ray should be obtained at 12 weeks and at the end of treatment. Patients should be followed after conclusion of harness treatment by an x-ray examination at 6 months of age with the hip held in both the "frog" and neutral positions.

13. What complications may occur with use of the Pavlik harness?

Osteonecrosis of the femoral head, failure of reduction, and femoral nerve praxia.

14. What is the treatment for a 6–9-month-old infant with a newly diagnosed hip dislocation?

If a hip dislocation is identified in this age group, two choices of treatment are available. One may use a Pavlik harness with the hope that over a period of 2–3 weeks the hip will reduce and may then be held in a reduced position by a more rigid brace. If this method fails, the second choice is a closed method of treatment. The established routine is to put the infant in traction for a short period of time with the hips flexed about 45°. Occasionally this is done at home, but generally it is done in the hospital. The position of the hip joint is followed sequentially during the traction period with radiographs. The femoral head initially rides high and lateral in relation to the acetabulum. The goal is to pull the femur downward to the point that the femoral head is at station zero, i.e., opposite the triradiate cartilage. Palpation for hip reduction is carried out every day or two during traction, and when treatment has brought the hip downward to an adequate relationship with the acetabulum, the child is examined under anesthesia. An arthrogram will make certain that the hip indeed enters the acetabulum properly, and frequently iliopsoas and adductor tenotomies are performed. The child is then placed in a well molded cast in the "safe" position, i.e., 90° of flexion and abduction of no more than 60° with the hips in a stable, reduced position. Casting is continued for as many months as the child is old, up to a maximum of 6 months.

15. What is the treatment for a 2-year-old child with a newly diagnosed hip dislocation?

A newly diagnosed hip dislocation in a 2-year-old child probably requires surgery. By this time the capsule of the hip and the musculature above the hip joint are shortened enough that a procedure must be performed to permit easy introduction of the femoral head into the acetabulum. The surgery, which is best done by a pediatric orthopedist, consists of femoral shortening, opening the acetabulum and introducing the femoral head, and then augmenting or repositioning the acetabulum and/or proximal femur through reconstruction.

16. What is the indication for open reduction of a developmentally dislocated hip?

The obvious indication is irreducibility by closed means. As a rule, open reduction of the hip joint involves acetabular augmentation if the hip is not stable after reduction. Acetabular modeling without augmentation at the time of operative reduction can be expected to progress only if the hip is well reduced and held in place, but potential improvement is not complete until the child is about 5 years old. If dysplasia persists after this age, augmentation and/or redirection of the acetabular roof is clearly necessary.

17. What is slipped capital femoral epiphysis (SCFE)?

SCFE is a common hip disorder that affects adolescents, most often between 12 and 15 years of age. Clinically, the femoral capital epiphysis of the hip displaces or "slips" off the femoral neck to a variable degree.

18. Describe the clinical features of a patient with SCFE.

The most frequent presenting complaint is a painful hip. Early on pain may be referred to the knee, and knee pain may be the sole presenting complaint. Pain is usually intermittent and gradual in onset. Some patients describe one or more episodes of trauma prior to diagnosis. Boys are affected approximately twice as frequently as girls. Physical examination reveals mild to severe pain on motion with limited internal rotation and abduction. Flexion of the hip results in obligatory external rotation of the thigh because of the abnormal relationship between the femoral head and neck.

19. What are the early radiographic features of SCFE?

In the earliest "preslip" stage, the only x-ray finding may be a subtle widening of the physis on the involved side when compared with the opposite hip. Hence it is important to obtain a view of the entire pelvis, not just the involved hip.

20. Describe the subsequent radiographic features of SCFE.

On the anteroposterior film the epiphysis displaces posteriorly and inferiorly. A rim of new bone formation is found at the posterior aspect of the neck adjacent to the femoral head. In addition, the femoral neck becomes uncovered by the femoral head anteriorly, producing the characteristic bony bump of the superior neck. A slip of less than one-third the width of the neck is considered grade I; a slip between 33 and 50% is grade II; and a slip > 50% is termed grade III. The severity of the condition may be determined by measuring the percentage of slip.

21. What is the treatment of SCFE?

Treatment is designed to stabilize the epiphysis on the femoral neck and to prevent further slipping, a goal generally achieved by inserting a single strong screw into the center of the epiphysis from the anterior aspect of the greater trochanter or femoral neck. Surgery should be performed without undue delay after diagnosis.

22. What are the complications of treatment for SCFE?

- Chronic and diminished range of motion
- Osteonecrosis
- Chondrolysis
- Degenerative arthritis
- Gait abnormalities

23. What is Legg-Calvé-Perthes (LCP) disease?

LCP disease is temporary interruption of the blood supply to the bony nucleus of the proximal femoral epiphysis with impairment of the epiphyseal growth and subsequent remodeling of revascularized, regenerated bone in the pediatric patient.

24. Describe the clinical presentation of a patient with LCP disease.

LCP disease may occur between the ages of 3 and 12 years, most commonly in children between 5 and 7 years of age. The disorder may be bilateral in up to 20% of patients; boys are affected 3–5 times more often than girls. Patients usually present with a limp accompanied by pain in the hip or referred to the thigh or knee and may report an associated traumatic event. The gait is usually described as Trendelenburg-type. Shortening of the extremity is rare. However, range of motion, especially abduction and internal rotation of the hip, is limited.

25. What is the etiology of LCP disease?

The etiology of the avascular changes in the femoral head of children with LCP disease remains unclear. This condition is different from the avascular necrosis of the femoral head that develops after a fracture or use of steroids. Theories include an endocrine- or trauma-induced loss of interosseous or extraosseous blood supply as well as perhaps a local manifestation of systemic epiphyseal disease.

26. Describe the radiologic findings in LCP disease.

In the early stages standard radiographs may remain normal. Technetium bone scans often provide evidence of disease in the early stages, but it is difficult to quantitate the information. Magnetic resonance imaging facilitates the early diagnosis and quantification of osteonecrosis and provides a clear picture of the articular cartilage.

27. Describe the classification of LCP disease.

Some confusion surrounds the treatment of LCP disease because of the lack of uniformity in classification systems. The following are currently in use:

1. The **Waldenström classification** is divided into two periods: (1) evolution and (2) healing and growth. The evolutionary period is characterized by (a) an initial stage in which the epiphysis is dense, patchy, and uneven, and (b) a second stage of fragmentation in which the epiphysis appears radiographically to be in pieces. In the period of healing the epiphysis becomes homogenous; the final period is distinguished by normal growth and reossification of the deformed femoral head.

2. The **Catterall classification** identifies four groups:
   (1) 25% of the femoral head in the anterior central region is involved.
   (2) Nearly 50% of the femoral head including the anterior lateral region is involved.
   (3) Approximately 75% of the femoral head is involved with the formation of a large sequestrum; the large medial pillar is usually uninvolved.
   (4) The entire femoral head is involved, with widespread collapse of the epiphysis.

3. The **Salter-Thompson classification** divides LCP disease into two groups on the basis of the extent of the subchondral fracture that defines the limit of underlying osteonecrosis and the presence or absence of an intact viable lateral margin of the femoral epiphysis:
   (1) Group A: a subchondral fracture line involves approximately one-half of the femoral head.
   (2) Group B: more than half of the femoral head involved; the fracture and the underlying avascular segment of the femoral head extend across more than one half the epiphysis.

28. Describe the prognostic factors and natural history in LCP disease.

1. Recovery without residual problems is more likely when the signs and symptoms of the disease develop before the age of 5 years. Patients older than 9 years at presentation almost universally have a poor prognosis.

2. Some question remains whether an increased amount of femoral head involvement correlates with a poorer result, but in general it is believed that this is true.

3. Patients who demonstrate lateral subluxation or extrusion of the femoral head are thought to have less likelihood of an ultimate good or excellent result.

4. Persistent loss of range of motion carries a poor prognosis.

5. Premature closure of the physis leads to poor results.

29. What are the goals of treatment of LCP disease?

The goal of treatment is a spherical, well-covered femoral head with a range of motion in the hip that approaches normal. The principles of treatment include maintenance of range of motion and acetabular containment of the femoral head during the active period of the process.

30. What treatment options are available for patients with LCP disease?

1. Patients should be instructed on range-of-motion exercises and work with a physical therapist.

2. Braces are used to abduct the leg to contain the femoral epiphysis in the acetabulum; they may be either non–weight-bearing or weight-bearing orthoses. They must be used for 18–24 months. Favorable results of brace treatment are limited.

3. Varus osteotomy of the proximal portion of the femur centers the femoral head more deeply within the acetabulum while maintaining the limb in a weight-bearing position.

4. Innominate osteotomy may be used to rotate the acetabulum into a position that better contains the head of the femur.

BIBLIOGRAPHY

1. Carney BT, Weinstein SL, Nuhe J: Long term follow up of slipped capital femoral epiphysis. J Bone Joint Surg 73A:667–674, 1991.
2. Catterall A: The natural history of Perthes' disease. J Bone Joint Surg 53B:37–53, 1971.
3. Coates CK, Paterson JM, Woods KR: Femoral osteotomy in Perthes' disease: Results at maturity. J Bone Joint Surg 72B:581–585, 1990.
4. Evans IK, Deluca PA, Gage JR: A comparative study of ambulator-abductor bracing and varus derotation osteotomy in the treatment of severe Legg-Calvé-Parthes disease in children over 6 years of age. J Pediatr Orthop 8:676–682, 1998.
5. Harding M, Harcke HT, Bowen JR, et al: Management of dislocated hips with Pavlik harness treatment and ultrasound monitoring. J Pediatr Orthop 17:189–198, 1977.
6. Kasser J (ed): Orthopedic Knowledge Update No. 5. Rosemont, IL, American Academy of Orthopedic Surgery, 1996, pp 355–357.
7. Kislic PJ: Congenital dislocation of the hip: A misleading term. J Bone Joint Surg 71B:136, 1989.
8. Salter RB, Thompson GM: Legg-Calvé-Perthes disease. J Bone Joint Surg 66A:479–489, 1984.
9. Wenger DR, Ward WT, Herring JA: Legg-Calvé-Perthes disease. J Bone Surg 73A:778–788, 1991.

55. ARTHRITIS OF THE HIP

Kim J. Chillag, M.D.

1. In the adult patient with chronic symptoms, what are the most common causes of hip arthritis?

The most common causes of chronic arthritic symptoms in the adult can be divided into two broad categories. The first is osteoarthritis, which is also called degenerative or idiopathic osteoarthritis. This category includes the majority of patients over the age of 50 years with chronic arthritic pain in the hip. The second broad category is inflammatory arthritis, which includes connective tissue diseases, such as rheumatoid arthritis, ankylosing spondylitis, systemic lupus erythematosus, and the crystalline-induced arthritides, such as gout and pseudogout.

2. The most common complaint of patients with arthritis of the hip is chronic pain. In the patient who presents with extreme acute pain, what etiologic factors must be considered?

The patient who presents with an acute onset of hip pain and no history of trauma should be assumed to have an infection of the hip until proved otherwise. The nature, duration, clinical course, and precipitating factors of the complaint should be considered in evaluation of the patient with acute hip pain. If no other cause is determined, an infection should be considered, and an aspiration of the joint should be performed.

If there is a history of trauma, such as a fall, and routine radiographs are normal, occult femoral neck fracture should be considered. The earliest confirmatory test is an MRI; radionuclide bone scanning is positive after several days.

3. How can the types of hip arthritis be differentiated?

The most common methods of differentiating the types of arthritis are the clinical history, physical examination, and radiographic evaluation. The typical radiographic changes in the common types of arthritis are listed below. If the diagnosis is still in question, serologic tests can be helpful; the common serologic tests are listed in the second table.

Radiographic Changes in Arthritis

DISEASE	FINDINGS
Degenerative joint disease	Joint space narrowing Bony sclerosis Osteophyte formation
Rheumatoid arthritis	Periarticular osteoporosis Joint erosions Loss of joint space Subluxation Ankylosis
Gout	Punched-out bone erosions
Pseudogout	Punctate linear calcification in hyaline and fibrocartilage
Infectious arthritis	No change (early), then osteoporosis Cartilage destruction and erosions if untreated (late)

Serologic Tests

DISEASE	TESTS	USUAL FINDINGS
Degenerative joint disease	Erythrocyte sedimentation rate (ESR) C-reactive protein (CRP) Complete blood count (CBC)	Normal
	Antinuclear antibody (ANA) Lupus erythematosus cell preparation (LE prep) Rheumatoid factor (RF)	Negative
Rheumatoid arthritis	ESR Red blood cell count White blood cell count (WBC) RF ANA	Elevated Mild anemia Mild leukocytosis (40%) Positive (80%) Positive (30%)
Gout	ESR Serum uric acid CBC	Elevated Elevated 95% Usually normal, occasionally mild leukocytosis
	ANA LE prep RF	Negative
Pseudogout	Same as above	Same as above, except serum uric acid is elevated in 30%
Infectious arthritis	ESR Blood cultures WBC	Elevated Positive Leukocytosis
	ANA LE prep RF	Negative

4. What nonsurgical treatments are available for patients with osteoarthritis or rheumatoid arthritis of the hip?

Especially early in the course of the disease, arthritis of the hip can be managed successfully by nonoperative means. Activity modification, weight loss, and walking aids, including canes, may significantly reduce the patient's symptoms. Nonsteroidal antiinflammatory drugs (NSAIDs) are the most frequently used pharmacologic agents for relief of symptoms. In the inflammatory arthritides, other medications are frequently prescribed, including corticosteroids.

5. What are the common side effects of NSAIDs?

As with any medications, side effects may occur. In the broad category of drugs that includes the common NSAIDs, gastrointestinal (GI) side effects are the most common serious complication. Peptic ulceration and GI bleeding have been reported with all of the NSAIDs. Minor GI problems such as dyspepsia also are common. Actual GI bleeding may occur in as many as 2–4% of patients treated with long-term therapy. The physician and patient should be alert to the symptoms of this complication. Other serious side effects, including hepatic and renal toxicity, may occur, and patients on long-term therapy should be monitored appropriately.

Recently, a new category of NSAIDs termed COX-2 inhibitors has become available. They may have a lower incidence of GI side effects.

6. What surgical procedures are used to correct osteoarthritis, the most common cause of hip arthritis?

Through the years many surgical procedures have been advocated for the treatment of osteoarthritis of the hip. As advancements have occurred, most of the procedures have been relegated to historical interest. Currently, arthrodesis, femoral or pelvic osteotomy, and total hip arthroplasty are the three commonly used procedures for treatment of osteoarthritis. The patient's age, activity level, overall health, other joint involvement, and specific radiographic presentation are considered in choosing the best surgical procedure.

7. Why consider alternatives to total hip arthroplasty, which is highly successful?

Alternatives to total joint arthroplasty are most often considered in young patients. Regardless of the advances that have been made in design and technique of total hip replacement, worrisome long-term results in young patients have been reported by numerous authors.

8. How is fixation of the prosthetic components achieved?

Excellent long-term fixation has been achieved using both methylmethacrylate (cement) fixation and porous or bone ingrowth (noncemented) fixation. The surgeon may use the patient's age, activity level, and bone quality in selecting the type of prosthesis.

9. What is the most common long-term complication of total hip replacement?

Aseptic loosening is the most common long-term complication of total hip replacement and is frequently associated with osteolysis. This was originally thought to be the result of cement failure, but also is seen after noncemented total hip replacement. The body's reaction to polyethylene particulate debris is now thought to be the prime cause of late aseptic loosening and osteolysis. Alternatives to metal on polyethylene bearing surfaces are in use and may eliminate this problem.

10. What is the infection rate following total hip replacement? Which patients are most at risk?

The prevalence of infection after total hip replacement of Medicare patients in the United States was approximately 2.3%. Patient factors associated with increased risk for infection include rheumatoid arthritis, diabetes mellitus, poor nutrition, obesity, oral steroid use, and previous surgery.

BIBLIOGRAPHY

1. Callaghan JJ, et al: Hip arthrodesis. A long-term follow-up. J Bone Joint Surg 67A:1328–1335, 1985.
2. Callaghan JJ: The clinical results and basic science of total hip arthroplasty with porous coated prosthesis. J Bone Joint Surg 75A:299–310, 1993.
3. Chandler HP, Reineck FT, et al: Total hip replacement in patients younger than thirty years old. J Bone Joint Surg 63A:1426–1434, 1981.
4. Door JD, Takei GK Connly JP: Total hip replacement in patients younger than thirty years old. J Bone Joint Surg 65A:474–479, 1983.
5. Hanssen AD, Rand JA: Evaluation and treatment of infection at the site of a total hip or knee arthroplasty. J Bone Joint Surg 80A:910–922, 1998.
6. Harris WH: The problem is osteolysis. CORR 311:46–53, 1995.
7. Jazrawi LM, Kummer FJ, DiCesare PE: Alternative bearing surfaces for total joint arthroplasty. J Am Acad Orthop 6(4):198–203, 1998.
8. Lane NE: Pain management in osteoarthritis: The role of COX-2 inhibitors. J Rheumatol 24:20–23, 1997.
9. Lipsky PE, Isakson PC: Outcome of specific COX-2 inhibition in rheumatoid arthritis. J Rheumatol 24:9–13, 1997.
10. Masterson EL, Masri BA, Duncan CP: Treatment of infection at the site of total hip replacement. J Bone Joint Surg 79A:1740–1749, 1997.
11. McCarthy GM, McCarty DJ: Intrasynovial corticosteroid therapy. Bull Rheum Dis 43:2–4, 1994.
12. McCoy TH, Salvati EA, Ranawat CS, et al: A fifteen year follow-up study of one hundred Charnley low-friction arthroplasties. Orthop Clin North Am 19:467, 1988.
13. Moreland JR, Gruen TA, Mai L, et al: Aseptic loosening of total hip replacement: Incidence and significance. In The Hip Proceedings of the Eighth Open Scientific Meeting of the Hip Society. St. Louis, Mosby, 1980.
14. Needleman P, Isakson PC: The discovery and function of COX-2. J Rheumatol 24:6–7, 1997.
15. Sells LL, German DC: An update on gout. Bull Rheum Dis 43:4–7, 1994.

56. AVASCULAR NECROSIS OF THE HIP

Kim J. Chillag, M.D.

1. What are the causes of avascular necrosis of the femoral head?

The most common cause of avascular necrosis is disruption of the blood supply to the femoral head from a displaced femoral neck fracture. The most common nontraumatic causes are excessive alcohol use and systemic steroid use. Other nontraumatic causes are sickle cell anemia, caisson disease, Gaucher's disease, and hyperlipidemia. Recent research indicates that a form of coagulopathy is a causative factor in many patients with avascular necrosis.

2. If one hip has been diagnosed with avascular necrosis, what is the likelihood that the opposite hip is involved?

Whether the opposite hip is symptomatic or asymptomatic, there is at least a 50% chance that is is already involved.

3. What symptoms are caused by avascular necrosis of the hip?

Early in the course of the disease, the patient may be asymptomatic. As the disease progresses, the patient complains of pain in the groin area. Later, severe pain, limp, and loss of hip motion occur.

4. Can other areas of the skeleton be affected by avascular necrosis?

Yes. The humeral head and the distal femur, particularly the medial femoral condyle, may be involved in 10–15% of patients with avascular necrosis of the hip.

5. What tests are most useful in the diagnosis and evaluation of avascular necrosis?

The most important test is routine AP and lateral x-rays of the affected hip. This test is the most cost-effective and may be sufficient alone.

Magnetic resonance imaging (MRI) is the most sensitive and specific test to evaluate the femoral head for the presence of avascular necrosis. MRI can detect the lesion before it is apparent on plain x-rays and allows the physician to quantitate the extent of femoral head involvement.

6. What is the original and most common classification system for avascular necrosis of the hip?

The most common classification system is the Ficat system, which is based on radiographic exposure of the femoral head.

Ficat System for Clinical and Radiographic Evaluation and Staging of the Hip in Avascular Necrosis of the Femoral Head

STAGE	SYMPTOMS	ROENTGENOGRAM	BONE SCAN
0	None	Normal	Decreased uptake
1	None/mild	Normal	Cold spot on femoral head
2	Mild	Density change in femoral head	Increased uptake
2A		Sclerosis or cysts, normal joint line, normal head contour	
2B		Flattening (crescent sign)	
3	Mild to moderate	Loss of sphericity, collapse	Increased uptake
4	Moderate to severe	Joint space, acetabular changes	Increased uptake

7. Has the classification system changed since MRI has become available?

Yes. Classification systems now use MRI of the femoral head to take into account the size of the lesion and amount of articular surface involved. These systems are more accurate and useful in determining prognosis and treatment. The University of Pennsylvania System is the most useful.

University of Pennsylvania System for Staging Osteonecrosis

STAGE	CRITERIA	STAGE	CRITERIA
0	Normal or nondiagnostic x-ray, bone scan, and MRI	IV	Flattening of femoral head A. Moderate (15% of surface and < 2 mm depression) B. Moderate (15–30% if surface or 2–4 mm depression) C. Severe (> 30% of surface or > 4 mm depression)
I	Normal x-ray: abnormal bone scan and/or MRI A. Mild (< 15% of femoral head affected) B. Moderate (15–30%) C. Severe (> 30%)		
II	"Cystic" and sclerotic changes in femoral head A. Mild (< 15% of femoral head affected) B. Moderate (15–30%) C. Severe (> 30%)	V	Joint narrowing and/or acetabular changes A. Mild B. Moderate } Average of femoral head involvement, as C. Severe } determined in stage IV, and estimated acetabular involvement
III	Subchondral collapse (crescent sign) without flattening A. Mild (< 15% of articular surface) B. Moderate (15–30%) C. Severe (> 30%)	VI	Advanced degenerative changes

8. What surgical procedures are recommended for treatment of avascular necrosis of the hip?

No single surgical procedure has been accepted for treatment of all patients with avascular necrosis of the hip. In the early stages, before collapse of the femoral head, core decompression with or without bone graft and osteotomy may be effective in preserving the femoral head. Variable results have been reported. In the later stages of the disease, when femoral head collapse has progressed, total joint arthroplasty is more frequently recommended.

BIBLIOGRAPHY

1. Aaron RK, Ciombor DM: Electrical stimulation, demineralized bone matrix, and bone morphogenic protein. Semin Arthroplasty 9:221–230, 1998.
2. Amstutz HC, Sparling EA, Grigoris P: Surface and hemi-surface replacement arthroplasty. Semin Arthroplasty 9:261–271, 1998.
3. Bauer TW, Plenk H: The pathology of early osteonecrosis of the femoral head. Semin Arthroplasty 9:192–202, 1998.
4. Cabanela ME: Femoral endoprostheses and total hip replacement for avascular necrosis. Semin Arthroplasty 9:253–260, 1998.
5. Calandruccio RA, Hungerford DS, Kenzora JE, et al: Symposium: Osteonecrosis of the femoral head. Contemp Orthop 14:119–162, 1987.
6. Camp JF, Colwell CW Jr: Core decompression of the femoral head for osteonecrosis. J Bone Joint Surg 68A:1313–1319, 1986.
7. Dutkowski JP: Miscellaneous nontraumatic disorders. In Canale ST (ed): Campbell's Operative Orthopaedics, 9th ed., St. Louis, Mosby, 1998, pp 787–855.
8. Hungerford DS: Bone marrow pressure, venography, and core decompression in ischemic necrosis of the femoral head. In The Hip: Proceedings of the Seventh Open Scientific Meeting of the Hip Society. St. Louis, Mosby, 1979, pp 175–181.
9. Jones JP: Etiology and pathogenesis. Semin Arthroplasty 9:184–191, 1998.
10. Santore RF: Intertrochanteric osteotomies for femoral head necrosis. Semin Arthroplasty 9:242–252, 1998.
11. Steinberg ME: Early diagnosis, evaluation, and staging. Semin Arthroplasty 9:203–212, 1998.
12. Steinberg ME: Core decompression. Semin Arthroplasty 9:213–220, 1998.
13. Sutker BD, Urbaniak JR: Grafting procedures. Semin Arthroplasty 9:231–241, 1998.

57. TOTAL HIP REPLACEMENT

Peter K. Buchert, M.D.

1. What is arthritis?

Arthritis is inflammation of the joint; in this case, inflammation of the hip joint.

2. What are the causes of arthritis?

- **Noninflammatory:** This category includes idiopathic and posttraumatic arthritis, congenital deformities (e.g., congenital hip dysplasia), and avascular necrosis.
- **Inflammatory:** The most common is rheumatoid arthritis; others include mixed connective tissue disease, lupus erythematosus, and psoriatic arthritis.

3. What are the clinical manifestations of hip arthritis?

Pain is the main symptom, but the patient also may demonstrate decreased walking distance, decreased range of motion, inability to sleep, and limp.

4. Why do patients commonly complain of groin pain?

The obturator nerve runs directly by the hip joint; therefore; it is irritated by the arthritis.

5. What are the common radiographic findings?

The most common findings are narrowing of the hip joint space, osteophyte formation, and subchondral cysts.

6. Why do the osteophytes form?

Once the auricular cartilage begins to degenerate, the ability of the cartilage to distribute stress begins to fail, and stress on the bone increases. The bone responds to increased stress by laying down increased bone (Wolff's law). Thus, more surface area is produced to cover the increased stress.

7. Why do subchondral cysts form?

In areas of very high stress, stress fractures occur. Because of continued pressure, the fractures cannot heal and cysts form. Once the stress is relieved (i.e., once a total hip replacement [THR] is properly done), the cysts usually heal and fill in with bone.

8. What conservative approach should be tried before recommending total hip replacement (THR)?

Most authors agree that antiinflammatory agents, cane, decreased activity, and weight loss (if appropriate) should be tried for at least 6 months before surgery is recommended.

9. On which side of the patient should the cane be used?

The cane should be in the hand opposite the involved hip to decrease the reactive force on the joint.

10. Besides THR, what other surgical procedures are sometimes offered?

Femoral osteotomies, while popular outside the United States, have not gained popularity here. Hip arthroscopy (unlike knee arthroscopy) has been shown to be of limited benefit.

11. What are the most popular surgical approaches to the hip?

The most popular are posterior, transtrochanteric, direct lateral, and anterior approaches. The posterior and direct lateral approaches are now the most popular. The advantages and disadvantages of each are listed in the table below.

Surgical Approaches to the Hip

APPROACH	ADVANTAGE	DISADVANTAGE
Posterior	Easy to do Easy to see femur Rarely trouble with limp	Harder to see acetabulum Increased rate of dislocation (usually)
Transtrochanteric	Easy to do Great exposure	Complication of trochanteric nonunion Limp
Direct lateral	Easy to do Good exposure Low dislocation rate	Limp Heterotopic bone
Anterior	Good exposure of acetabulum	Hard to get femoral component Hard to do

12. What characteristics do modern cemented components have in common?

- Made of super alloys (cobalt-chrome or titanium alloys).
- Smooth edges with no sharp corners.
- Fill at least one-half of the diameter of the femoral canal.
- Some sort of texturing proximally to encourage cement attachment to stem.
- Cobalt chrome heads for articulation.

13. Describe the modern cement technique.
Modern cement technique consists of distal femoral plugging, use of a cement gun to fill the canal from distal to proximal, and pressurization of the cement. In addition, most surgeons recommend either vacuum mixing or centrifugation to decrease porosity of the cement. Metal backing of the polyethylene acetabular component does not appear to help long-term results.

14. Why did cementless prostheses come into vogue in the mid 1980s?
Although cemented hips did well for older people, many studies showed less than optimal results for younger people.

15. What size should the pores be to facilitate bone ingrowth?
Most authors agree that the pore size should be between 200–500 microns.

16. How much porous ingrowth is enough?
No one knows. Certainly, the more porous the surface, the more likely ingrowth will occur. However, the more porous surface that is available, the more likely there is to be stress shielding, and the harder it would be to remove a well-fixed stem if the need should arise.

17. Why are cementless acetabular components so popular?
Although cement techniques on the femoral side have greatly improved the long-term results, the results of cemented acetabular components have failed to show similar improvements.

18. What design characteristics should a cementless acetabular component have?
The component should be circular in shape, fully porous coated, and placed in a press-fit (tight) fashion. The necessity and advisability of screw reinforcement is under debate.

19. What size head and liner should be used?
Most experts agree that a 26- or 28-mm head provides the least amount of wear. At least 6 mm of polyethylene in the socket should be available.

20. What is the Dorr classification of bone stock?
While looking at a lateral radiograph of the proximal femur, Dorr classified the amount of funnelization of the metaphysis. A maximal funnel represented good bone stock and was classified as A. If no funnel was present, the classification was C. The intermediate classification was B. Cementless THR results directly correlated with the classification (A is optimal).

BIBLIOGRAPHY

1. American Academy of Orthopaedic Surgeons: Orthopaedic Knowledge Update 2, 3, 4.
2. Balderston RA: The Hip. Philadelphia, Lea & Febiger, 1992, pp 393–452.
3. Harkess JW: Arthroplasty of hip. In Canale ST (ed): Campbell's Operative Orthopaedics, 9th ed. St. Louis, Mosby, 1998, pp 296–381.
4. Tullos HS (ed): American Academy of Orthopaedic Surgeons Instructional Course Lectures, Vol XL, 1991, pp 117–160.
5. Zimlich RH: Current status of anticoagulation therapy after total hip and total arthroplasty. J Am Acad Orthop Surg 4:54–62, 1996.

58. COMPLICATIONS OF TOTAL HIP REPLACEMENT

Peter K. Buchert, M.D.

INTRAOPERATIVE COMPLICATIONS

1. What is the vascular effect of insertion of the cement?
The cement is a potent vasodilator and thus causes hypotension (and can cause immediate death). It is important that the patient remain well hydrated throughout the procedure.

2. What nerves can be injured? What are the common mechanisms of injury during total hip replacement (THR)?
The most common nerve injury is to the sciatic nerve. Injury is usually caused by retractors on the nerve, but it may result from lengthening a shortened extremity. The femoral nerve can be injured by an anterior retractor. The obturator nerve is rarely injured but may be at risk from a poorly placed retractor.

3. When putting in screws for an acetabular component, what quadrant is to be avoided?
In the anterior superior quadrant (some say the anterior quadrant) the femoral vein and artery are located immediately on the other side of the bone of the acetabular and may be easily injured by a drill or screw.

4. What factors lead to intraoperative femoral fractures?
The most common factors are (1) failure to ream straight down the canal; (2) attempts to put too large a component down the canal; (3) attempts to pound the component down the canal too rapidly without allowing the viscoelastic nature of the bone to accept the component (bone expands with time); and (4) failure to appreciate preoperative deformities or distal tightness of the canal.

IMMEDIATE POSTOPERATIVE PERIOD (IN THE HOSPITAL)

5. What is the incidence of thrombophlebitis in untreated patients?
The incidence in most studies is around 50%.

6. What measures are available to decrease the incidence of thrombophlebitis?
• Early mobilization
• Sequential compression stockings
• Anticoagulation (warfarin, aspirin, heparin, dextran, low–molecular-weight heparin)

7. What position should the patient avoid to minimize the possibility of posterior dislocation of the THR?
The patient should avoid flexion and internal rotation of the hip.

8. What are the most common organisms causing infections in THR?
The two most common organisms are *Staphylococcus epidermidis* and S*taphylococcus aureus*. Whereas *S. aureus* was previously the more common of the two, most authors believe that *S. epidermidis* is more common now.

9. What known factors decrease the incidence of infection?

The factors known to decrease infection rates are (1) prophylactic antibiotics, (2) decreased traffic in the patient's room, and (3) rapid filtration of the air. Ultraviolet light, exhaust suits, and laminar flow also may decrease infection rates.

10. How long may it take for preoperative infection to manifest clinically?

It may take as long as 1 year before a low-virulent organism finally manifests itself.

LONG-TERM COMPLICATIONS

11. What is the most common long-term complication?

Loosening that causes pain is the most common complication.

12. How can one determine if a component is loose on radiographs?

Radiographic evidence of loosening includes (1) migration of the component, (2) fracture of the cement, and (3) a 2-mm lucent line completely surrounding the prosthesis.

13. What is osteolysis?

Osteolysis is a severe absorption of bone around the prosthesis mediated by collagenases, prostaglandins, and proteases.

14. What is thought to be the initiating factor in osteolysis?

Debris from polyethylene wear is thought to be the initiating factor. When the polyethylene of the acetabular liner wears, it goes down to the femur, around the edges of the cup, or through the screw holes of the cup.

15. How can one minimize polyethylene debris?

Four factors minimize polyethylene debris: (1) proper head size (26–68 mm); (2) maximal polyethylene thickness (at least 6 mm); (3) better metal for the head, possibly zirconium or ceramic; and (4) better grade of polyethylene.

16. How can late hematogenous infections be prevented?

Preventive strategies include (1) prophylactic antibiotics for dental work, nonclean operations, and urologic manipulations, and (2) aggressive treatment of systemic infections.

17. How can heterotopic bone be prevented in high-risk patients?

The best and easiest method of prevention is radiation. A single dose of 600 rads 2–3 days after surgery is recommended. Indomethacin also may be used.

BIBLIOGRAPHY

1. American Academy of Orthopaedic Surgeons: Orthopaedic Knowledge Update 2, 3, 4.
2. Balderston RA: The Hip. Philadelphia, Lea & Febiger, 1992, pp 393–352.
3. Fitzgerald RH: Infected total hip arthroplasty: Diagnosis and treatment. A comprehensive review. J Am Acad Orthop Surg 3:249–262, 1995.
4. Harkess JW: Arthroplasty of hip. In Canale ST (ed): Campbell's Operative Orthopaedics, 9th ed., St. Louis, Mosby, 1998, pp 381–424.
5. Lotke PA (ed): Postoperative Infections in Orthopaedic Surgery. American Academy of Orthopaedic Surgeons, 1992, pp 35–46.
6. Pritchard DJ (ed): Instructional Course Lecture, vol. 45. American Academy of Orthopaedic Surgeons, 1996, pp 171–198.
7. Tullos HS (ed): American Academy of Orthopaedic Surgeons Instructional Course Lectures, Vol XL, 1991, pp 177–160.

59. REVISION OF TOTAL HIP REPLACEMENT

Bradley K. Vaughn, M.D., FACS

1. What are the mechanisms of failure of total hip replacement?

1. **Aseptic loosening** is due to poor patient selection, modulous mismatch between implant and bone, generation of wear debris, or fixation failure.

2. **Infection** may be decreased by the use of prophylactic antibiotics, laminar flow, ultraviolet lights, and exhaust systems. The incidence varies from 0.4–1.5%.

3. **Dislocation** is caused by component malposition, component impingement, sepsis, and patient factors such as senility, noncompliance, alcoholism, and revisional surgery. The surgical approach is also important; a posterior approach is associated with a higher dislocation rate than an anterior approach. The incidence of dislocation is 1–10%.

4. **Heterotopic ossification** is usually associated with revision operations. The incidence is higher in patients with previous heterotopic ossification, ankylosing spondylitis, diffuse idiopathic skeletal hyperostosis (DISH syndrome), and Paget's disease. Current prophylactic treatment favors single-dose radiation therapy of 700 rads. Indomethacin has been used, but diphosphonates usually do not work.

5. **Unstable fractures** about the total hip replacement should undergo internal fixation if the implant is not loose. If the implant is loose, revision arthroplasty should be performed.

6. **Component breakage** is not a contemporary problem, because components are now made of superstrength metals and with stronger designs.

7. **Particle generation** has caused concern about dissimilar metals and corrosion at the interface of modular head-neck components, which may result in component fracture.

8. **Osteolysis** is focal endosteal erosion due to wear debris or particle disease (polyethylene, metal, or cement). It may occur in both cemented and noncemented forms.

2. What are the current problems with wear?

Wear in total hip arthroplasty may occur at any interface: the articulating surface, modular connections, and fixation interfaces. All biomaterials can wear: methacrylate, polyethylene, metallic alloys, and bone. Accumulation of wear debris in periarticular tissues results in a foreign-body reaction that is linked to bone resorption. Migration may occur with gross wear. Systemic accumulation also may occur, but the consequences are unknown. Factors affecting wear include polyethylene thickness (early designs with less than 6 mm of polyethylene show increased wear), head diameter (a large head in a small metal-backed acetabulum leads to increased polyethylene wear), and properties of the polyethylene. Metal backing of the acetabular component causes thinning of the acetabular polyethylene. In addition, hemispherical polyethylene liners fit the metal shell better than cylindrical designs. The locking mechanism is also important to prevent polyethylene wear within the metal shell. Recently, more wear problems have been reported secondary to heightened awareness and longer service of the implant.

3. Describe the symptoms of patients with failed total hip arthroplasty.

Patients frequently complain of pain. Start-up pain results when the patient must stand and place weight on the prosthesis before beginning to walk. Patients feel that they must seat the prosthesis into a stable position so that it will bear their full weight during stance phase. Patients sometimes have night pain. Patients with infection have pain daily and certainly complain of night pain. Deformity may be noted, especially external rotation and shortening of the lower extremity.

4. What is the technique of component removal?

1. **Acetabular component removal.** The strategy for component removal should include the selection of an appropriate surgical approach to maximize visualization and access, while

minimizing risk to the adjacent neurovascular structures of the hip joint. Thin, curved osteotomes may be used to disrupt the cement prosthesis interface. Extraction devices may be embedded into the polyethylene. Levering against the thin, attenuated bony columns should be avoided, because a fracture may occur. High-speed burs may be used to divide well-fixed cups. Cement may be removed from the acetabulum by fragmenting the cement with sharp osteotomes or a high-speed bur. Special caution is required when the cement and the anchor hole protrude into the acetabulum and pelvis, because vascular structures may be entrapped; in such cases, a preoperative arteriogram or contrast CT should be considered.

    2. **Femoral component removal.** Cement overhanging the bone should be removed. A slap hammer, vice grips, or bone tamps may be used to remove the cement in a retrograde fashion. Broken stems must be removed by creating an anterior perforation hole, removing the proximal portion, and using the controlled perforation for retrograde removal of the distal portion. The femoral cement is removed with hand instruments for fragmentation, such as high-speed drills or ultrasonic equipment. The cement fails under tension. Ultrasonic instruments may be used at all levels of the femur. Precoated or porous stems require special caution. The long distal cement mantel may require window or controlled perforation or an osteotomy.

5. Describe the classification of acetabular defects developed by the American Academy of Orthopaedic Surgeons.
    1. Segmental defects
       • Peripheral (rim)
       • Central (medial)
    2. Cavitary defects
       • Superior
       • Anterior
       • Posterior
       • Medial (protrusio)
    3. Combined defects (cavitary and segmental), which are the most common
    4. Pelvic discontinuity
    5. Arthrodesis

6. Describe the principles of acetabular reconstruction.
    1. Restore the center of rotation.
    2. Restore bony continuity and integrity of the acetabulum.
    3. Contain the prosthesis.
    4. Contain the graft.
    5. Use rigid graft fixation.
    6. Secure prosthetic fixation.

7. Describe acetabular reconstruction.
    Preoperative planning includes templating to determine the size and to find the center of rotation. The contralateral hip should be used, if normal. Special studies may be required, such as an arthrogram to rule out sepsis, arteriography, or contrast CT to study vascular structures in cases of protruded components or cement. An attempt should be made to classify the deficiencies postoperatively.

    Bone grafting may be used to feel the defect. The graft depends on the type of deficiency. Bulk graft may be used for segmental and large cavitary defects, whereas particulate graft is preferred for cavitary defects. Small defects may heal spontaneously. The sources of bone include autograft from the iliac crest, allograft femoral heads, femoral condyles, or acetabula. The defect also may be filled with a custom prosthesis or oblong cups. Cement may be used to fill smaller defects. Pelvic discontinuity needs to be repaired with reconstruction plates.

    For **severe deficiencies**, trochanteric osteotomy or plating may be performed in patients with an anteroposterior column defect, as necessary. Triradiate exposure may be used for anterior column disruption or whole acetabular allograft. Anterior, trochanteric slide, direct lateral, or posterior approaches may be used, depending on the preoperative defect.

With **segmental and large cavitary defects**, the component may be unstable in the host bone. In this case, structural graft is required. Allograft using femoral heads or distal femoral condyles are fixated with K-wires or Steinmann pins. The defect is reamed, as well as the allograft, to size the acetabulum. Fixation is performed with screws and/or plates directed along the weight-bearing forces. The graft is then prepared for the acetabular component, which is usually placed in a noncemented mode. The goals of acetabular grafting are to restore hip mechanics and bone stock. Many studies of hip revision indicate that failed grafts were performed with poor graft preparation, poor bed preparation, and poor internal fixation.

8. What are the options for reconstruction of the femur?

Indications for cemented fixation include an intact cortex and intact intramedullary content, advanced age (75 years or older), metabolic bone disease, low activity level, and limited life expectancy. Cementless fixation may be used in patients who have lost the intramedullary content of the femur but have an intact cortex as well as in patients in whom the proximal femur is destroyed. Cementless fixation is also desirable in younger patients with no significant medical history, medium or high activity expectations, and absence of significant metabolic bone disease. Porous coating should be used to stabilize the prosthesis in a rotatory and axial fashion.

9. Outline the incidence of fracture associated with total hip arthroplasty.

Intraoperative Fractures	Incidence (%)
Cemented primary arthroplasty	1–3.2
Cemented revision	3–12
Uncemented primary arthroplasty	3–28
Uncemented revision	3–46
Postoperative Fractures	
Primary cemented arthroplasty	0.6
Uncemented primary arthroplasty	0.4
Cemented revision	2.8
Uncemented revision	1.5

10. How are femoral fractures classified?

Type 1: proximal to stem tip
Type 2: spiral, proximal, and distal to stem tip
Type 3: distal to stem tip

11. What factors contribute to femoral fractures?

• Osteoporosis
• Need for removal of cement and implant
• Bone preparation mistakes
• Oversizing the implant
• Overzealous insertion

12. What measures can be taken to prevent femoral fractures?

Prevention includes preoperative planning and radiographs to avoid femoral perforation; prophylactic cerclage wires when fracture is possible; cleaning of the canal of residual cement to avoid fracture during reaming; and bypassing cortical defects or stress fractures by two femoral canal diameters.

13. Discuss the treatment of femoral fractures.

Most **intraoperative fractures** are proximal and minor. A routine cerclage is advisable for treatment.

Postoperative fractures have high complication rates. Closed treatment gives variable results with a higher nonunion rate. The malunion rate is lower with revision or open reduction and internal fixation. Treatment options include cerclage wire, Ogden plates, bone grafts or struts, long-stemmed prosthesis, and cement. Postoperative fracture management includes partial non–weight-bearing strategies and casting. Most patients require open reduction and internal fixation or revision of the prosthesis if it is loose or if the fracture is unstable.

14. Describe the management of infected total hip arthroplasty.

The incidence of infection is approximately 1%. Prophylactic antibiotics are the most important factor in reducing the rate of deep sepsis. The organism is usually gram-positive; 90% are staphylococci. Organisms with increased virulence include the methicillin-resistant *Staphylococcus aureus*, gram-negative bacilli, group D streptococci, and enterococci. The incidence is increased in patients who have had previous hip surgery, including fracture or total hip arthroplasty. Treatment options include:

1. Surgical debridement in acute infections (less than 2–3 weeks after arthroplasty)
2. Antibiotic suppression in patients with limited life span
3. Prosthetic removal, organism-specific antibiotics, and reimplantation of the prosthesis
4. Resection arthroplasty or arthrodesis

One-stage reimplantation has a 77% success rate with antibiotic-impregnated cement. Delayed reimplantation, which is more common, involves removal of the prosthesis and cement followed by a period of parenteral antibiotics. Reimplantation delayed from 3 months to 1 year has been shown to have a success rate of approximately 88%. If the reconstruction is delayed longer than 1 year, the rate of recurrence is 7.1%. If the reimplantation is done within the first year, the rate of recurrence is 26%. In patients infected with an organism of increased virulence the time frame between debridement and reimplantation should be prolonged. The Hospital for Special Surgery in New York reports that a 6-week time frame is adequate for eradication of infection and improves the functional outcome. The success rate of this protocol is 92%.

15. What are the results of revision hip total arthroplasty?

With acetabular revision, cementless, ingrown sockets are useful in all types of deficiencies. Results show re-revision of 2.5–8% during a 2–7 year follow-up. With massive acetabular allografts, 17% of the porous cups migrated within 2 years. Although bipolar acetabular components have high early rates of migration and failure, they may be indicated in the elderly or inactive patient with a nonstable ingrowth socket. Cemented revision of the socket acetabular component shows a re-revision ranging from 0–30% during a follow-up for 2–10 years. The loosening in patients with allografts has been reported as 0–62%. Radiolucent lines may be seen in the cemented component but do not necessarily indicate failure.

Cemented femoral components have high radiolucent rates and loosening compared with most cementless revisions. A re-revision rate of 4.5–10% was observed in patients followed for 4–10 years; loosening was apparent on radiographs in 12–64%. The results of cementless femoral components depend greatly on prosthetic stability, bone stock deficiency, prevention of interoperative fracture, and type of implant chosen for a specific deficiency. Re-revision rates of 3–10% were observed in patients followed for 2–8 years. Radiographic lucency is as high as 37%. Studies of the cortical strut allograft for femoral bone grafting report a rate of 80–90% union during an average of 2–5 year follow-up. Rigid fixation and maximal host–graft contact have been shown to increase union. In patients who have had an entire proximal femoral allograft, union at the graft–host junction has been shown to be 77%, but the incidence of infection approaches 5%.

Improved results may be seen with careful preoperative planning, proper prosthetic selection, provision of necessary equipment and inventory with back-up, and use of long stems (both cementless and cemented). Surgical technique should show wide exposure, preserve proximal bone, avoid fracture and perforation, expose defects, and ensure implant stability.

BIBLIOGRAPHY

1. Bartel DL, Bicknell VL, Wright TM: The effect of conformity, thickness, and material on stresses in ultra-high molecular weight components for total joint replacement. J Bone Joint Surg 68A:1041–1051, 1986.
2. Callaghan JJ, Elder SH, Stranne SK, et al: Revision arthroplasty facilitated by ultrasonic tool cement removal. J Arthroplasty 7:495–500, 1992.
3. Christensen CM, Seger BM, Schultz RB: Management of intraoperative femoral fractures associated with revision total hip arthroplasty. Clin Orthop 248:177–179, 1989.
4. Collier JP, et al: Mechanisms of failure of modular prostheses. Clin Orthop 285:129–139, 1992.
5. Cornell CN, Ranawat CS: Survivorship analysis of total hip replacements. Results in a series of active patients who were less than fifty-five years old. J Bone Joint Surg 68A:1430–1434, 1986.
6. D'Antonio JA, Capello WN, Borden LS, et al: Classification and management of acetabular abnormalities in total hip arthroplasty. Clin Orthop 243:126–137, 1989.
7. Eftekhar NS, Nercessian O: Incidence and mechanism of failure of cemented acetabular component in total hip arthroplasty. Orthop Clin North Am 19:557–566, 1988.
8. Emerson RH, Head WC, Berklacich FM, Malinin TI: Noncemented acetabular revision arthroplasty using allograft bone. Clin Orthop 249:30–43, 1989.
9. Engh CA, Glassman AH, Griffin WL, Mayer JG: Results of cementless revision for failed cemented total hip arthroplasty. Clin Orthop 249:30–43, 1989.
10. Fitzgerald RH Jr: Treatment of the infected total hip arthroplasty. In Lotke PA (ed): Postoperative Infections in Orthopaedic Surgery: Prevention and Treatment. AAOS Monograph Series, 35-8, 1992.
11. Garvin KL, Salvati EA, Fitzgerald RH Jr, et al: Reconstruction of the infected total hip and knee arthroplasty with gentamicin-impregnated Palacos® bone cement. In Heckman JD (ed): American Academy of Orthopaedic Surgeons Instructional Course Lectures 42:293–302, 1993.
12. Hall RM: Wear of polyethylene acetabular components in total hip arthroplasty. An analysis of one hundred and twenty-eight components retrieved at autopsy or revision operations. J Bone Joint Surg 80A:764–765, 1998.
13. Head WC, et al: Presented at the 59th Annual American Academy of Orthopaedic Surgeons Meeting, Washington, DC, 1992.
14. Head WC, Emerson RH, Cuellar AD: Cortical strut allografts for femoral reconstruction in revision hip arthroplasty. Semin Arthroplasty 4(1):9–15, 1993.
15. Head WC, Wagner RA, Emerson Jr RH, Malinin TI: Revision total hip arthroplasty in the deficient femur with a proximal load-bearing prosthesis. Clin Orthop 298:119–126, 1994.
16. Johansson JE, McBroom R, Barrington TW, Hunter G: Fractures of the ipsilateral femur in patients with total hip replacement. J Bone Joint Surg 69A:1435–1442, 1981.
17. Kavanaugh BF, Ilstrup DM, Fitzgerald RH: Revision total hip arthroplasty. J Bone Joint Surg 67A:517–526, 1985.
18. Kavanaugh BF, Fitzgerald RH: Multiple revisions for failed total hip arthroplasty not associated with infection. J Bone Joint Surg 69A:1435–1442, 1981.
19. Kavanaugh BF, Berry D, Ilstrup DM, et al: Ten-year follow-up of cemented revision total hip replacement. Presented at the 60th Annual American Academy of Orthopaedic Surgeons Meeting, San Francisco, 1993.
20. Keating EM, Ritter MA, Farris PM: Structures at risk from medially placed acetabular screws. J Bone Joint Surg 72A:509–511, 1990.
21. Klapper RC, Caillouette JT, Callaghan JJ, Hozaack WJ: Ultrasonic technology in revision joint arthroplasty. Corr 285:147–154, 1992.
22. Mallory TH: Preparation of the proximal femur in cementless total hip revision. Clin Orthop 235:47–60, 1988.
23. Masri BA, Campbell DG, Garbuz DS, Duncan CP: Seven specialized exposure for revision hip and knee replacement. Orthop Clin North Am 29:229–240, 1998.
24. McCarthy JC, Mattingly DA, et al: Revising the deficient femur with a modular femoral component. Presented at the 60th Annual American Academy of Orthopaedic Surgeons Meeting, San Francisco, 1993.
25. McDonald DJ, Fitzgerald RH Jr, Ilstrup DM: The two-stage reconstruction of a total hip arthroplasty because of infection. J Bone Joint Surg 71A:828–834, 1989.
26. McGann W, Mankin HJ, Harris WH: Massive allografting for severe failed total hip replacement. J Bone Joint Surg 68A:1–12, 1986.
27. Morrey BF, Kavanagh BF: Complications with revision of the femoral component of total hip arthroplasty. Comparison between cemented and uncemented techniques. J Arthroplasty 7:71–79, 1992.
28. Morrey BF, Trousdale RT: Uncemented femoral revision of total hip arthroplasty. Presented at the 60th Annual American Academy of Orthopaedic Surgeons Meeting, San Francisco, 1993.

29. Paprosky WG, Jablowsky WS, Mangus RG: Cementless femoral revision in the presence of severe proximal bone loss using diaphyseal fixation. Presented at the 60th Annual American Academy of Orthopaedic Surgeons Meeting, San Francisco, 1993.

30. Paprosky WG, Perona PG, Lawrence JM: Acetabular defect classification and surgical technique in revision total hip arthroplasty. Six-year follow-up. Presented at the 60th Annual American Academy of Orthopaedic Surgeons Meeting, San Francisco, 1993.

31. Rubash HE, Sinha RK, Shanbhag AS, Kim SY: Pathogenesis of bone loss after total hip arthroplasty. Orthop Clin North Am 29:173–186, 1998.

32. Sydney SN, Mallory TH: Controlled perforation: A safe method of cement removal from the femoral canal. Corr 253:168–172, 1990.

33. Weber KL, Callaghan JJ, Goetz DD, Johnston RC: Revision of a failed cemented total hip prosthesis with insertion of an acetabular component without cement and a femoral component with cement. A five to eight-year follow-up study. J Bone Joint Surg 78A:982–994, 1996.

60. ALTERNATIVES TO TOTAL HIP ARTHROPLASTY: OSTEOTOMY

Joseph Yao, M.D.

1. What are the goals of hip osteotomy?

In prevention of osteoarthritis, the goal of osteotomy is to restore anatomy to as normal a state as possible and thereby to eliminate excessive load to the joint caused by abnormal joint mechanics. In the case of limited joint damage (e.g., osteonecrosis with partial femoral head involvement), the goal is to direct a more normal part of the joint into the weight-bearing area. Such goals may be accomplished by osteotomy of the pelvis, femur, or both.

2. What common conditions may be treated by hip osteotomy?

Hip osteotomy is used for treatment of osteoarthritis, osteonecrosis, slipped capital femoral epiphysis, Legg-Calvé-Perthes disease, and congenital hip dysplasia (CHD). The first four entities involve the femoral head and are treated by femoral osteotomy. CHD involves acetabular deformity and is treated with pelvic osteotomy; concurrent femoral deformity is treated with femoral osteotomy. CHD rarely involves primary femoral deformity; hence, it is generally not treated by isolated femoral osteotomy.

3. List the desirable clinical characteristics for hip osteotomy.

- Young age with life expectancy greater than the expected survivorship of a primary total hip replacement (e.g., generally less than 50 years old)
- Lack of obesity
- Occupation other than heavy labor
- Good joint range of motion
- Mild degree of symptoms

4. What are the desirable radiographic characteristics for hip osteotomy?

- Good cartilage space
- Correctable malalignment
- Impingement and joint incongruity that can be improved by altering acetabular or femoral alignment
- Preoperative radiographs showing hip joint capable of being positioned in the desired postoperative alignment (e.g., radiograph taken with the hip abducted that demonstrates improved joint congruity and joint space)

5. What part of the femur is usually osteotomized in hip osteotomy?
Intertrochanteric region.

6. What are the major disadvantages of osteotomy in the femoral neck area?
Avascular necrosis of the femoral head and chondrolysis.

7. List the major types of femoral osteotomy.

1. Flexion	4. Valgus
2. Extension	5. Rotational (e.g., Sugioka osteotomy)
3. Varus	6. Combinations of the above

8. What are the indications for flexion osteotomy?
Indications for flexion osteotomy include hip extension contracture, osteonecrosis with anterior involvement and posterior sparing of the femoral head, and full range of hip extension preoperatively. The apex of the osteotomy is located posteriorly so that the shaft of the femur is flexed and the proximal femur is extended.

9. What are the indications for extension osteotomy?
Indications for extension osteotomy include hip flexion contracture and deficient anterior acetabular coverage (e.g., as seen frequently with CHD). The apex of the osteotomy is located anteriorly so that the shaft of the femur is extended and the proximal femur is flexed.

10. What are the indications for varus osteotomy?
Indications for varus osteotomy include relative valgus neck–shaft angle (i.e., > 135°), lateral joint space disease, and an enlarged and congruent joint space with the leg abducted on preoperative radiographs. Results are best if the femoral head is spherical and acetabular dysplasia is minimal.

11. What are the indications for valgus osteotomy?
Indications for valgus osteotomy include relative varus neck–shaft angle, medial joint space disease, and and enlarged and congruent joint space with the leg adducted on preoperative radiographs. The medial femoral head osteophyte is rotated superiorly to a weight-bearing location.

12. What are the indications for rotational osteotomy?
CHD is often associated with increased femoral neck anteversion. Derotation of the femoral neck into a more normal degree of anteversion may be combined with angular osteotomy. Rotational osteotomy also assists in moving osteonecrotic segments of femoral head away from the weight-bearing aspect of the joint.

13. Describe the role of medial or lateral displacement of the femoral shaft in combination with varus or valgus osteotomy.
Varus and valgus osteotomies change the center of femoral head rotation and hence alter the mechanical alignment of the lower extremity. Varus osteotomy displaces the center of hip rotation medially and should be combined with medial displacement of the femoral shaft to maintain the lower extremity mechanical axis; this technique avoids overloading the medial compartment of the ipsilateral knee. Valgus osteotomy displaces the center of hip rotation laterally and should be combined with lateral displacement of the femoral shaft; this technique avoids overloading the lateral compartment of the ipsilateral knee.

14. What is the effect of osteotomy on leg lengths?
Varus osteotomy usually shortens the limb at least 1 cm, whereas valgus osteotomy generally lengthens the limb. However, valgus osteotomy may shorten the limb by as much as 2 cm if a closing wedge is used.

15. Describe preoperative planning for femoral osteotomy.

Fluoroscopy and radiographs are used to assess whether a limb can be placed in a position that will improve hip joint space and congruity. The appropriate degree of angular and rotational correction can then be determined. Tracings are used to determine optimal locations for the os-teotomy and hardware, the size of wedge resection, and the possible need for femoral shaft dis-placement. Radiographs can determine the degree of femoral head involvement in cases of osteonecrosis. Femoral angular osteotomy may be appropriate when < 33% of the femoral head is involved on the anteroposterior (AP) radiograph or when the necrotic angle is < 200°.

16. What is the most common indication for pelvic osteotomy?

CHD, which involves deficient coverage of the femoral head laterally and often anteriorly.

17. What is the goal of pelvic osteotomy?

The goal is to improve femoral head coverage by the acetabulum.

18. Describe preoperative planning for pelvic osteotomies.

Radiographs should include an AP view of the pelvis and a false-profile (faux-profil) view taken with 20° of rotation while the patient is standing. Some patients have nearly normal-ap-pearing hips on AP pelvis radiographs, whereas the false-profile view demonstrates anterior sub-luxation of the femoral head. AP and lateral center-edge (CE) angles are measured to assess femoral containment. Lateralization of the femoral head can be assessed. Computed tomographic (CT) scans provide three-dimensional reconstructions to help in visualizing acetabular deficien-cies and the results of different osteotomies.

19. What is the role of pelvic osteotomy in a young patient (second or third decade) with a congruent hip joint and deficient femoral head coverage?

Pelvic osteotomy can be used to redirect the acetabulum without altering its shape or capac-ity. Improved femoral head coverage is then achieved. Osteotomy should be done early before significant arthritis develops.

20. Give examples of redirection osteotomies.

The Salter osteotomy can increase the CE angle by 20–30° in children, but only about 10° of improvement can be expected in patients older than 10 years. The Salter osteotomy allows cor-rection in only one direction. Double osteotomy (Sutherland and Greenfield) and triple os-teotomy (Steel) can be used in patients with preoperative CE angles of 0–15°. However, such osteotomies essentially create an unstable setting similar to a pelvic fracture. The dial osteotomy involves separating the acetabulum from the pelvis and rotating it in the appropriate direction; it can accomplish almost any degree of correction, but it is a technically difficult operation. The peri-acetabular osteotomy (Ganz) also corrects any degree of acetabular coverage deficiency and also allows the acetabulum to be medialized. The periacetabular osteotomy is done from inside the pelvis and is slightly easier to perform than the dial osteotomy.

21. Does pelvic osteotomy have a role in patients in whom hip arthritis has already developed?

Yes. A simple shelf procedure that consists of bone-grafting the superior-lateral acetabulum may be used in cases of congruous acetabular hypoplasia. The Chiari osteotomy may be consid-ered as a salvage procedure in patients with deficient femoral head coverage and arthritis. This osteotomy should be considered only if there is no congruous portion of acetabulum to rotate su-periorly; often an intact portion of acetabulum, located posteriorly and inferiorly, can be rotated superiorly.

22. What is the Chiari osteotomy?

An osteotomy is created just cephalad to the superior hip joint capsule. The osteotomy is angled from the distal anterolateral to the proximal posteromedial aspect. The acetabular (distal) fragment is abducted and medialized. An iliac crest bone graft is placed just cephalad to the hip capsule over the uncovered femoral head. The interposed superior-lateral joint capsule assumes a weight-bearing role. A triangular bony defect is created anteriorly by the osteotomy. Iliac crest bone graft is placed into the bony defect to serve as a buttress and to prevent anterior instability.

CONTROVERSIES

23. How does hip osteotomy influence subsequent total hip arthroplasty (THA)?

Pelvic osteotomy may simplify later THA by allowing the acetabulum to be reconstructed in a more normal position and by reducing the need for acetabular bone-grafting. Femoral osteotomy is generally done at the intertrochanteric level and consequently may make femoral preparation for THA more difficult. Therefore, angular corrections accomplished by femoral osteotomy should be limited to 15–20°. A custom-made femoral prosthesis or intraoperative femoral osteotomy may be necessary for successful THA in cases of severe alteration of proximal femoral anatomy due to previous reconstructive femoral osteotomy.

24. Is pelvic osteotomy warranted in young patients in view of the fact that later THA will probably be more difficult as a result of the altered anatomy?

Osteotomy has an important role, especially in young patients. Although excellent clinical results can be expected after THA, there are long-term problems, such as component wear and stress-shielding. Osteotomy is a particularly desirable alternative in young patients with early arthritis. In appropriate cases, osteotomy can alter the mechanisms of the hip joint and thereby arrest or reverse a degenerative process that would progress if left untreated. A major benefit of osteotomy is to delay the need for THA until the patient is older.

BIBLIOGRAPHY

1. Aronson J: Osteoarthritis of the young adult hip: Etiology and treatment. Instr Course Lect 35:119. St. Louis, Mosby, 1986.
2. Atsumi T, Kuroki Y: Modified Sugioka's osteotomy: More than 130 degrees posterior rotation for osteonecrosis of the femoral head with large lesion. Clin Orthop 334:98, 1997.
3. Bombelli R: Osteoarthritis of the Hip, 2nd ed. Berlin, Springer-Verlag, 1989.
4. Boos N, Krushell R, Ganz R, Muller M: Total hip arthroplasty after previous proximal femoral osteotomy. J Bone Joint Surg 79B:247, 1997.
5. Chiari K: Medial displacement osteotomy of the pelvis. Clin Orthop 98:55, 1974.
6. Gotuh E, Inao S, Okamoto T, Ando M: Valgus-extension osteotomy for advanced osteoarthritis in dysplastic hips. Results at 12 to 18 years. J Bone Joint Surg 79B:609, 1997.
7. Matsuno T, et al: Modified Chiari osteotomy: A long term followup study. J Bone Joint Surg 74A:470, 1992.
8. Millis MB, Poss R, Murphy SB: Osteotomies of the hip in the prevention and treatment of osteoarthritis. Inst Course Lec 41:145. Park Ridge, IL, American Academy of Orthopedic Surgeons, 1992.
9. Morgensen BA, Zoega H, Marinko P: Late results of intertrochanteric osteotomy for advanced osteoarthritis of the hip. Acta Orthop Scand 51:85, 1980.
10. Pauwels F: Biomechanics of the Normal and Diseased Hip. Berlin, Springer-Verlag, 1976.
11. Poss R: Current concepts review: The role of osteotomy in the treatment of osteoarthritis of the hip. J Bone Joint Surg 66A:144, 1984.
12. Poss R: Intertrochanteric osteotomy in osteoarthritis of the hip. Inst Course Lec 35:129. St. Louis, Mosby, 1986.
13. Schatzker J: The intertrochanteric osteotomy. Berlin, Springer-Verlag, 1984.

61. ALTERNATIVES TO TOTAL HIP ARTHROPLASTY: ARTHRODESIS

Joseph Yao, M.D.

1. What are common indications for hip arthrodesis?

The ideal clinical setting for hip arthrodesis is a unilaterally painful hip with greatly restricted range of motion in older adolescents or young adults, particularly if their occupation involves heavy labor.

2. What common hip problems may require treatment with hip arthrodesis?

- Osteonecrosis of the femoral head
- Osteoarthritis secondary to congenital hip dysplasia (CHD)
- Joint destruction due to tuberculosis and pyogenic septic arthritis
- Posttraumatic arthritis
- Previously failed total hip replacement, especially after infection by a highly virulent organism

3. What is the most common indication for hip arthrodesis in children?

Infection of the hip.

4. Name the major prerequisites to hip fusion.

The patient must have a normal lumbosacral spine, contralateral hip, and ipsilateral knee. These joints should be checked by examination and radiographs. Because an immobile hip that has undergone arthrodesis places increased stresses on these joints, the clinical results of hip arthrodesis are compromised if they are diseased.

5. Describe the optional position in which to perform arthrodesis on a hip.

Flexion of 30–40°, adduction of 0–5°, and external rotation of 0–7°.

6. What are the consequences of performing arthrodesis on a hip in an abducted position?

- Increased incidence of pain in the back and knee
- More degenerative changes on radiographs of the knee
- A more pronounced limp

7. What is the advantage of using internal fixation?

Internal fixation helps to ensure maintenance of the arthrodesis position obtained at surgery and decreases the duration of immobilization in a spica cast after surgery. In some cases, it eliminates the need for postoperative spica cast immobilization and permits earlier mobilization of the patient.

8. Describe the common methods for hip arthrodesis.

One of the most common methods of hip arthrodesis uses an AO cobra head plate spanning the pelvis and the proximal femur. Another method uses screws or pins passing through the femoral head and neck into the pelvis. The use of intramedullary nails transfixing the pelvis to the intramedullary canal of the femur also has been described.

9. What is the role of osteotomy in hip arthrodesis?

Pelvic and femoral osteotomies have been used by some surgeons in an attempt to maximize contact at the site of arthrodesis. Schneider described a pelvic osteotomy that allowed the femoral head to be medialized. He believed that the osteotomy increased bony contact between pelvis and femur. Subsequent cadaver studies did not confirm the increased bony contact that Schneider hypothesized. Charnley described central dislocation of the femoral head through the acetabulum to increase bony contact. Charnley's osteotomy had the advantages of avoiding distortion of the pelvis and reducing blood loss compared with Schneider's pelvic osteotomy. Others have used proximal femoral osteotomies to enhance bone contact at the arthrodesis site. Subtrochanteric osteotomy with adduction of the femoral shaft has the effect of abducting the hip and thus provides a larger contact area for arthrodesis.

10. Describe the role of bone grafts in hip arthrodesis.
Bone grafts have been used to improve the chances of successful arthrodesis. Iliac crest bone grafts can be packed into the arthrodesis site. Various techniques of transferring vascularized bone grafts to the arthrodesis site have been described. Davis transferred a portion of the anterior ilium along with the attachments of the tensor fascia lata and the anterior portions of the gluteus medius and minimus muscles to the arthrodesis site. Ranawat transferred a larger piece of anterior ilium with attachments of the tensor fascia lata, anterior portions of the gluteus medius and minimus, rectus femoris, and sartorius muscles. Kostuik transferred the greater trochanter with its attached gluteal muscles to the posterior aspect of the arthrodesis site.

11. Describe a relatively simple method to maintain the desired portion of the hip before use of internal fixation in hip arthrodesis.
Blasier et al. described a technique that uses a vacuum-splint beanbag to support the lower extremity. The patient is placed in the lateral decubitus position with the involved hip facing the ceiling. One beanbag is placed beneath the patient to maintain the body in the lateral position. A second beanbag is placed between the legs. After the involved leg is placed in the desired arthrodesis position, the beanbag between the legs is evacuated of air, thereby maintaining the desired position. The patient is then prepared and draped, and the arthrodesis procedure is completed.

12. What long-term results should a patient expect after hip arthrodesis?
Preoperative hip pain is generally relieved. About 70% of patients can walk more than 1 mile and sit comfortably for 2 hours after hip arthrodesis. Patients also should be able to drive an automatic transmission car. They generally cannot run or jog.

13. What are the effects of hip arthrodesis on other joints?
About 60% of patients have pain in the ipsilateral knee, 75% have anteroposterior laxity, and 80% have mediolateral laxity of the ipsilateral knee. About 60% of patients experience back pain, and 25% have pain in the contralateral hip.

14. What effect does hip arthrodesis have on contralateral total hip replacement?
Mechanical loosening of a total hip replacement probably occurs at a higher rate when the opposite hip has undergone arthrodesis.

15. What effect does hip arthrodesis have on an ipsilateral total knee replacement?
Loosening rates for the total knee replacement are not increased. However, there is an increased incidence of knee stiffness and the need for postoperative manipulation of the total knee replacement.

16. What are the major potential complications associated with hip arthrodesis?
Injury to blood vessels and nerves can occur during surgical exposure or during insertion of internal fixation. The internal fixation devices may loosen or fracture. Rates of pseudarthrosis range from 0–50%, with reported figures most commonly between 15 and 25%. Femur fractures occur in 5–15% of patients. Variable amounts of leg length shortening may occur, necessitating the use of a shoe lift. Accelerated degenerative changes may occur in the back, contralateral hip, and ipsilateral knee.

17. What are the major indications for converting a hip arthrodesis to a total hip arthro-plasty?
  • Low back pain
  • Pain in the ipsilateral or contralateral knee or in the contralateral hip
  • Severe gait abnormality secondary to bilateral hip arthroplasty

18. How does conversion of a hip arthrodesis to a total hip arthroplasty affect pain in adjacent joints?
  Pain is improved in the back (76% of patients), knee (35% of patients), and contralateral hip (12% of patients).

19. What is one of the most important determinants of a successful conversion of a hip arthrodesis to a total hip arthroplasty?
  The condition of the gluteus medius muscle.

20. How does the anticipated future conversion to a total hip arthroplasty affect the choice of hip arthrodesis technique?
  The surgical technique should minimize injury to the gluteus medius muscle. The use of a cobra head plate requires greater soft-tissue dissection and hence involves the potential for greater disruption of the gluteus medius muscle than the use of screws placed through the femoral neck and head into the pelvis. It is best to avoid altering pelvic or femoral anatomy, if possible, as well as creating pelvic or femoral osteotomies.

21. What are the clinical results of total hip arthroplasty after hip arthrodesis?
  The postoperative flexion arc averaged 87° in the review by Kilgus et al. Leg-length discrepancy improved by an average of 2.5 cm. The need for supportive walking devices decreased after surgery. Patients regained strength slowly, sometimes for as long as 5 years postoperatively. Patients who have spontaneous hip arthrodesis and no subsequent surgeries until total hip arthroplasty may have results comparable to those in patients who have primary total hip arthroplasty for more common causes of hip arthrosis. Failure of total hip arthroplasty after hip arthrodesis is more common in patients ≤ 50 years of age at the time of conversion, patients with two or more previous hip operations, and patients with an injury to the hip.

CONTROVERSY

22. Is it better to offer hip arthrodesis or total hip replacement to a young patient with isolated arthritis of one hip?
  The treatment of isolated hip arthritis in a young patient is a difficult problem. Hip arthrodesis generally provides a painless and stable joint for many years. The patient can bear weight on the arthrodesed limb without concern about limiting the degree of activity. A hip arthrodesis can be converted to a total hip arthroplasty in the future when the patient is older and less active. The disadvantages of arthrodesis include leg-length discrepancy, an immobile joint, and pain in adjacent joints with long-term follow-up. Total hip arthroplasty relieves pain associated with an arthritic joint and preserves joint motion. Usually leg lengths can be restored to almost normal after total hip arthroplasty. The major problem with total hip arthroplasty in a young patient is the generation of prosthetic wear debris over time. Wear rates may be accelerated in young patients because they have higher activity levels than older patients. Significant osteolysis may result from wear debris in joints. Osteolysis makes future reconstruction much more difficult and also may lead to fracture. Stress-shielding of bone by stiffer metal femoral prostheses leads to bone loss over time. Subsequent revision total hip arthroplasties are associated with a greater incidence of complications and poorer clinical results. Both hip arthrodesis and total hip arthroplasty have advantages and disadvantages. Hip arthrodesis still has a role in the treatment of arthritis in young patients despite the improving technology associated with hip arthroplasty. However, as

more patients become familiar with hip arthroplasty, it is often difficult to convince them to choose hip arthrodesis.

BIBLIOGRAPHY

1. Amstutz HC, Sakai DN: Total joint replacement for ankylosed hips. J Bone Joint Surg 57A:619, 1975.
2. Barnhardt T, Stiehl JB: Hip fusion in young adults. Orthopedics 19:303, 1996.
3. Blasier RB, Holmes RH: Intraoperative positioning for arthrodesis of the hip with the double beanbag technique. J Bone Joint Surg 72A:766, 1990.
4. Callaghan JJ, Brand RA, Pedersen DR: Hip arthrodesis: A long-term follow-up. J Bone Joint Surg 67A:1328, 1985.
5. Charnley J: Stabilization of the hip by central dislocation. J Bone Joint Surg 37A:514, 1955.
6. Duncan CP, Spangehl M, Beauchamp C, McGraw R: Hip arthrodesis: An important option for advanced disease in the young adult. Can J Surg 38(Suppl 1):539, 1995.
7. Garvin KL, Pellicci PL, Windsor RE, et al: Contralateral total hip arthroplasty or ipsilateral total knee arthroplasty in patients who have a long-standing fusion of the hip. J Bone Joint Surg 71A:1355, 1989.
8. Kilgus DJ, Amstutz HC, Wolgin MA, Dorey FJ: Joint replacement for ankylosed hips. J Bone Joint Surg 72A:45, 1990.
9. Kostuik JP: Arthrodesis of the Hip. In Amstutz HC (ed): Hip Arthroplasty. New York, Churchill Livingstone, 1991.
10. Murrell GA, Fitch RD: Hip fusion in young adults using a medial displacement osteotomy and cobra plate. Clin Orthop 300:147, 1994.
11. Schneider R: Hip arthrodesis with the cobra head plate and pelvic osteotomy. Reconstr Surg Traumatol 14:1, 1974.
12. Strathy GM, Fitzgerald RH: Total hip arthroplasty in the ankylosed hip. J Bone Joint Surg 70A:963, 1988.

62. PELVIC FRACTURES

Donald J. Walla, M.D.

1. What are the most common causes of pelvic fractures?

The automobile is responsible for most fractures of the pelvis in all age groups except for people over 60 years of age, for whom falls at home lead to the majority of pelvic fractures.

2. What clinical findings are present in a patient with a fractured pelvis?

A patient with a fractured pelvis may present with pain, tenderness, difficulty with ambulation, crepitus, ecchymosis, and swelling of the pelvis or perineum. Exerting posterior pressure on the iliac crests of a supine patient produces pain at the fracture site, because the pelvic ring is opened. Compressing the pelvic ring in a side-to-side direction by pressure on the iliac wings may be painful. Pain also may be elicited by downward pressure on the symphysis pubis.

3. On what does the stability of the pelvic ring depend?

The stability of the pelvic ring depends on both bony and ligamentous structures. The anterior portion of the pelvic ring does not participate in normal weight bearing, nor is it essential for maintenance of pelvic stability. The posterior arch (consisting of the sacrum, sacroiliac (SI) joints and ilia) serves as the weight-bearing portion of the pelvis. The posterosuperior SI ligaments connecting the iliac tuberosities to the sacrum provide most of the ligamentous stability to the SI joints.

4. What is meant by a stable pelvic fracture?

Pelvic fractures that do not involve the pelvic ring or that have minimal displacement of the pelvic ring are considered stable.

5. Name and describe the most commonly used mechanical classification scheme for pelvic fractures.

Pennal and Tile's classification of pelvic disruptions into three separate patterns is based on the presumptive injurious force primarily responsible for the disruption.

1. The **anteroposterior compression (open book)** injury hinges the pelvis open on the intact posterosuperior SI ligaments. It is not grossly unstable.

2. The **lateral compression injury** occurs as a result of a direct force to the iliac crests. It may be stable or unstable, depending on the magnitude of force and the degree of disruption of the posterior pelvic arch.

3. **Vertical shear injuries** result from forces through the femur directed perpendicularly to the pelvic ring and cause disruption of the SI joint or unimpacted fractures through the sacrum or ilium. The hemipelvis is unstable both rotationally and vertically. Displacements of 1 cm of the SI joint or 0.5 cm vertically of the hemipelvis are signs of instability.

6. What radiographic studies are useful in evaluating a patient with a pelvic fracture?

A complete baseline radiographic evaluation would include anteroposterior, 40° cephalad (outlet), 40° caudad (inlet), and 45° oblique projections of the pelvis. Further radiographic studies include computed tomographic (CT) scans and possible three-dimensional imaging. Push-pull or stress radiographs may be used to predict stability of a fractured pelvis.

7. What are the basic treatment principles for stable pelvic fractures?

The basic principles or treatment of pelvic fractures include fracture healing and rapid rehabilitation. Most pelvic fractures are stable and treated nonoperatively, initially with bed rest and protected ambulation.

8. What are the basic treatment principles for unstable fractures?

All pelvic fractures should be assessed for instability and displacement. Complications of unstable fractures may lead to later instability and nonunion, which in turn may lead to complaints of sacroiliac pain, leg-length discrepancy, painful sitting, and functional impairment. Women may have problems with parturition and dyspareunia. When instability is defined, the preferred treatment is surgical stabilization.

9. What is the indication for provisional stabilization of pelvic fractures?

Provisional fixation is indicated for patients with lesions that increase the pelvic volume and all unstable fractures. Application of a pelvic clamp or external fixator frame plus a supracondylar femoral traction pin reduces the pelvic volume, partially stabilizes the bones and soft tissues, and reduces the amount of bleeding and pain from the pelvis and facilitates nursing care.

10. What is the role of an external fixator in the treatment of pelvic fractures?

The traditional external fixator uses two or three pins in each iliac crest. The pins are joined by an anterior frame. The pelvic clamp and external skeletal fixator may restore adequate stability to a partially stable open book fracture; however, neither can restore adequate stability to the unstable pelvic fracture.

11. Define definitive internal fixation treatment of unstable pelvic fractures.

Definitive internal fixation should be done only by surgeons experienced with these techniques. The timing of surgery is dependent on the general state of the patient, but as a general rule it should be done as early as safety allows (usually within the first 5–7 days). Neurologic monitoring is desirable, as is use of a cell saver device; hemorrhage in open pelvic surgery can be massive. Prophylactic antibiotics are essential. It is important to avoid operating through crushed or contused skin or soft tissues, which helps to determine the choice of surgical approach. The specific incisional site should be based on the soft tissue injury and pelvic fracture pattern.

12. What is a Malgaigne fracture?

Malgaigne fractures usually refer to unstable fracture-dislocations of the pelvis. A simple definition includes all pubic fractures of both the superior and inferior pubic rami or pubic symphysis dislocation in conjunction with an ipsilateral posterior disruption that involves a sacral fracture, an iliac fracture, or a sacroiliac dislocation. Such injuries may lead to cephalad migration of the fragment containing the hip joint and thus to a leg-length discrepancy. Current treatment options favor surgical stabilization, including open reduction and internal fixation (ORIF) of the disrupted segments. Stabilization with external fixation in combination with ORIF is also an option.

13. Discuss the initial measures in management of a patient who has sustained a high-energy pelvic fracture.

Emergency resuscitative protocols are frequently involved, including control of intrapelvic bleeding, which can lead to shock and ultimately to death. Volume replacement by intravenous crystalloid solutions and whole blood, use of MAST suits, angiography, transarterial embolization, vascular repair, and surgical stabilization of unstable pelvic fractures are other considerations.

14. What potential injuries are associated with high-energy pelvic fractures?

High-energy pelvic trauma carries a significant risk of associated injury to the neurologic, urologic, gynecologic, gastrointestinal, and vascular systems as well as to the skin and subcutaneous tissues.

15. What common urologic and gynecologic injuries are associated with pelvic fractures?

Pelvic fractures may lead to disruption of the urethra and bladder by direct laceration or by tension stresses. Intravenous pyelograms, transurethral cystograms, and retrograde urograms are specialized radiographic exams useful in evaluating the extent of genitourinary injuries.

16. What types of gastrointestinal injuries are associated with high-energy pelvic fractures?

Perforations of the large and/or small bowel and lacerations of the rectum may occur. When a rectal laceration is present, a diverting colostomy should be considered.

17. What types of neurologic injuries are associated with severe pelvic fractures?

Fractures of the sacrum may lead directly to neurologic injury, whereas pelvic fracture or displacement may lead indirectly to nerve root and peripheral nerve-stretch injuries. A complete baseline neurologic exam, including a rectal evaluation, is necessary.

18. What treatment is necessary for uncontrolled hemorrhage in the patient with a pelvic fracture?

Management of uncontrolled hemorrhage from a pelvic fracture requires both general surgical and orthopedic approaches. Abdominal injuries are associated with 22–45% of pelvic fractures. Peritoneal lavage is useful in evaluating the presence or absence of intraabdominal bleeding. Laparotomy is usually required in the hemodynamically unstable patient who exhibits unstable pelvic fracture or dislocation. Immediate pelvic stabilization by either internal or external fixation may stabilize the retroperitoneal hemorrhage. If bleeding is not controlled, one must consider the possibility of a coagulopathy, disseminated intravascular coagulation (DIC), or hemorrhage from a major vessel. If hemorrhage from a major vessel is suspected, pelvic angiography is the next step.

19. What is the overall mortality rate associated with pelvic fractures?

The mortality rate for open pelvic fractures is 30–50% compared with 10–30% for closed pelvic fractures. Major causes of death related to open pelvic fractures are (1) hemorrhage and (2) sepsis and/or renal failure.

20. What complications are associated with pelvic fractures in children?

Several unique features are associated with pelvic fractures in children, including displacement of the pelvic ring through the triradiate cartilage with lateral compression injury; undergrowth of the hemipelvis in association with SI joint injury and subsequent fusion; and pelvic deformity with leg-length discrepancy in unreduced vertical shear fractures.

BIBLIOGRAPHY

1. Chapman MW: Fractures of the pelvic ring and acetabulum in patients with severe polytrauma. Instr Course Lect 3:591–593, 1990.
2. Guyton JL: Fractures of hip, acetabulum, and pelvis. In Canale ST (ed): Campbell's Operative Orthopaedics, 9th ed., St. Louis, Mosby, 1998, pp 2252–2279.
3. Helfet DL: Open reduction internal fixation of the pelvis. Techn Orthop 4:67–78, 1990.
4. Perry JF: Pelvic open fractures. Clin Orthop 151:41–45, 1980.
5. Peters PC Jr, Bucholz RW: The assessment of pelvic stability following pelvic ring disruptions. Techn Orthop 4:52–59, 1990.

63. ACETABULAR FRACTURES

Donald J. Walla, M.D.

1. What radiographs are best suited for evaluation of acetabular fractures?

The acetabular fracture is best evaluated on anteroposterior (AP) views of the pelvis and hip and 45-degree oblique views of the pelvis. CT scans are also useful in most patients.

2. What is meant by the anterior and posterior columns of the acetabulum?

The anterior or iliopubic column runs obliquely downward, inward, and anteriorly from the anterior part of the superior iliac crest to the pubic symphysis. The posterior of ilioischial column descents downward from the level of the angle of the greater sciatic notch to the ischial tuberosity.

3. What is meant by a transverse acetabular fracture?

Transverse fractures involve both the anterior and posterior columns and divide the innominate bone into a superior segment that contains the acetabular roof and intact ilium and an inferior segment that consists of the ischiopubic bone.

4. How are acetabular fractures classified?

The Letournel classification includes ten types of fracture. In the five elementary or simple fractures, a part or all of one column of the acetabulum has been detached. Elementary fractures include (1) posterior column fractures, (2) anterior column fractures, (3) anterior wall fractures, (4) posterior wall fractures, and (5) transverse fractures.

The five complex associated fractures include at least two of the simple fractures: (1) fractures of the posterior column and posterior wall, (2) associated transverse and posterior wall fractures, (3) T-shaped fractures, (4) associated anterior and posterior hemitransverse fractures, and (5) fractures of both columns.

5. What are the goals of acetabular fracture management?

The goals are to restore motion of the hip, to mobilize the patient, and to avoid posttraumatic arthritis. An imperfect reduction with as little as 1–2 mm of displacement may lead to osteoarthritis. Bony fragments within the hip joint and injury of articular cartilage may lead to early posttraumatic arthritis.

6. What are the basic treatment principles of acetabular fractures?
As with any articular injury, the goal is to restore function and prevent late osteoarthritis, the most common long-term complication. Most osteoarthritis is caused by imperfect reduction, and residual displacements as small as 1–2 mm, particularly in weight-bearing surfaces, may lead to degenerative changes. Other common causes are incarcerated bony fragments or articular surface damage that is not evident radiographically.

7. Can acetabular fractures be life-threatening?
An acetabular fracture is usually not life-threatening. Massive pelvic hemorrhage occurs usually from associated pelvic injuries and rarely from displaced acetabular fragments.

8. What types of treatment are used to manage acetabular fractures?
Nonoperative treatment is a consideration for nondisplaced acetabular fractures as well as transverse fractures and minimally displaced two-column fractures. Traction of the affected leg should be maintained for 4–8 weeks to obtain fracture healing. Open reduction and internal fixation (ORIF) of displaced fractures of the acetabulum have become the standard of care.

9. Does timing of surgical treatment of acetabular fractures make a difference?
Urgent surgical treatment is necessary when a patient has an anterior or posterior dislocation that cannot be reduced by closed means. A delay of 2–3 days with the patient maintained in distal femoral traction is appropriate for all other fractures. A delay longer than 10 days makes reduction more difficult, and by 3 weeks callus formation significantly complicates reduction.

If such delays are unavoidable, open reduction and internal fixation should be undertaken in younger patients. In older patients, particularly those with complex fractures, surgery may be deferred with the anticipation that total joint replacement may be required later.

10. How are acetabular fractures stabilized surgically?
Various surgical exposures are available, depending on the location of the fractures. One should select an approach that allows the complete operation to be performed and stabilization of the fractures with a combination of screws and plates. The exposure also should allow exploration of the joint surface when necessary. The most common surgical exposures are (1) the Kocher-Langenbeck, (2) the ilioinguinal, (3) the extended iliofemoral, and (4) the triradiate incisions.

11. What complications are associated with operative management of acetabular fractures?

Infection	Heterotopic bone formation
Sciatic nerve palsy	Posttraumatic arthritis
Thrombophlebitis	Avascular necrosis of the femoral head

12. What are the principles of postoperative management of open reduction and internal fixation of acetabular fractures?
Closed suction drainage and antibiotic therapy is used for 48 hours. Passive motion of the hip is initiated after drain removal and crutch walking with limited weightbearing starts as soon as pain is diminished. Eight weeks after internal fixation, weightbearing is increased progressively as long as the fracture shows evidence of healing.

13. What are the causes of sciatic nerve palsy?
The sciatic nerve may be injured by initial trauma or by retraction of the nerve during a posterior surgical approach to the acetabulum.

14. What are the causes of heterotopic bone formation or myositis ossificans?
Ectopic bone formation usually occurs after an extended iliofemoral approach, which provides lateral exposure of the innominate bone. This complications can be minimized by use of Indocin or postoperative low-dose irradiation.

15. How can the risks of postoperative infections be minimized?
The incidence of wound infection can be reduced by careful manipulation of the soft tissues, use of profuse antibiotic irrigation, perioperative intravenous antibiotics, hemostasis, and suction drains.

16. How can the risk of thrombophlebitis be minimized?
A patient may be fitted with compression stockings and sequential compression devices. Heparin or Coumadin may be used for anticoagulation.

17. What is the significance of the superior gluteal artery?
The superior gluteal artery may be incarcerated in fractures that communicate with the greater sciatic notch. It also may be injured during a surgical approach, resulting in massive bleeding and possibly ischemic necrosis of the gluteal musculature.

18. What is the treatment for heterotopic ossification?
Removal of established ectopic bone may be considered if it inhibits motion of the hip joint. The removal is usually done 12–18 months after the initial surgery when there is less likelihood of recurrent ectopic bone formation.

19. What should be done if a bony fragment is evident on radiographs after ORIF of an acetabular fracture?
The fragment(s) should be removed.

20. What is the infection rate after ORIF of displaced acetabular fractures?
The infection rate is 2–4%.

BIBLIOGRAPHY

1. Frymoyer JW (ed): Orthopaedic Knowledge Update 4. American Academy of Orthopedic Surgeons, 1993.
2. Guyton JL: Fractures of hip, acetabulum, and pelvis. In Canale ST (ed): Campbell's Operative Orthopaedics, 9th ed., St. Louis, Mosby, 1998, pp 2234–2252.
3. Letournel E: Classification and evaluation of acetabular fractures. Techn Orthop 4(4)5–23, 1990.
4. Mears DC, Gordon RG: Internal fixation of acetabular fractures. Techn Orthop 4(4):36–51, 1990.
5. Pennal GF, et al: Results of treatment of acetabular fractures. Clin Orthop 151:115–124, 1980.
6. Rockwood CA, Green DP, Bucholz RN, et al (eds): Fractures, 4th ed. Philadelphia, J.B. Lippincott, 1996.

64. HIP DISLOCATIONS AND FEMORAL HEAD FRACTURES

Samar K. Ray, M.D., FRCS

1. What is a hip dislocation?
The hip joint is a ball-and-socket type of joint: the acetabulum is the socket and the head of the femur is the ball. It is one of most stable joints in the body because of the deep acetabular cavity, the spherical concentric head of the femur, strong capsular ligaments, and massive surrounding muscles. The head of the femur may get displaced in relation to the acetabulum from severe trauma, causing dislocation.

2. Why is a hip dislocation so important?
Hip dislocation causes immediate, profound disability and, if not treated properly, may cause life-long disability due to complications such as as avascular necrosis and early degenerative arthritis in the joint.

3. What important features must be remembered in the initial evaluation of a patient with hip dislocation?

Because hip dislocation occurs from high-energy trauma, such as motor vehicle or pedestrian accidents, patients may have other life-threatening injuries. In 35–40% of cases, other severe injuries occur, including craniofacial, chest, abdominal, and other musculoskeletal injuries. An estimated 50% of patients have fractures in other parts of the body.

4. What are the principles of treatment?
- Careful evaluation of the patient for associated injury
- Immediate closed reduction with assessment of stability and reduction
- Careful radiographic evaluations, including postreduction computed tomography (CT), if necessary, for evaluation of congruency of reduction and associated fractures of the femoral head or acetabulum.

5. Discuss the classification of hip dislocations.

Hip dislocations are divided into three types: anterior, posterior, or central dislocation. Classification depends on the position of the femoral head in relationship to the acetabulum. In anterior dislocation, the femoral head rests anterior to the coronal plane of the acetabulum, perhaps with associated fractures of the acetabulum or femoral head. In posterior dislocations, the femoral head rests posteriorly to the coronal plane of the acetabulum. Posterior dislocations may occur with fracture of the posterior acetabular rim, the acetabular floor, or the femoral head. In central of fracture dislocation, a fracture is present on the inner wall of the acetabulum with inward displacement of the femoral head.

6. What is the most common dislocation?

Only 10–15% of all hip dislocations are anterior. Posterior dislocations occur in 85–90% of cases.

7. How are posterior and anterior dislocations differentiated clinically?

In a posterior dislocation, the lower extremity is flexed, adducted, and internally rotated at the hip. In anterior dislocations, the extremity is slightly shortened, abducted, and externally rotated.

8. What types of anterior dislocations are seen?

Anterior dislocations may be classified as superior or inferior. Both types result from abduction and external rotation. Superior dislocations occur in extension, whereas inferior dislocations occur in flexion.

9. What neurovascular structures are in jeopardy with anterior dislocations?

Trauma to the femoral artery, vein, and nerve has been reported in superior and open anterior dislocations.

10. Describe the treatment for anterior dislocations of the hip.

Early diagnosis with prompt closed reduction under general anesthesia is the treatment of choice. If multiple attempts at closed reduction fail, open reduction is necessary.

11. What maneuvers must be done to reduce anterior dislocations of the hip?

Most clinicians believe that elements of longitudinal traction, adduction of the hip, and internal rotation are needed. Stimson's gravity method has sometimes been used for reduction. The patient lies in a prone position with the affected leg placed in a downward position. Traction is placed longitudinally, and the pelvis is stabilized. Internal and external rotation and abduction are then used to reduce the dislocation.

12. What are the complications of anterior dislocations?

Early complications include neurovascular compromise of the femoral artery, vein, or nerve, which occur mainly with the superior anterior dislocation. Inferior dislocations do not have a high incidence of compromise. Anterior hip dislocations may be irreducible by closed means. Obstructions to closed reduction include fractures and iliopsoas and rectus muscles. Late complications include posttraumatic arthritis, aseptic necrosis, and recurrent dislocations.

13. What is the incidence of aseptic necrosis after anterior dislocation of the hip?

Aseptic necrosis, which is less common in anterior than in posterior dislocation, is reported in approximately 5–8% of the cases. Aseptic necrosis may appear from 2–5 years after dislocation.

14. What is the mechanism of injury of posterior dislocation?

Posterior dislocation is usually related to high-energy trauma. The mechanism of injury is usually force applied to the flexed knee in an abducted position, as often occurs when the knee strikes the dashboard in an automobile accident.

15. Describe the clinical findings in posterior dislocation.

The limb is shortened, internally rotated, and adducted. Sciatic nerve injury may be seen in 10–14% of patients. Associated fractures of the femoral head and femoral shaft are common. Knee ligament injuries also are seen because of the high-energy trauma.

16. What anatomic areas should be carefully scrutinized on the radiographs?
- The femoral head for fracture.
- The acetabulum for fracture.
- The femoral neck for nondisplaced fractures that may displace when closed reduction is attempted.

17. With posterior dislocation and associated acetabular fractures, is stability of the joint an issue?

Studies have shown that fragments < 20–25% of the acetabular wall usually do not affect hip stability, whereas those > 40% result in instability and recurrent dislocations.

18. What radiographs should be taken in patients with suspected dislocations?
- Anteroposterior (AP) radiograph
- Oblique lateral view of the pelvis
- Posterior oblique view of the pelvis
- Lateral film of the hip to show the position of the fragments

19. What other radiographic studies are indicated?

Radiographs must be taken postoperatively to show the adequacy of reduction, the presence or absence of fragments in the joint, and the accuracy of reduction of associated femoral head and acetabular fracture fragments. CT scans may be helpful in patients suspected of having loose fragments in the joint, incomplete reduction of the fractured femoral head fragment, or soft-tissue interposition.

20. What is the method of treatment for posterior dislocations without fractures?

The Allis reduction maneuver involves traction at the level of the knee at 90° with internal and external rotation of the extremity and progressive extension.

21. What is the postoperative treatment for dislocation of the hip?

Postoperative treatment involves gentle traction until the hip is pain-free, usually from several days to 2 weeks. General passive range of motion is begun. Spica cast and immobilization after reduction are not used. Controversy exists as to when the hip can safely bear weight.

Opinions range from 2 weeks to 12 months after reduction. Most authors state that weightbearing may resume with crutches when pain and spasm disappear.

22. **What are the indications for open reduction in posterior dislocations of the hip?**
   • To remove loose fragments from the joint.
   • To restore joint stability and joint congruity by open reduction and internal fixation of large fragments.
   • To ensure the accuracy of the reduction.

23. **What complications may occur in posterior fracture dislocations of the hip?**
   1. Approximately 10% of patients have **sciatic nerve palsy,** usually involving the peroneal component. In patients with simple dislocations, reduction removes the pressure on the nerve, and recovery usually is complete. If sciatic nerve deficit occurs after reduction, surgical exploration is indicated.
   2. **Irreducible posterior dislocations** occur in 3–16% of patients with simple dislocations usually because of buttonholing of the femoral head through the hip capsule or interposition of the piriformis muscle and tendon. Nonconcentric reductions are usually caused by fracture fragments; surgical removal is necessary.
   3. Approximately 20% of patients have significant **knee injuries,** involving collateral or cruciate ligaments. Most often the posterior cruciate ligament is injured. Because the injury is related to an anterior blow to the tibia, posterior lateral instabilities are found.
   4. **Recurrent dislocations** usually occur in patients with a posterior fracture; they also may be associated with paralysis and sepsis.
   5. **Myositis ossificans,** which develops in approximately 2% of patients, is related to muscle damage and hematoma formation.
   6. The incidence of **aseptic necrosis** may be diminished significantly by reduction within 6 hours. Delay greater than 12 hours results in a high incidence of avascular necrosis.
   7. **Posttraumatic degenerative arthritis** develops in approximately 35% of patients with posterior fracture dislocation of the hip. The severity of the initial trauma is usually the major factor in determining the development of posttraumatic arthritis. Posttraumatic arthritis is found approximately twice as often in fracture dislocations as in simple dislocations.

24. **Describe the femoral head fractures that are seen with dislocations.**
   Femoral head fractures were classified by Pipkin in four categories:
   Type 1: Femoral head fracture caudad to the fovea centralis, which is the most inferior portion of the femoral head.
   Type 2: Femoral head fracture from inferior to superior to the fovea centralis.
   Type 3: Type 1 or 2 with associated femoral neck fracture.
   Type 4: Type 1, 2, or 3 with associated acetabular fracture.

25. **List the treatment options for central fracture dislocation at the acetabulum.**
   • Traction with or without closed reduction of the femoral head
   • Open reduction and internal fixation
   • Primary arthroplasty
   • Primary arthrodesis

BIBLIOGRAPHY

1. Frymoyer JW (ed): Hip Trauma. Orthopedic Knowledge Update. Rosemont, IL, American Academy of Orthopaedic Surgeons, 1993, pp 525–537.
2. Guyton JL: Fractures of the hip, acetabulum, and pelvis. In Canale ST (ed): Campbell's Operative Orthopaedics, 9th ed. St. Louis, Mosby, 1998, pp 2224–2234.
3. Rockwood CA, Green DP, Bucholz RW (eds): Rockwood and Green's Fractures in Adults, vol. II, 3rd ed. Philadelphia, J.B. Lippincott, 1991, pp 1574–1625.

65. FEMORAL NECK FRACTURES

Michael J. Schmidt, M.D., and Randall D. Neumann, M.D.

1. What are the major risk factors contributing to the occurrence of hip fractures?

Individuals at risk include urban Caucasian women who are of slight build and physically inactive. Other significant risk factors include a history of excessive alcohol intake, use of psychotropic medications, senile dementia, and history of previous hip fracture.

2. What is osteoporosis?

Osteoporosis is a disease process associated with aging and inactivity; it is characterized by decreased bone mass with normal mineralization and results in loss of bone strength.

3. Does osteoporosis contribute to the incidence of hip fractures?

By decreasing bone strength, osteoporosis increases the likelihood of fracture from minor trauma such as falls.

4. What is the effect of hip fractures on mortality rates?

In general, the mortality rate increases during the first year after a hip fracture. After 1 year, the mortality rate returns to normal for age- and sex-matched controls.

5. What are the two major types of femoral neck fractures?

The two major types of neck fractures are **nondisplaced/impacted** and **displaced.**

6. What are the signs and symptoms of an impacted femoral neck fracture?

- Groin pain referred down the medial thigh, sometimes to the level of the knee
- Antalgic gait
- Limitation of hip motion

7. What are the signs and symptoms of displaced femoral neck fractures?

Generalized pain occurs in the hip region with the thigh in external rotation and abduction. Slight shortening of the extremity is often present.

8. What major medical complications may result from femoral neck fractures and subsequent surgical management?

Deep venous thrombosis, pulmonary embolism, and infection.

9. What is the major cause of hip fractures in young adults?

High-energy trauma resulting from motor vehicle accidents or falls from heights.

10. Do femoral neck and femoral shaft fractures occur together?

Ipsilateral (same side) femoral neck and femoral shaft fractures occur in about 2.5–6% of all femoral shaft fractures.

11. What is the recommended treatment for nondisplaced/impacted femoral neck fractures?

The recommended treatment is usually surgical, consisting of internal fixation with 3 or 4 parallel, cannulated lag screws. The procedure can be performed through a small incision or percutaneously.

12. What is the recommended treatment for displaced femoral neck fractures?

In general, prompt closed or open reduction with internal fixation is recommended in the younger, active patient. Hemiarthroplasty or total hip arthroplasty is generally recommended for the older, less active patient whose physiologic age is > 70 years. Younger patients with Parkinson's disease, dementia, or psychosis also are candidates for hemiarthroplasty.

13. What are the major bony complications after internal fixation of displaced femoral neck fractures?
- Nonunion (10–30% of patients)
- Avascular necrosis (15–33%)
- Late segmental collapse (7–27%)

14. What are the major bony complications after treatment of displaced femoral neck fractures with hemiarthroplasty?
- Hip pain secondary to acetabular erosion and prosthetic loosening
- Hip dislocation
- Femur fractures
- Heterotopic ossification

15. What is avascular necrosis?
Avascular necrosis is a phenomenon that occurs early after femoral neck fracture and results in the actual death of bone in the femoral head secondary to ischemia.

16. What is late segmental collapse?
It refers to the collapse of subchondral bone and articular cartilage overlying avascular necrotic bone resulting in joint incongruity, subsequent degenerative joint disease, and pain.

17. Do all patients who develop avascular necrosis after femoral neck fracture later develop late segmental collapse?
No. After adequate reduction and internal fixation, portions of the femoral head that develop avascular necrosis may revascularize and repair before stresses on the hip joint result in collapse of the necrotic area.

18. What are the two most important factors in decreasing the occurrence of nonunion or avascular necrosis after femoral neck fracture?
The two most important factors are prompt, anatomic fracture reduction and stable internal fixation. Acceptable reduction may include up to 15° of valgus angulation (valgus impacted fracture) and < 10° of anterior or posterior angulation.

19. What is the treatment for ipsilateral femoral neck and shaft fractures?
The femoral neck fracture takes precedence. Treatment should include anatomic reduction with stable internal fixation. Avascular necrosis occurs in up to 20% of cases.

20. What are the indications for performing a total hip arthroplasty after a femoral neck fracture?
Indications include displaced femoral neck fractures in patients > 60 years old with rheumatoid arthritis, preexisting osteoarthritis or degenerative joint disease, and Paget's disease or pathologic fractures with associated acetabular involvement.

21. What problems arise with the patient when performing a total hip arthroplasty after femoral neck fracture?
In one study, 21% had perioperative medical complications, which included an extremely high incidence (10%) of dislocation. Both complication rates are higher than for patients undergoing total hip arthroplasty for arthritis, who showed good long-term function and survival.

22. Which of the four ascending cervical arteries (anterior, medial, posterior, and lateral) provide the major source of blood supply to the femoral head and neck?
The lateral ascending branches arising from the lateral femoral circumflex artery.

23. What prophylactic measures are useful in preventing thromboembolic disease after hip fractures?

Prophylactic measures include aspirin (particularly in male patients), warfarin, and dextran alone or in combination with dihydroergotamine. Low-dose intravenous heparin alone or in combinations with dihydroergotamine and intermittent pneumatic compression stockings also have proved useful in reducing the incidence of thromboembolic disease.

24. What diagnostic tools are useful in evaluating patients with suspected nondisplaced stress fractures or impacted fractures of th femoral neck?

Useful diagnostic tools include anteroposterior pelvic and lateral radiographs, bone scans, and tomograms. If a fracture is not confirmed by these methods, radiographs should be repeated in 10–14 days.

25. Can fractures of the femoral neck occur in younger patients without significant trauma?

Yes. The most common patients are amenorrheic female athletes, especially runners, who develop pain and subsequent stress fractures. Such fractures also may occur bilaterally.

BIBLIOGRAPHY

1. Canale ST (ed): Campbell's Operative Orthopaedics, 9th ed. St. Louis, Mosby, 1998.
2. Frymoyer JW: Orthopaedic Knowledge Update-4. Rosemont, IL, American Academy of Orthopaedic Surgeons, 1993.
3. Koval KJ, Zuckerman JD: Hip fractures: I. Evaluation and treatment of intertrochanteric fractures. J Am Acad Orthop Surg 2:150–156, 1994.
4. Koval KJ, Zuckerman JD: Hip fractures: I. Overview and evaluation and treatment of femoral neck fractures. J Am Acad Orthop Surg 2:141–149, 1994.
5. Lee BP, Berry DJ, Harmsen WS, Sim FH: Total hip arthroplasty for the treatment of an acute fracture of the femoral neck: Long-term results. J Bone Joint Surg Am 80:70–75, 1998.
6. Peljovich AE, Patterson BM: Ipsilateral femoral neck and shaft fractures. J Am Acad Orthop Surg 6:106–113, 1998.
7. Poss R: Orthopaedic Knowledge Update-3. Rosemont, IL, American Academy of Orthopaedic Surgeons, 1990.
8. Rockwood CA, Green DP, Bucholz RW, Heckman JD (eds): Rockwood and Green's Fractures in Adults, Vols. 1 and 2, 4th ed. Philadelphia, J.B. Lippincott, 1996.
9. Voss L, DaSilva M, Trafton PG: Bilateral femoral neck stress fractures in an amenorrheic athlete. Am J Orthop 26:789–792, 1997.
10. Wosinsky PR, Johnson KD: Ipsilateral femoral neck and shaft fractures. Clin Orthop 92:81–90, 1995.

66. INTERTROCHANTERIC FRACTURES

Michael J. Schmidt, M.D., and Randall D. Neumann, M.D.

1. What is an intertrochanteric fracture of the hip?

An intertrochanteric fracture of the hip is an extracapsular fracture that occurs along a line between the greater and lesser trochanters with variable comminution.

2. Which is more common in the elderly: intertrochanteric fracture, subtrochanteric fracture, or femoral neck fractures?

In one study, 47% were intertrochanteric, 23% were subtrochanteric, and 37% were femoral neck fractures.

3. What clinical signs and symptoms are associated with an intertrochanteric fracture of the hip?
- Swelling and pain in the hip region
- Ecchymosis over the greater trochanter
- Marked shortening of the extremity with as much as 90° of external rotation deformity

4. What diagnostic tools are necessary to evaluate an intertrochanteric fracture?
An anteroposterior radiograph, preferably in internal rotation, and a lateral radiograph.

5. Evans' classification divides intertrochanteric fractures into two main types, depending on the direction of the fracture. What are the characteristics of a type I fracture?
The type I fracture extends upward and outward from the lesser trochanter. Fracture stability is obtained by anatomic medial-cortical reduction.

6. What are the characteristics of type II fractures?
The fracture line is in reversed obliquity or extends downward from the lesser trochanter. Type II fractures retain a degree of instability secondary to a tendency of the distal segment or femoral shaft to displace medially.

7. What is a four-part intertrochanteric fracture?
A four-part intertrochanteric fracture is composed of four major fracture fragments, including the femoral head neck, greater trochanter, lesser trochanter, and femoral shaft.

8. Which major muscle groups create indirect forces that contribute to the formation of a four-part intertrochanteric fracture?
The iliopsoas muscle on the lesser trochanter and the abductor muscles on the greater trochanter.

9. What is the Singh index?
The Singh index is a classification system that measures the degree of osteoporosis in the proximal femur based on radiographic evaluation of the trabecular patterns.

10. Are intertrochanteric fractures stable?
Not always. Unstable intertrochanteric fractures result from comminution of the posteromedial cortical buttress of the distal fragment, fracture extension into the subtrochanteric area, and reverse oblique fractures. Unstable fractures may account for 50–65% of all intertrochanteric fractures.

11. What is the recommended treatment for intertrochanteric fractures?
Most intertrochanteric fractures are treated by sliding hip compression screws after closed reduction. Calcar replacement prostheses are used in selective cases involving severe comminution.

12. How is closed reduction of intertrochanteric fractures achieved before internal fixation?
The patient is positioned supine on a fracture table, and the physician applies longitudinal traction, slight abduction, and usually slight external rotation to the hip under anesthesia.

13. What are the advantages of a sliding hip compression screw for fixation of an intertrochanteric fracture?
The sliding hip compression screw may be used to treat both stable and unstable intertrochanteric fractures, because it provides secure fixation of the head and neck fragment to the distal fragment and allows controlled impaction at the fracture site. Therefore, its use decreases the risk of fixation failure compared with rigid nail-plate devices and allows earlier mobilization and weightbearing.

14. What is medial displacement osteotomy?

Medial displacement osteotomy is a reduction technique for unstable intertrochanteric fractures involving medial displacement of the distal segment or femoral shaft in hopes of achieving better mediocortical stability. This technique was commonly used in conjunction with rigid nail-plate fixation devices.

15. Is medial displacement osteotomy useful in conjunction with sliding screw compression devices?

In general, anatomic reduction of unstable intertrochanteric fractures results in less shortening and better stability and is preferred over medial displacement osteotomy.

16. Sideplate angles of the sliding hip compression screw device are available in 5°-increments, ranging from 130–150°. Which sideplate angles are most commonly used for fixation of intertrochanteric fractures?

The 135°- and 150°-angle sideplates are used most commonly.

17. What are the advantages and disadvantages of using a 150°-angle sideplate?

Theoretical advantages include close approximation of resultant forces across the hip joint, which facilitates sliding, fracture impaction, and reduction in the moment arm on the device, thus reducing the risk of implant failure. Disadvantages include difficulty with the insertion of the lag screw into the center of the femoral head and neck and the need for a diaphyseal insertion point, which may cause a greater stress-riser effect than the 135°-angle device.

18. What are the advantages and disadvantages of the 135°-angle plates?

Advantages include easy insertion of the compression screw into the central portion of the femoral head and neck and a metaphyseal insertion point that causes less of a stress-riser effect than the diaphyseal insertion points required with 150°-angle plates.

19. What position of the lag screw within the femoral head and neck provides the most secure fixation?

Central position of the lag screw within the femoral head and neck to within 1 cm of subchondral bone is usually recommended. Short of this position, a posteroinferior position is acceptable.

20. The strength of the fracture-implant combination is determined by which five variables?
- Degree of osteoporosis
- Fragment geometry
- Adequacy of reduction
- Implant design
- Placement of the implant

21. What complications are seen with the internal fixation of intertrochanteric fractures?

1. Device failure, including plate fatigue fracture and lag screw cutting out of the femoral head posteriorly and superiorly
2. Malunion with shortening and rotation
3. Nonunion
4. Avascular necrosis
5. Infection

22. How are calcar replacement prostheses used in the treatment of intertrochanteric fractures?

Calcar replacement prostheses are used primarily to salvage fixation failure of an intertrochanteric fracture when repeat open reduction and internal fixation are not possible. Their use as a primary prosthetic replacement for treatment of unstable intertrochanteric fractures is controversial; they should be confined to patients with severe osteoporosis that renders proximal fixation with any device questionable.

23. Complications of unstable intertrochanteric fractures can be significantly decreased by what two measures?

Stronger implants and restoration of the posteromedial cortical buttress.

24. Are nonunions of intertrochanteric fractures common?

No. Because intertrochanteric fractures occur in cancellous bone with good blood supply, the actual incidence of nonunion is reported to be < 2%.

25. Does avascular necrosis occur in association with intertrochanteric fractures?

Rarely. The actual incidence is ~ 0.8%.

BIBLIOGRAPHY

1. Canale ST (ed): Campbell's Operative Orthopaedics, 9th ed. St. Louis, Mosby, 1998.
2. Frymoyer JW: Orthopedic Knowledge Update-4. Rosemonth, IL, American Academy of Orthopaedic Surgeons, 1993.
3. Koval KJ, Zuckerman JD: Hip fractures: I. Evaluation and treatment of intertrochanteric fractures. J Am Acad Orthop Surg 2:150–156, 1994.
4. Michelson JD, Myers A, Jinnah R, et al: Epidemiology of hip fractures among the elderly. Risk factors for fracture type. Clin Orthop 311:129–135, 1995.
5. Poss R: Orthopaedic Knowledge Update-3. Rosemont, IL, American Academy of Orthopaedic Surgeons, 1990.
6. Rockwood CA, Green DP, Bucholz RW, Heckman JD (eds): Rockwood and Green's Fractures in Adults, Vols. 1 and 2, 4th ed. Philadelphia, J.B. Lippincott, 1996.

67. SUBTROCHANTERIC FEMUR FRACTURES

James T. Canedy, M.D.

1. What is a subtrochanteric fracture?

A subtrochanteric fracture occurs between the lesser trochanter and a point 5 cm distal to the lesser trochanter.

2. Who is most susceptible to hip fractures?

Three distinct categories of people are susceptible to hip fractures:

1. The elderly population (especially white women > 50 years of age, who account for approximately 80% of all hip fractures);

2. Patients (usually young, with normal bones) who have sustained high-energy trauma such as motor vehicle accidents, falls from a height, or gunshot wounds; and

3. Older patients with impending pathologic fracture due, for example, to multiple myeloma or metastatic cancer.

3. What percentage of falls in the elderly result in proximal femur fractures?

One percent of falls in the elderly result in hip fractures. However, such falls make up 40% of nursing home admissions, and more than 90% of hip fractures are caused by falls.

4. What work-up is appropriate for a recent fall and proximal femur fracture?

The work-up should include electrocardiogram, x-rays of the pelvis, hip, proximal femur, and chest. CBC, electrolytes, BUN, serum creatinine and blood glucose, liver function analysis, and stool guiac are usual laboratory tests.

5. What underlying medical conditions may a history of falls indicate?

The differential diagnosis should include dehydration, urinary tract infection, malnutrition, orthostatic hypotension, neoplasm, and cardiac and neurologic disease.

6. Which measures may prevent falls in the elderly?
- Encouraging patients to report falls
- Rubberized mats on bathroom floors and slippers with nonslip soles
- Grab bars near bathtubs and toilets
- An obstacle-free path to the bathroom at night
- Night-lights for better visibility
- An external hip protector for dissipation of energy may reduce the risk of hip fractures in the nursing home population
- Evaluation for adequate nutrition

7. What are the main causes of proximal femur fracture in young populations?
The quality of a young person's bone requires a much more violent injury, such as a motor vehicle accident or a fall from a height, to sustain a fracture. The bone is able to absorb more energy; therefore, the fracture tends to be more severe and difficult to treat.

8. What associated medical problems contribute to proximal femur fractures in the elderly?
Associated medical problems such as coronary artery disease, cardiac arrhythmias, and diabetes may cause dizziness and syncope that result in falls and associated proximal femur fractures. Osteoporosis, which is probably the most important factor in development of a hip fracture, places white elderly women at highest risk.

9. What factors are responsible for a slower rate of union and a higher rate of nonunion in subtrochanteric fractures?
The subtrochanteric area of the femur is composed mainly of cortical bone, which is often comminuted in fractures. Less vascularity and fracture surface are available for healing in cortical bone than in cancellous bone (e.g., intertrochanteric fractures). The large mechanical stresses in the subtrochanteric area may result in failure of internal fixation devices before bony union occurs.

10. How are subtrochanteric fractures classified?
Several classification systems are based on the area of the fracture. Fielding bases his system on distance at or below the lesser trochanter. The incidence of complications after treatment increases as the fracture becomes more distal. Seinsheimer's classification is based on the number of major fragments and the location and shape of fracture lines. The higher grade fractures extend into the intertrochanteric region and have a high level of comminution. Others categorize subtrochanteric fractures as stable or unstable. In stable subtrochanteric fractures it is possible to reestablish bone-to-bone contact in the medial and posterior cortexes. In unstable fractures the medial cortical apposition is not attainable because of comminution or fracture obliquity.

11. Describe the treatment options for subtrochanteric fractures.
Patients may be treated operatively or nonoperatively. In the past nonoperative treatment resulted in high rates of morbidity and mortality. Nonoperative treatment includes traction, hip spica cast, and a cast-bracing technique. Operative treatment includes the use of plate and sliding hip screws or intramedullary devices.

12. What operative treatment is used for treatment of subtrochanteric fractures?
Many devices are available. The most common are a plate and screw assembly, intramedullary devices, and sliding hip screws. Sliding compression hip screws and plates have difficulty withstanding the stresses placed at the subtrochanteric region with weightbearing. In the past they have had a higher incidence of plate fracture and nonunion at the fracture site. When feasible, intramedullary devices are generally the treatment of choice; they are usually done with image intensification and essentially closed treatment of the fracture with a proximal incision.

13. What is an intramedullary device? What are its advantages?
The center of the proximal femur is hollow and filled with cancellous bone and fat. An intramedullary nail acts as an internal splint. The nail is generally completely circular, or it may be slotted. A proximal incision in the trochanteric region gives access to the medullary canal. The

nail is driven proximally to distally and holds the fracture fragments in place until the fracture heals. Often early weightbearing is allowed. Intramedullary rods, the most stable form of fixation, are the treatment of choice in pathologic fracture.

14. What is the most common cause for nonunion of a subtrochanteric fracture?
Lack of stability at the fracture site and comminution.

15. Should bone grafting be used in the treatment of subtrochanteric fractures?
Supplementary bone graft is used in patients with severe comminution along the medial cortex; it is especially useful in patients with a medial gap after fracture fixation.

16. What are the most common early complications of proximal femur fractures?
Acute blood loss and hypovolemia are initial considerations, especially in younger patients who experience more violent trauma. Third space blood loss may account for a significant drop in blood volume. Other significant injuries in young patients include knee ligament disruption, associated spinal or pelvic fractures, and nerve or vessel damage. Complications associated with trauma and requiring subsequent bed rest may include deep venous thrombosis, pneumonia, and urinary tract infection if a Foley catheter is in place.

FEMORAL SHAFT FRACTURES

17. What is the mechanism for femoral shaft fractures?
Most femoral shaft fractures require major trauma, including motor vehicle and motorcycle accidents, falls from heights, and gunshot wounds. Patients who have pathologic bone due to osteoporosis, tumor, or osteomyelitis may sustain a fracture. Stress fractures rarely occur.

18. Why is a femoral shaft fracture considered an emergency?
Femoral shaft fractures result from significant trauma and often are associated with multiple injuries. Early treatment may prevent medical as well as orthopedic complications.

19. What is the appropriate mechanism of transportation of a patient with proximal femur fracture, either from the accident scene or from an initial emergency room visit?
The patient should be transported by ambulance; intravenous access is crucial because of the possibility of initial blood loss. A form of longitudinal traction and/or strapping is appropriate for comfort and prevention of additional injury.

20. How are femoral shaft fractures classified?
No classification is universally accepted. Femoral shaft fractures generally are categorized by the amount of soft-tissue injury, geographic location, fracture geometry, fracture comminution, and associated injury. Geographic classification includes three categories: proximal third, midshaft, and distal third. Categories based on geometric shape with a major fracture line include transverse, oblique, spiral, and segmental. Classification as an open or closed injury depends on whether the bone has broken through the skin. Distinction should be made between minimal and moderate comminution at the fracture site.

21. What is the incidence of ligamentous injuries with ipsilateral femoral shaft fractures?
The incidence of ligamentous injuries about the knee is as high as 5%. It is easy to miss a ligamentous injury, because the patient is in a great deal of pain. Deformity of the leg is common, and there may be no easy way to test the stability until the fracture is internally reduced or has healed.

22. What is the incidence of ipsilateral femoral neck and femoral shaft fracture?
The incidence is 5%. The most common area is the femoral neck, but other sites are also possible. Pelvic radiographs should be routine in patients with a femoral shaft fracture to rule out femoral neck and intertrochanteric fracture, hip dislocation, and acetabular or pelvic fracture.

23. What are the common immediate complications associated with femoral shaft fractures?

Vascular injuries occur in 2% of patients with femoral shaft fractures. Even without an arterial injury, bleeding may be significant and lead to hypovolemia. Arteriograms are indicated for any fracture related to penetrating trauma and in patients with suspected arterial injury. Because ligamentous injuries are associated with femoral shaft fractures, careful palpation of collateral ligaments and joint spaces is necessary. Nerves escape injury with most fractures of the femoral shaft, although the incidence of nerve injury is higher with penetrating trauma, such as stab wound or gunshot wounds.

24. What types of treatment are available for femoral shaft fractures?

Treatment may be either nonoperative with casting or operative with internal fixation. Balanced skeletal traction is a good option in pediatric patients, followed by treatment with spica cast and immobilization. In adults internal fixation is the treatment of choice; intramedullary nails are preferred for subtrochanteric femoral shaft fractures. Traction followed by a cast brace is not as commonly used as in the past. External fixation is used in open, contaminated femoral shaft fractures.

25. What is the initial treatment of choice for an open femur fracture?

An open femur fracture should be treated as an emergency with initial debridement and irrigation of the fracture site, appropriate antibiotic coverage, and initial cultures. Primary internal fixation continues to be controversial.

26. Can internal fixation be used with an open fracture of the femur?

Two options are available with an open shaft fracture. The first consists of debridement, irrigation, delayed wound closure, and skeletal traction, followed by fracture stabilization in 7–10 days. Multiple injuries dictate the necessity for stabilization. The severity of the wound also dictates the appropriateness of internal fixation. Wounds with minimal contamination may be treated with internal fixation with no significant increase in risk of wound infection after debridement. Patients with grossly contaminated wounds and vascular injuries should be treated on an individual basis.

27. What is a Kirchner wire traction pin? How is balanced skeletal traction used?

The Kirchner wire traction pin is a small pin that is inserted under sterile techniques through the distal femur or proximal tibia with care to avoid the neurovascular structures. This technique allows application of longitudinal skeletal traction, which extends the bone fragments to full length, and helps to control pain and to diminish bleeding. An intramedullary device should not be inserted unless the bone fragments are extended to length or the fracture is acute. Balance suspension is any form of sling below the leg to align the fracture fragments and to prevent undue pressure on any one area of the leg. When the fracture fragments show evidence of callus or new bone formation, a cast brace or hip spica cast is applied.

28. Describe the technique for closed intramedullary rodding of the femur.

The patient is placed on the fracture table with image intensification for proximal and distal visualization. An incision is made over the greater trochanter, and dissection is taken down to the piriformis tendon, which is the entrance into the canal. A guidewire is placed through the proximal fragment and across the fracture site into the distal fragment, which is then reamed until cortical bone is exposed on both sides of the fracture site. The rod is then driven across the fracture site until it is level with the proximal bone.

29. What surgical techniques are used when the femur is highly comminuted?

One option is longitudinal traction, which has the disadvantages of prolonged bed rest and the need for a hip spica cast. Longitudinal traction is no longer used frequently. Also available are intramedullary rods with screws that lock above and below the fracture site, allowing the fracture fragments to life in near-anatomic position. Plate and screw techniques are less satisfying for severely comminuted fractures; reduction of the involved comminuted fragments is difficult.

30. What are the complications from intramedullary rod reduction of femur fractures?

Intraoperative nerve damage may result from either a stretch injury due to excessive traction or direct compression due to poor positioning of the patient. A sciatic nerve is the most frequently stretched. Incidence of infection is approximately 1% in closed femoral nailings. Open wounds treated with intramedullary nailing have a higher incidence of infection. Vascular injury generally does not occur during intramedullary nailing but may be found in 2% of acute femoral shaft fractures. Any fracture of the femoral shaft that has not healed by 6 months clearly qualifies as a delayed union. A union rate of 95% is generally obtained within 20 weeks. Nonunion may occur, especially when the intramedullary device fails.

31. What is the role of external fixation of femoral shaft fractures?

The most appropriate indication for an external fixator is a highly comminuted, open fracture of the midshaft of the femur. An external fixator allows repeated debridement of the leg to facilitate soft-tissue coverage as well as early mobilization; it also can be applied quickly in a limited open procedure. External fixation is often complicated by knee stiffness, pin tract infection, and delayed union.

32. What is the treatment of ipsilateral femoral neck and shaft fractures?

Ipsilateral femoral neck and shaft fractures should be treated with internal fixation. Several devices allow internal fixation of the femoral shaft with intramedullary nail and proximal screw fixation through the nail. The screws go through the lateral femoral cortex, through the nail, and into the femoral neck to stabilize the femoral neck fracture.

BIBLIOGRAPHY

1. Canale ST (ed): Campbell's Operative Orthopaedics, 9th ed. St. Louis, Mosby, 1998.
2. McElbinney J, Lauritzen JB, Petersen MM, Lund B: Falls and the elderly. Arch Am Acad Orthop Surg 2:1998.
3. Lauritzen JB, Petersen MM, Lund B: Defective external hip protectors on hip fractures. Lancet 341: 11–13, 1993.
4. Orthopaedic Knowledge Update 1, Home Study Syllabus. Rosemont, IL, American Academy of Orthopaedic Surgeons, 1984.
5. Orthopaedic Knowledge Update 3, Home Study Syllabus. Rosemont, IL, American Academy of Orthopaedic Surgeons, 1990.
6. Orthopaedic Knowledge Update 4, Home Study Syllabus. Rosemont, IL, American Academy of Orthopaedic Surgeons, 1993.

VIII. The Knee

68. EVALUATION OF THE INJURED KNEE

Christeen S. Kaga, M.D.

1. The evaluation of the injured knee begins with a detailed history. What are the important aspects of the history?

1. Mechanism of injury: the position of the knee at the time of injury, the weight-supporting status, the force applied (either direct and external or indirect and generated by the patient's momentum), and the position of the extremity after the injury are all important.

2. Pop or snap felt or heard: associated with ACL injury, meniscal injury, or patellar subluxation.

3. Swelling: intraarticular swelling or effusion within the first 2 hours after trauma suggests hemarthrosis, whereas swelling that occurs overnight is an indication of acute traumatic synovitis.

4. Pain: location, severity, type.

5. Instability: was there a sensation of the knee slipping out of joint, giving way, or deforming with weight bearing?

6. Past history: previous injury or problems before current injury.

7. Miscellaneous: is the patient able to walk or continue playing?

2. What are the causes of an acute hemarthrosis?
- Rupture of the ACL or PCL
- Peripheral meniscus tear
- Intraarticular fracture
- Tear in the deep portion of the joint capsule

3. What are the general principles of a knee examination?
The physical exam should be complete, precise, systematic, and carried out as soon after the injury as possible. Both lower extremities should be completely undressed to allow comparison. Always examine the uninjured knee first to obtain a baseline for comparison and to allay the patient's fear. Observe the patient standing, walking, sitting, and lying down.

4. Classify and describe disruptions of ligamentous structures.
Grade I: mild sprain—a tear of a minimal number of fibers of the ligament with localized tenderness but no instability.

Grade II: moderate sprain—disruption of more ligamentous fibers with more loss of function and more joint reaction with mild-to-moderate instability.

Grade III: severe sprain—a complete disruption of the ligament with resulting marked instability.

5. The severity of a grade III sprain is categorized further by the degree of instability demonstrated during stress testing. Describe the categories.
- 1+ instability: separation of joint surfaces by 5 mm or less
- 2+ instability: 5–10 mm of separation
- 3+ instability: ≥ 10 mm of separation

6. What is the terrible triad of O'Donoghue?
Medial meniscus tear
Rupture of the ACL
Rupture of the medial collateral ligament (MCL)

7. The general overview of the patient should include what points?
• Height
• Weight
• Body build
• Muscular tone
• Overall alignment of both knees (varus or valgus)
• Amount of disability estimated by observing the patient walking and making transfers
• Alignment of adjacent joints, such as the tibia, foot, and hip (e.g., presence of external or internal tibial torsion, pes planus, pelvic obliquity)

8. What functional tests should be performed?
Basic tests include squatting, kneeling, duck waddling, stationary jog, and fast jog. The leaning hop test is an excellent way to check functional instability. The patient first holds the unaffected leg in abduction (producing a valgus thrust to the knee) and then hops on the affected leg in clockwise and counterclockwise directions. When the patient crosses the unaffected leg in front of the affected leg, the same maneuver places a varus stress to the knee.

9. What general evaluations of the lower extremity must be recorded?
1. Circumferential measurements of the thigh, vastus medialis obliquus (VMO) area, mid-patellar area, and midcalf
2. Active range of motion (AROM) and passive range of motion (PROM) of both knees
3. Hamstring, quadriceps, and heelcord tightness
4. Hip and ankle of both sides
5. Note pain caused by forced extension, flexion, or varus or valgus motion
6. Neurovascular status of the lower extremity

10. What details of swelling should be noted?
• Whether it is intraarticular or extraarticular
• Location of extraarticular swelling
• Degree of swelling—mild, moderate, severe
• Severe injuries often present with little intraarticular swelling, because the blood escapes from the joint and into the soft tissues.

11. What are the important points in evaluation of the extensor mechanism?
1. Inspect the quadriceps femoris muscles for atrophy, tenderness, and tone. Note dysplasia of the VMO.
2. Palpate the quadriceps and patellar tendons for integrity and tenderness.
3. Identify the position of the patella (midline, subluxed, or dislocated).
4. Note the height of the patella. Patella alta (high-riding) is associated with subluxation and patella baja (low-riding) with chondromalacia.
5. Note the mobility of the patella and presence or absence of the apprehension test.
6. Note retropatellar grating, which may or may not be associated with pain.
7. The medial joint line (MJL) and lateral joint lines (LJL), patellar tendon, anterior fat pad, and tibial tubercle are examined for tenderness and size.

12. How do you perform or demonstrate an apprehension sign? What is its significance?
The patient's leg is supported at 30° of flexion by the examiner's leg, thus guaranteeing the appropriate amount of flexion, muscle relaxation, and reassurance of the patient. A firm, laterally directed force is applied to the medial border of the patella, subluxating it laterally, while applying

a small amount of passive flexion to the knee. The test is positive if the patient experiences acute apprehension, as if the patella were about to dislocate. A positive test is associated with acute and subacute subluxation or dislocation of the patella.

13. How do you measure the Q angle? What is its significance?

The quadriceps angle is formed by two lines, one projecting from the anterosuperior iliac spine to the midpatella and the second from the midpatella to the tibial tubercle. The angle is measured while the quadriceps is contracted. The average Q angle in men is 10°; in women, 15°. The Q angle is not diagnostic of any particular patellofemoral disorder; however, an increased angle should be viewed as an indication of a potential force that may act to subluxate or dislocate the patella.

14. Why is palpation important?

All anatomic structures are palpated for tenderness and swelling; palpation helps to localize the site of injury, especially when done early. The following are a few examples of the anatomic area and associated injury:

Medial joint line—medial meniscus tear
Lateral joint line—lateral meniscus tear
Medial femoral condyle, pes anserinus, MJL, posterior oblique ligament (POL; posterior one-third of medical capsular ligament)—anteromedial rotatory instability (AMRI)
Iliotibial tract, lateral collateral ligament—anterolateral rotatory instability
Medial retinaculum—patellar dislocation
Medial tibia—medial tibial plateau fracture
Quadriceps tendon—quadriceps rupture
Patellar tendon—patellar tendon rupture

15. Classify knee joint instability resulting from ligamentous injury.
  I. One-plane instability (simple or straight)
    A. One-plane medial
    B. One-plane lateral
    C. One-plane posterior
    D. One-plane anterior
  II. Rotary instability
    A. Anteromedial (AMRI)
    B. Anterolateral (ALRI)
      1. In flexion
      2. Approaching extension
    C. Posterolateral (PLRI)
    D. Posteromedial
  III. Combined instability
    A. Anterolateral/posterolateral
    B. Anterolateral/anteromedial
    C. Anteromedial/posteromedial

This classification attempts to describe the instability by the direction of the tibial displacement and, when possible, by structural deficits, thus it is anatomic. One-plane medial instability means that the tibia moves abnormally away from the femur on the medial side, whereas anteromedial instability means that the tibia rotates anteriorly and externally and moves away from the femur on the medial side. The classification becomes more complex when attempts are made to include anatomic or structural deficits. One-plane and rotary instabilities are usually understandable, although some of the implied structural deficits are still debatable. Combined instabilities, however, rarely are either clearly defined or consensual, and each orthopedic surgeon has to satisfy personal beliefs about what structures are specifically damaged and their relative degree of involvement in the instability.

ONE-PLANE INSTABILITY

16. How do you perform an abduction or valgus stress test at 30° and 0°? What is their significance?

With the patient supine on the examining table, the knee to be examined is placed on the side of the table and flexed to 30°. One hand is placed about the lateral aspect of the knee and the other supports the ankle. Abduction or valgus stress is applied gently to the knee while the hand at the ankle externally rotates the leg slightly. Note stability with the knee flexed to 30°. Bring the knee into full extension and repeat the gentle rocking or valgus stressing with a gentle swinging motion.

Instability at 30° of flexion indicates injury limited to the medial compartment ligaments (tibial collateral ligament, medial collateral ligament, medial capsule, or any combination of the above).

Instability to valgus stress at 0° indicates injury to the posterior structures of the knee (posterior capsule and/or posterior cruciate ligament) and medial structures. Both are examples of one-plane medial instability.

17. How do you perform an adduction or varus stress test at 30° and 0°? What is their significance?

The adduction or varus stress test is carried out in a manner similar to the valgus stress test after examining the normal knee. Adduction or varus stress is applied by changing the hand to the medial side of the knee and applying an adduction or varus force. Examination should be done both in full extension and in 30° of flexion. In addition, with the patient's hip abducted and externally rotated and the knee flexed, the heel of the injured leg is placed on the opposite knee (figure-of-four position), and the lateral aspect of the knee is palpated for a taut narrow band consisting of the fibular collateral ligament (FCL). When the FCL is torn, it is not as prominent as on the uninjured knee.

Varus instability at 30° suggests injury to the lateral compartment ligaments (lateral [fibular] collateral ligament, iliotibial tract, and lateral capsule). With any injury to the lateral aspect of the joint or any varus-producing injury, the integrity of the peroneal nerve must be examined closely.

One-plane lateral instability with the knee in extension is apparent on the adduction or varus stress testing when the knee opens on the lateral side. This indicates disruption of the lateral capsular ligament, the lateral collateral ligament, the biceps tendon, the iliotibial band, the arcuate-popliteus complex, the popliteofibular ligament, the anterior cruciate ligament, and, often, the posterior cruciate ligament.

One-plane instability with the knee in extension, whether medial or lateral, is a major instability approaching the severity of a dislocation.

18. Which tests assess the integrity of the ACL? How are they performed?

The tests for anterior instability include the Lachman test and the anterior drawer test, which are performed at 90° in neutral rotation. For the Lachman test place the patient supine on the examining table with the involved extremity to the side of the examiner. Position the involved extremity in slight external rotation, with the knee between 20–30° of flexion; stabilize the femur with one hand; and apply firm pressure to the posterior aspect of the proximal tibia, lifting it forward in an attempt to translate it anteriorly. Anterior translation of the tibia associated with a soft or a mushy endpoint indicates a positive test.

The anterior drawer test at 90° is performed in neutral, internal, and external rotation. With the patient supine on the examining table, flex the hip to 45° and the knee to 90°, placing the foot on the tabletop. Sit on the dorsum of the foot to stabilize it, and place both hands behind the knee to feel for relaxation of the hamstring muscles. Then gently and repeatedly pull and push the proximal part of the leg anteriorly and posteriorly, noting the movement of the tibia on the femur. Perform the test in three positions of rotation, initially with the tibia in neutral position. A positive test denotes ACL insufficiency. Next perform the test with the foot externally rotated 30° to rotate the medial tibia anteriorly. A positive drawer test indicates anteromedial rotatory instability (AMRI). Now internally rotate the foot 30° and repeat the test. This position may tighten the PCL enough to obliterate an otherwise positive anterior test.

One-plane anterior instability is present when the tibia moves forward on the femur during the anterior drawer test in neutral position. This instability indicates that disrupted structures include the ACL, lateral capsular ligament (partial or complete), and medial capsular ligament (partial or complete). In this type of instability the test becomes negative as the tibia internally rotates, because in this position the PCL becomes taut.

19. How is PCL injury tested?
  A posterior drawer test is performed in a similar fashion to the anterior drawer test, except that a posterior force is applied on the proximal tibia, again in neutral position as well as internal and external rotation. Posterior movement of the tibia on the femur demonstrates posterior instability when compared with the normal knee. It is sometimes difficult to interpret whether the tibia is abnormally moving too far anteriorly or too far posteriorly. Careful attention to the neutral position or unstressed reduction point avoids misinterpretation. This misinterpretation can be prevented by carefully palpating the relationship between the femur and tibia of both knees simultaneously. Place both knees in the position for a posterior drawer test with the patient supine and the hips flexed 45° and the knees flexed 90°. Place a thumb on the anteromedial joint line of each knee. Normally the anterior aspect of the tibia can be palpated as a 10-mm anterior step-off in relation to the anterior aspect of the medial femoral condyle. A posterior drop back with decreased prominence of the tibial margin compared to the opposite knee indicates injury to the posterior cruciate ligament. When posterior instability is present, the tibia, as sighted across the horizon of the flexed knee, visibly sags posteriorly from the effects of gravity, producing the "gravity sign," "posterior sag," or "drop-back sign."
  One-plane posterior instability is apparent when the tibia moves posteriorly on the femur during the posterior drawer test. Such instability indicates disruption of the PCL, the arcuate ligament complex (partial or complete), and the posterior oblique ligament complex (partial or complete).
  The posterior cruciate ligament can also be evaluated by the quadriceps active test. With the patient supine, support the relaxed limb with the knee flexed to 90° in the drawer test position. It is important to adequately support the thigh so that the patient's muscles are completely relaxed. Have the patient execute a gentle quadriceps contraction to shift the tibia without extending the knee. At this 90° angle the patellar ligament in the normal knee is oriented slightly posterior, and contraction of the quadriceps does not result in an anterior shift. If the posterior cruciate has ruptured, the tibia sags into posterior subluxation and the patellar ligament is then directed anteriorly. Contraction of the quadriceps muscle in a knee with a posterior or cruciate ligament deficiency results in an anterior shift of the tibia of ≥ 2 mm.
  From such abnormal anatomic findings one can see that severe grades of instability—that is, severe varus, valgus anterior, or posterior instability—are accompanied by additional central or peripheral ligamentous deficiencies. Most, therefore, are accompanied by rotary instabilities as well.

ROTARY INSTABILITIES

20. Rotary instabilities result when the PCL remains intact to serve as the axis about which the tibial plateaus rotate under the femur. Anteromedial rotary instability (AMRI) is apparent when stress testing produces anterior and external rotation of the medial plateau of the tibia as the joint opens on the medial side. Which tests are positive in AMRI? Which structures are likely to be disrupted?
  Positive tests include the anterior drawer at 90° with the leg externally rotated and the abduction stress test at 30°. Positive tests imply disruption of the medial capsular ligament, the tibial collateral ligament, the posterior oblique ligament, and the anterior cruciate ligament.

21. In anterolateral rotary instability, the lateral tibial plateau subluxates forward on the femur as the knee approaches extension. This implies disruption of the ACL and lateral capsular ligament. Which tests for ALRI are positive? How are they performed?
  1. **Jerk test (Hughston and Losee):** Perform the test with the patient supine and the examiner supporting the lower extremity, flexing the knee to 90°, and internally rotating the tibia.

When the right knee is examined, grasp the foot with the right hand and internally rotate the tibia while exerting a valgus stress with the left hand over the proximal end of the tibia and fibula. Then extend the knee gradually, maintaining the internal rotation and valgus stress. When the test is positive, subluxation of the lateral femorotibial articulation becomes maximal at about 30° of flexion; then, as the knee extends further, spontaneous relocation occurs. The relocation takes the form of a sudden jerk.

2. **Lateral pivot shift test (Macintosh):** Lift the foot with the knee extended, internally rotate the leg, and apply a valgus stress to the lateral side of the leg in the region of the fibular neck with the opposite hand. Slowly flex the knee while valgus and internal rotation are maintained. If the test is positive, a subluxation will occur at 30–40° of flexion as the iliotibial band passes posterior to the center of rotation of the knee and provides the force that reduces the lateral tibial plateau on the lateral femoral condyle.

3. **Flexion rotation drawer test (Noyes):** With the patient supine and the knee at 0° (not hyperextended), lift the leg upward, allowing the femur to fall back and rotate externally. This results in anterolateral tibial subluxation as the starting position for the test. While the knee is flexed, the tibia moves backward and the femur rotates internally, causing the joint to reduce when the test is positive.

4. **Anterolateral drawer test:** With the patient supine, the knee flexed at 90°, and the foot resting on the table, apply an anterior and internal rotation stress to the proximal tibia. The test is positive if the lateral tibial plateau subluxates anteriorly and internally.

22. Posterolateral rotary instability (PLRI) is apparent when stress testing produces posterior rotation of the lateral tibial plateau in relation to the femur with lateral opening of the joint. This implies disruption of the popliteus tendon, the arcuate ligament complex (partial or complete), the lateral capsular ligament, and at times stretching or loss of integrity of the PCL. Which tests are useful in diagnosing PLRI? How are they performed?

1. **External rotation recurvatum test:** Perform this test with the patient supine and compare it with the normal knee. Lift the affected extremity by the large toe and evaluate any external rotation of the tibia, posterior displacement of the tibia, or recurvatum. Check for peroneal nerve injury.

2. **Reverse pivot shift (Jacob):** The lateral tibial plateau shifts from a position of posterior subluxation to a position of reduction as the knee is extended under valgus stress with the foot held in external rotation. The plateau subluxates again as the knee is flexed in the opposite manner. Position the patient supine on the examining table. To test the right knee, face the patient and lift the foot and ankle with your right hand, resting it on the right side of your pelvis. Support the lateral side of the calf with the palm of your left hand on the proximal fibula. Bend the knee to 70–80° of flexion. At this position, externally rotate the foot and the leg to cause the lateral tibial plateau to subluxate posteriorly in relation to the lateral femoral condyle. This position is seen as a posterior sag of the proximal tibia. Now allow the knee to straighten, using nothing more than the weight of the leg. Lean slightly against the foot and transmit an axial load through the leg. Apply a valgus stress to the knee, using your iliac crest as a fulcrum. As the knee approaches 20° short of full extension, feel and observe the lateral tibial plateau moving anteriorly in a jerklike shift from a position of posterior subluxation and external rotation into a position of reduction and neutral rotation.

3. **Posterolateral drawer test:** The posterolateral drawer test is performed with the patient supine and the hip flexed 45°, the knee flexed 80°, and the tibia in 15° external rotation. With the foot flexed, perform posterior drawer testing.

4. **Tibial external rotation test:** When an injured knee is tested for posterolateral instability, external rotation of the tibia on the femur is measured at both 30° and 90° of knee flexion. The test can be performed with the patient supine or prone. The medial border of the foot in its neutral position is used as a reference point for external rotation. At the chosen knee flexion angle, forcefully externally rotate the foot. Measure the degree of external rotation of the foot relative to the axis of the femur and compare it with the opposite leg. Measure external rotation by the foot-thigh angle. Additionally palpate the tibial plateaus to determine

whether the external rotation is caused by the lateral medial tibial plateau moving anteriorly (AMRI). A 10° difference between knees is pathologic.

23. How is posteromedial rotary instability (PMRI) diagnosed?
Posteromedial rotary instability is present when, with stress testing, the medial tibial plateau rotates posteriorly in reference to the femur, with medial opening of the joint.This implies disruption of the medial collateral ligaments, the medial capsular ligament, the posterior oblique ligament, the posterior cruciate ligament, and the medial portion of the posterior capsule, plus stretching or major injury to the semimembranosus insertions. The anterior cruciate ligament also may be injured.

COMBINED INSTABILITIES

24. What is the most common combined instability?
Combined anterolateral-anteromedial instability.

25. Why are the combined rotary instabilities so clinically important?
Failure to recognize a combined instability may result in inadequate surgery or surgery that aggravates the missed instability. Correcting only one aspect of a combined instability has no chance of restoring normal function.

26. What radiographs should routinely be taken to evaluate an acute injury?
Anteroposterior (AP), lateral, and sunrise views of the patella and the notch or tunnel view.

27. What important information can be gained from the above views?
The sunrise view evaluates patellofemoral instability frequently associated with dislocations and acute medial ligamentous disruptions. In children avulsions of osteocartilaginous portions of the intercondylar eminences are much more common than cruciate ligament disruptions. In adults pieces of bone occasionally are avulsed from the femoral condyle or from the tip of the fibula where the collateral ligament inserts. Occasionally a fragment from the back of the tibia may be seen in a PCL disruption. Small fragments along the medial or lateral tibial joint line suggest avulsion of the capsular ligament at that location (lateral capsular sign). Stress radiographs are necessary in all apparent ligamentous disruptions of the knee in patients whose distal femoral and proximal tibial epiphyseal plates are still open to rule out epiphyseal separation.

28. How are first-degree sprains treated?
Treatment is symptomatic, with relative rest, ice, compression, and rehabilitation. Return to normal function and activities should be rapid.

29. How are second-degree sprains treated?
Second-degree sprains require protection. Although the remaining untorn portion of the ligament may stabilize the knee to routine stress testing, the strength of the ligament has been significantly impaired. Such patients are best treated with a cast brace or a controlled motion brace allowing full, protected motion for 4–6 weeks. Recovery usually can be expected, with no residual laxity once the rehabilitation program has been completed.

30. How are third-degree sprains treated?
Third-degree sprains often require surgical treatment, depending on severity and type of instability. The proper treatment for each patient must be selected depending on other factors such as age, general health, associated injuries, activity demands, and patient desires.

31. What is the difference between ligament repair and ligament reconstruction?
Repair of ligaments of the knee refers to surgical treatment of acute injuries, whereas reconstruction usually refers to surgical treatment of ligamentous laxity several months after injury.

BIBLIOGRAPHY

1. Carson WG: Diagnosis of extension mechanism disorders. Clin Sports Med 4:231–245, 1985.
2. Hughston JC, Andrews JR, Cross MJ, et al: Classification of knee ligament instabilities. Part I. The medial compartment and cruciate ligaments. J Bone Joint Surg 58A:159, 1976.
3. Hughston JC, Andrews JR, Cross MJ, et al: Classification of knee ligament instabilities. Part II. The lateral compartment. J Bone Joint Surg 58A:173, 1976.
4. Jenson JE, Conn RR, Hazelrigg G, Hewett JE: Systematic evaluation of acute knee injuries. Clin Sports Med 4:295–312, 1985.
5. Miller RH: Knee injuries. In Canale ST (ed): Campbell's Operative Orthopedics, 9th ed. St. Louis, Mosby, 1998, pp 1113–1299.
6. Rockwood CA, Green DP, Bucholz RW, Heckman JD (eds): Rockwood and Green's Fractures, vol. II, 4th ed. Philadelphia, J.B. Lippincott, 1996.

69. MENISCAL INJURIES

Christeen S. Kaga, M.D.

1. Name several functions of the menisci.

The menisci, which have reached their highest level of development in humans, are essential to the normal function of the knee joint. Their specific contributions include joint filler, joint lubrication by helping to distribute synovial fluid and aiding the nutrition of articular cartilage, joint stability (especially rotary), absorption of shock and energy (load transmission), and sparing the articular cartilage from compressive loads.

2. Describe the microstructure of the menisci and its relation to injury.

The menisci are composed of dense, tightly woven collagen fibers arranged in a pattern that is highly elastic and able to withstand compression. The major orientation of collagen fibers in the meniscus is circumferential; radial and perforating fibers are also present. The arrangement of the collagen fibers determines to some extent the characteristic patterns of meniscal tears. Collagen fibers function primarily to resist tensible forces along the directions of the fibers. The normal tensile stresses on the menisci are in the longitudinal axis. Because the predominant fiber pattern is in this plane, tears are not unusual. The small number of peripheral radial collagen bundles is inadequate to prevent longitudinal tears when the force is substantial. Likewise, horizontal cleavage tears occur because of the paucity of vertically oriented fibers.

3. Why is the lateral meniscus injured less often than the medial meniscus?

The lateral meniscus is smaller in diameter, thicker in periphery, wider in body, more mobile, attached to both cruciate ligaments, and stabilized posteriorly to the medial femoral condyle and popliteus muscle.

4. What is the vascular supply of the menisci?

The vascular supply to both menisci originates predominantly from the medial, lateral, and geniculate vessels (both inferior and superior). Branches give rise to a perimeniscal capillary plexus that supplies the peripheral border of the meniscus throughout its attachment to the joint capsule. The depth of peripheral vascular penetration is 10–30% of the width of the medial meniscus and 10–25% of the width of the lateral meniscus.

5. How does this vascular supply affect healing and repair of the meniscus?

Only the most peripheral injuries are capable of healing, because the body of the meniscus is relatively avascular.

6. What is the usual mechanism of injury for a meniscal tear?
Rotational force as the flexed knee moves toward an extended position.

7. What is the most common meniscal tear?
Longitudinal tear of the posterior horn of the medial meniscus is the most common tear. However, increased use of the arthroscope has made more thorough inspection of both menisci possible; medial and lateral meniscus tears are believed to occur with almost equal frequency.

8. Draw the main types of meniscal tears.

bucket handle   longitudinal   flap   transverse   horizontal

9. Name common symptoms of a torn meniscus.

Pain	Locking	Swelling
Catching	Giving away	Popping

10. List signs and tests that help diagnose a meniscal tear.

Joint line tenderness	Quadriceps atrophy
Effusion	Positive McMurray test
Lack of complete knee extension	Positive Apley grind test

11. How do you perform a McMurray test?
With the patient supine and the knee acutely and forcibly flexed, the examiner checks the medial meniscus by palpating the posteromedial margin of the joint with one hand while grasping the foot with the other hand. Keeping the knee completely flexed, the leg is externally rotated as far as possible; then the knee is slowly extended. As the femur passes over a tear in the meniscus, a painful click or pop is felt or heard if the test is positive. The lateral meniscus is checked by palpating the postero-lateral margin of the joint, internally rotating the leg as far as possible, and slowly extending the knee while listening and feeling for a click. A negative McMurray test does not rule out a tear.

12. How is the grinding test as described by Apley performed?
With the patient prone the knee is flexed to 90°, and the anterior thigh is fixed against the examining table. The foot and leg are then pulled upward to distract the joint and rotated to place rotational strain on the ligaments; when ligaments are torn, this part of the test is usually painful. Next, with the knee in the same position, the foot and leg are pressed downward and rotated as the joint is slowly flexed and extended; when a meniscus is torn, popping and pain localized to the joint line may be noted.

13. What radiographic studies may be helpful?
Anteroposterior (AP), lateral, intercondylar notch, and sunrise views of the patella should be routine to exclude osteocartilaginous loose bodies, osteochondritis dissecans, and other internal derangements that may mimic a torn meniscus. Other diagnostic studies helpful in evaluating the menisci include arthrography, CT, and MRI.

14. Name other conditions that produce signs and symptoms that mimic meniscal lesions.

Chondromalacia	Ligamentous lesions	Synovial chondromatosis
Patellofemoral arthritis	Loose bodies	Ganglion cysts
Synovitis	Osteochondritis dissecans	Plicas
Fat pad lesions	Degenerative arthritis	

15. What is the most common congenital meniscal anomaly?

A discoid lateral meniscus, which tears more frequently than a normal lateral meniscus.

16. Does nonsurgical treatment have a place in the management of mensical tears?

Yes. An incomplete meniscal tear or a small (5 mm) stable peripheral tear with no other pathologic condition, such as a torn anterior cruciate ligament, can be treated nonsurgically with predictably good results. Meniscal tears that cause infrequent and minimal symptoms can be treated with rehabilitation and restricted activity.

17. What surgical options are available for a torn meniscus?

Two surgical options are available: (1) Total or partial meniscectomy, done arthroscopically or as an open procedure, and (2) suture of a peripheral tear, performed arthroscopically or as an open procedure.

BIBLIOGRAPHY

1. Canale ST (ed): Campbell's Operative Orthopedics, 9th ed. St. Louis, Mosby, 1998.
2. Henning CE, Lynch MA: Current concepts of meniscal function and pathology. Clin Sports Med 4:259–265, 1985.
3. Rockwood CA, Green DP, Bucholz RW, Heckman JD (eds): Rockwood and Green's Fractures in Adults, vol. 2, 4th ed. Philadelphia, J.B. Lippincott, 1996.

70. ANTERIOR CRUCIATE LIGAMENT INJURIES

Randall D. Neumann, M.D., and David E. Brown, M.D.

1. Describe the anatomy of the anterior cruciate ligament.

The anterior cruciate ligament (ACL) is an intraarticular structure that traverses the joint attaching the tibia and the femur. It consists of multiple longitudinal fascicles that insert proximally on the medial aspect of the lateral femoral condyle and distally on the anterior tibial plateau. These fascicles are described as fanning out as they approach the tibial insertion. The ACL provides the primary restraint to anterior displacement of the tibia. The intact ACL is a secondary stabilizer to varus and valgus stress.

2. Describe the different mechanisms for anterior cruciate ligament injuries in contact sports.

1. **Clipping injury.** The most common injury to the ACL is associated with a valgus load and external rotation of the tibia on the femur. The mechanism of injury is often associated with damage to the medial collateral ligament and a medial meniscus.

2. **Hyperextension.** The second most common injury pattern is associated with meniscal tears in approximately 30% of the patients. Contact hyperextension injuries also may damage the posterior cruciate ligament (PCL) and posterior capsule.

3. **Direct blow.** In this pattern of injury, the knee is flexed, as often seen in dashboard and turf injuries. A direct blow to the anterior portion of the knee results in tear of the PCL and possible tear of the ACL.

4. **Varus load on the flexed knee.** This pattern may injure the ACL along with the posterior lateral complex, resulting in anterior instability with posterior lateral instability.

3. Describe the mechanism of ACL injuries in noncontact sports.

1. **Skiing injuries.** The classic cause of knee injury in downhill skiers is a forward fall in which the inside edge of the ski is caught in the snow, placing the knee in external rotation and valgus stress. A second injury mechanism is the so-called "boot-induced" injury, resulting from a

backward fall. With the skier's center of gravity posterior to the boot, the back of the boot causes an anteriorly directed force onto the tibia. When coupled with significant quadriceps contraction (the skier attempts to right himself), the ACL undergoes tension failure.

2. **Deceleration injuries with increased quadriceps contraction.** Anterior force on the proximal tibia is caused by tremendous quadriceps contraction. Such injuries may be seen in basketball and football players who suddenly decelerate to change direction.

3. **Hyperextension.** Noncontact ACL injuries also are seen with hyperextension injury in basketball players (e.g., in rebounding) and in gymnasts during the dismount.

4. What percent of patients with acute knee injuries and hemarthrosis have an ACL tear?
70%.

5. What is the ratio of ACL to PCL injuries?
There are approximately 9 ACL injuries for every PCL injury in sports.

6. Describe the history given by the patient who sustains an acute disruption in the ACL.
Most patients claim that the knee "gave way," "buckled," or "popped out" at the time of injury. The mechanism of injury includes clipping, hyperextension, and direct blows. Noncontact injuries may be due to twisting and cutting. Swelling is usually immediate in onset and maximizes within the first 2–3 hours after injury. Most patients have immediate and profound disability with guarded or painful range of motion and the inability to ambulate.

7. What is the significance of the history of hearing or feeling a "pop"?
The pop results from a tear of a ligament, tendon, or meniscus. It is often heard by fellow athletes.

8. Describe the physical examination in a patient with suspected tear of the ACL.
The examination should start with evaluating the normal knee for a "built-in" comparison. Some patients have excessive hypermobility or generalized ligamentous laxity that must be taken into account when evaluating knee laxity. The knee should be inspected for areas of ecchymosis, swelling, effusion, or tenderness. Range of motion should be evaluated. Flexion and extension are frequently compromised because of the large amount of effusion following injury. Ligament stability testing is performed and should include a minimum of the Lachman test, anterior drawer, pivot shift, posterior drawer, external rotation measurement, and varus and valgus stability testing.

9. What is the most reliable test during physical examination for an anterior cruciate ligament injury?
The Lachman test.

10. How is the Lachman test performed?
The Lachman test is performed in approximately 15–30° of flexion. The femur is stabilized with the examiner's hand. The opposite hand is used to apply an anteriorly directed force to the posterior tibia while stabilizing the femur. The examiner senses any tibial displacement and compares it with the uninvolved knee. The endpoint may be graded as either firm, marginal, or soft. The Lachman test may be graded as 1+ (0–5 mm displacement), 2+ (5–10 mm displacement), or 3+ (> 10 mm displacement). Excessive anterior displacement compared with the normal side, especially when coupled with a marginal or soft endpoint, usually signifies a torn ACL.

11. What is the anterior drawer test?
The anterior drawer test is performed with the patient's knee at 90° of flexion with muscular relaxation. The hip is flexed at 45°. A smooth, steady pull is placed in an anterior direction on the posterior portion of the tibia. The test is generally done with the foot in neutral position, 15° of external rotation, and 15° of internal rotation. In a positive test, increased anterior step-off occurs between the femoral condyle and tibial plateau.

12. What is the pivot shift test?

The pivot shift describes the anterior subluxation of the lateral tibial plateau on the femoral condyle. With the patient in the supine position and relaxed, the knee is examined in full extension. The tibia is rotated internally, with one hand grasping the foot and the other hand applying a mild valgus stress at the level of the knee joint. Then, with flexion in the knee to approximately 20–30°, a jerk is suddenly experienced at the anterolateral corner of the proximal tibia. The patient also may feel the anterior subluxation and comment that it is the same feeling that occurred when the knee was injured or, in chronic cases, when it is continually injured. The result is graded as 0 (absent), 1+ (mild), 2+ (moderate), or 3+ (severe).

13. What is the differential diagnosis for an acute hemarthrosis?

Ligamentous tear (e.g., ACL, PCL, or deep collateral ligament)	Peripheral meniscal tear
	Capsular tear
Osteochondral fracture	Patellar dislocation

14. Describe the radiographic findings in an acute ACL injury.

Anteroposterior, lateral, intercondylar notch, and patellofemoral (sunrise) views are recommended for initial evaluation of acute knee injuries. In the isolated ACL tear, such studies are generally interpreted as normal.

15. What is a Segond fracture?

A Segond fracture is an avulsion fracture of the inferior lateral capsule adjacent to the tibia. It is highly suggestive of an injury to the ACL but is seen in only about 6% of the cases.

16. Describe the radiographic appearance of a chronic ACL tear.

In most cases of chronic ACL tear, degenerative changes with narrowing of the medial and lateral joint space are seen. Osteophytes may be present along the intercondylar portion of the femur, on the tibial spines, and along the medial or lateral joint margins. Femoral osteochondral lesions or loose bodies are often present.

17. What is the best diagnostic radiographic test for ACL tears?

Magnetic resonance imaging (MRI) is the best diagnostic test. The advantages of an MRI include its noninvasive nature, lack of radiation, and ability to image in any plane and to detect nonosseus injuries such as ligament, meniscal, or articular damage. A complete tear is visualized on both T1- and T2-weighted images as a discontinuity in the ligament, with fluid filling the defect. MRI is also helpful in assessing fractures, medial and lateral collateral ligament injuries, PCL injuries, and meniscal injuries.

18. What is a KT-1000?

The KT-1000 (MedMetric, San Diego, CA) is a measuring system that documents anteroposterior tibial displacement by tracking the tibial tubercle in relation to the patella. Studies using the KT-1000 have shown that a side-to-side difference > 3 mm of anterior displacement at 20 lbs predicts an ACL deficiency with 94% accuracy.

19. What treatment options are available for acute isolated ACL tears?

Conservative nonoperative treatment, repair, repair and augmentation, extraarticular reconstruction, and intraarticular reconstruction.

20. What factors should be considered when discussing treatment for patients with an ACL injury?

Presence or absence of other pathology involving the knee	Level of activity
	Degree of instability
Age of the patient	Associated ligamentous injuries

21. Can ACL injuries be left untreated?

Yes. Many physiologically older patients with a low activity level, no associated injuries, and only mild symptoms may be treated conservatively and nonoperatively.

22. What type of patient generally requires reconstruction of the ACL?

Physiologically young patients with high demands on the knee generally require reconstruction. Demands include the ability to cut, jump, accelerate, and decelerate. Patients with associated meniscal lesions, who often continue to be symptomatic, also may require reconstruction.

23. Is surgical repair of the ACL a treatment option?

No. Studies have indicated that primary repair of the injured ACL results in persistent laxity and instability of the knee.

24. Describe an intraarticular vs. extraarticular reconstruction for ACL loss.

Intraarticular reconstruction tries to reproduce the anatomic ACL. The donor tendon spans the intercondylar notch from the anatomic insertion and origin of the ACL. An extraarticular reconstruction uses structures on the lateral side of the knee to simulate the ACL. Typical extraarticular reconstructions include those of Andrews, Steadman, and Arnold. The goal of an extraarticular procedure is to correct anterolateral rotatory instability or to prevent anterior subluxation of the lateral tibial plateau in relation to the lateral femoral condyle. Such procedures surgically stabilize the iliotibial tract so that the excessive lateral excursion of the tibia is halted. Their success has been limited. With the advent of arthroscopically assisted ACL intraarticular reconstructions, the extraarticular procedures are performed less often; however, they may be indicated for the unstable, skeletally immature patient.

25. What appropriate autografts are used for substitution and reconstruction of the ACL?

1. Central one-third patellar tendon
2. Semitendinosus tendon (hamstring)
3. Quadriceps tendon

26. What are the advantages and disadvantages of using the central one-third patellar tendon graft for ACL reconstruction?

Advantages of the central one-third patellar tendon graft are high initial tensile strength, stiffness, and fixation strength. Disadvantages include patellofemoral pain, patellar tendinitis, fracture, and patellar tendon rupture.

27. What are the advantages and disadvantages of using hamstring tendons for ACL reconstruction?

The major advantages of harvesting the semitendinosus tendon grafts are lower surgical morbidity during graft harvest and lower incidence of donor risk complications. The disadvantages are lower tensile strength and stiffness and less fixation strength compared with the patellar tendon graft.

28. What associated surgical procedures may be done at the same time as ACL reconstruction?

Meniscus repair or excision and removal or fixation of osteochondral loose bodies are the most common concomitant procedures performed at the time of ACL reconstruction. If associated ligament pathology is present, appropriate repair or reconstruction is indicated. Generally, medial collateral ligament injuries are allowed to heal before arthroscopic ACL reconstruction.

Meniscal repair or excision may need to be performed before the ACL reconstruction if the meniscus is causing a mechanical block to regaining full extension after injury. This type of staged surgical reconstruction has led to a dramatically lower rate of flexion contracture following reconstruction.

29. Describe the procedure for an ACL reconstruction using the central one-third patellar tendon autograft.
1. Diagnostic arthroscopy.
2. Meniscus repair or excision.
3. ACL stump excision.
4. Lateral superior expansion notchplasty.
5. Graft harvest and preparation (some surgeons prefer to perform this at the beginning of the procedure).
6. Placement of appropriately sized tibial tunnel centered 7 mm in front of the posterior cruciate ligament. This center point is usually at, or slightly posterior to, the anterior horn of the lateral meniscus.
7. Placement of an appropriately sized tibial bone tunnel centered 6–7 mm in front of the "over-the-top" position, high and posterior in the intercondylar notch (this position would be at 12:30 to 1:00 in a left knee).
8. Secure fixation of the graft in both bone tunnels. Usually performed with interference screw fixation. Acceptable alternatives include many other types of soft-tissue fixation methods.
9. Careful evaluation of graft fixation, stability, and impingement-free range of motion.
10. Standard wound closure over drains.

30. What are the complications of ACL reconstruction?
Complications include infection, thrombophlebitis, skin necrosis, hemarthrosis, sensory nerve damage, reflex sympathetic dystrophy, and arthrofibrosis. The most common problems include failure to regain full extension or flexion, patellofemoral complications (e.g., chondromalacia and fracture), graft impingement, and graft failure.

31. Does a narrow notch increase the risk for ACL injury?
Yes. Patients who had a narrow notch (< 15 mm) measured during ACL reconstruction have a significantly higher risk for contralateral ACL injury.

32. What are the reasons for loss of full extension after cruciate surgery?
1. **Lack of full preoperative extension.** Patients should regain complete extension before reconstruction. This may be achieved with physical therapy time or arthroscopic removal of mechanical blocks to extension.
2. **Anterior tibial placement** of the graft causing roof impingement.
3. **Cyclops lesion.** This nodular abundance of fibrous tissue lying anterior to the tibial portion of the graft impinges on the anterior notch, which may be caused by roof impingement.
4. Infrapatellar contracture syndrome.

33. What is arthrofibrosis?
Arthrofibrosis is a complication of cruciate surgery. This syndrome involves contracture of the retropatellar fat pad and patellar tendon. Patients present with severe postoperative pain, diminished patellar mobility, and failure to gain extension and flexion. The best initial treatment is aggressive physical therapy. Attempts at surgical intervention have met with limited success.

34. Describe the natural history of the ACL-deficient knee.
Patients may report pain related to activity or giving-way episodes, described as either buckling or feeling as if the knee would not hold the patient's weight. Giving-way episodes occur in 17–65% of patients, often in association with strenuous activities; they may not be present during activities of daily living. Recurrent swelling is common after strenuous or prolonged activity; it also may be an early sign of developing osteoarthritis.

35. In patients with chronic ACL insufficiency, what percentage develop meniscal tears?
Between 65 and 91%, with approximately 20% of tears involving both the medial and lateral menisci.

36. What should be done for the patient who ruptures an anterior cruciate ligament graft?

If the individual desires to remain active, revision reconstruction may be performed. Appropriate graft choices include all forms of autogenous graft not previously used, including contralateral knee autografts. In some instances, patellar or Achilles allografts are used. Reconstruction with synthetic tissue such as Gortex, Dacron, or Xenografts has largely been abandoned because of high failure rates.

CONTROVERSIES

37. What is the best graft choice for ACL reconstruction?

This remains a mildly contested issue. As noted in questions 26 and 27, each major graft choice has advantages and disadvantages. There appears to be very little difference in outcome regardless of the graft choice. The graft choice is frequently made in accordance with the surgeon's particular preference or training.

38. Should continuous passive motion (CPM) be used after ACL reconstruction?

The use of CPM seems limited to situations in which individuals are at high risk for restriction of range of motion after surgery, including associated surgical procedures such as meniscus or ligament repairs. In uncomplicated anterior cruciate ligament reconstruction, postoperative CPM use allows an earlier return of range of motion. One month after surgery, there is no statistically significant difference between groups who either did or did not use CPM.

39. Are cryotherapy devices indicated after ACL reconstruction?

Yes. Cryotherapy devices, whether manual or mechanical, reduce pain and swelling in the knee after surgery. Patients use less postoperative pain medicine and have fewer side effects (e.g., narcotic-related nausea).

40. Can ACL reconstruction be safely performed in an outpatient setting?

Yes. Patients who are educated and prepared for the immediate postoperative period can safely be managed at home after ACL reconstruction. This results in cost savings to both the patient and the payer.

41. How should you treat the pediatric patient with a torn ACL?

If the pediatric ACL injury is a tibial spine avulsion fracture, reduction and fixation are performed by either open or arthroscopic methods.

A controversy occurs when a midsubstance ACL disruption occurs in a pediatric patient with widely open physes. Options include activity restriction and bracing until physes are closed, extraarticular reconstructions, standard intraarticular reconstruction, or modified intraarticular reconstruction methods. If the physes are nearly closed, standard intraarticular reconstruction methods may be employed.

Extraarticular reconstructions eventually fail in pediatric patients as they do in the adult. However, this may be a compromise for the young athlete who insists on remaining athletically active. A better alternative may be a modified intraarticular reconstruction in which a smaller groove is made in the anterior tibia for tibial ACL placement and the femoral "over-the-top" method is used for femoral positioning and fixation.

42. In a severe knee injury in which both the ACLs and PCLs are torn in midsubstance and require reconstruction, should both be reconstructed at the same time?

Generally not. PCL reconstruction coupled with appropriate capsular and collateral ligament repairs are performed at the index procedure. After knee range of motion, stability, and muscle control is achieved, an arthroscopic ACL reconstruction is performed.

BIBLIOGRAPHY

1. Clancy WG, Nelson DA, Reider B, et al: Anterior cruciate ligament reconstruction using one-third of the patellar ligament, augmented by extraarticular tendon transfers. J Bone Joint Surg 64A:352, 1982.
2. DeHaven KE: Diagnosis of acute knee injuries with hemarthrosis. Am J Sports Med 8:9–14, 1980.
3. Fu FH, Shulte KR: Anterior cruciate ligament surgery 1996. State of the art? Clin Orthop 325:19–24, 1996.
4. Kaborn DN, Johnson BM: The natural history of the anterior cruciate ligament-deficient knee. Clin Sports Med 12:625–636, 1993.
5. Kartus J, Stener S, Lindahl S, et al: Ipsilateral or contralateral patellar tendon graft in anterior cruciate ligament revision surgery. A comparison of two methods. Am J Sports Med 26:449–504, 1998.
6. Noyes FR, Mooar PA, Matthews DS, et al: The symptomatic anterior cruciate deficient knee: I. The long term functional disability in athletically active individuals. J Bone Joint Surg 65A:154–162, 1983.
7. Pressman AE, Letts RM, Jarvis JG: Anterior cruciate ligament tears in children: An analysis of operative versus non-operative treatment. J Pediatr Orthop 17:505–511, 1997.
8. Scarson WG: The role of lateral extra-articular procedures for anterolateral rotatory instability. Clin Sports Med 7:751–772, 1988.
9. Schaefer RK, Jackson DW: Arthroscopic management of the cruciate ligaments. In McGinty JB, et al (eds): Operative Arthroscopy. New York, Raven Press, 1991, pp 389–416.
10. Shelbourne KD, Davis TJ, Klootwyk TE: The relationship between intercondylar notch width of the femur and the incidence of anterior cruciate ligament tears. A prospective study. Am J Sports Med 26:402–408, 1998.
11. Shelbourne KD, Nitz PA: The O'Donoghue triad revisited: Combined knee injuries involving anterior cruciate and medial collateral ligament tears. Am J Sports Med 19:474–477, 1991.
12. Shelbourne KD, Wilckens JH, Mollabashy A, et al: Arthrofibrosis in acute anterior cruciate ligament reconstruction. The effect of timing of reconstruction and rehabilitation. Am J Sports Med 19:332, 1991.
13. Swenson TM, Fu FH: Anterior cruciate ligament reconstruction: Long-term results using autograft tissue. Clin Sports Med 12:709–722, 1993.

71. POSTERIOR CRUCIATE LIGAMENT INJURIES

David E. Brown, M.D.

1. Describe and discuss the anatomy of the posterior cruciate ligament.

The posterior cruciate ligament (PCL) does not have as discrete a bundle arrangement as the anterior cruciate ligament (ACL). Many authors, however, describe an anterolateral (largest) bundle and a posteromedial bundle. The presence of the ligament of Humphrey (45% of individuals) and ligament of Wrisberg (35% of individuals) is variable; if present, however, they may account for up to one-third of the diameter of the PCL.

The femoral attachment area resembles a half circle, thus causing differential bundle tightening with knee motion. The anterolateral bundle tightens with flexion, whereas the posteromedial bundle tightens in extension. The femoral attachment of the PCL is approximately 25 mm in length and 8 mm in width from anterior to posterior, with its center point 6–8 mm from the anterior articular edge when the knee is flexed. The tibial attachment site, which is nearly circular, is 12 mm in width and takes up most of the central sulcus on the posterior aspect of the tibial plateau.

2. What are the relative size and diameter of the PCL?

The PCL previously was thought to be twice the size and strength of the ACL. Recent studies, however, have demonstrated that the PCL is only 40–50% larger than the ACL.

3. What is the incidence of PCL tears?

Injury to the PCL is thought to occur in approximately 3–5% of all knee ligament injuries. The incidence appears to be rising slightly because of improved imaging techniques (MRI), improved techniques of physical examination, and greater knowledge of PCL injuries.

4. **What common mechanisms of injury may cause a PCL tear?**
   - Fall on flexed knee with the foot in plantar flexion
   - Dashboard knee (motor vehicle accident with the knee flexed and the tibia forced posteriorly on impact)
   - Hyperflexion
   - Hyperextension (usually in combination with other ligament injuries)

5. **What is the most important test for evaluating PCL injuries?**
   The 90° posterior drawer test is the most important. The patient is supine, the hip is flexed 45°, and the knee is flexed 90°. Force is applied from anterior to posterior on the proximal tibia. Excessive motion in an anterior to posterior direction is a positive test indicative of PCL injury. A grade I posterior drawer reflects 5 mm of movement. At maximal posterior displacement, the tibial condyles are still anterior to the femoral condyles. A grade II posterior drawer reflects 5–10-mm posterior displacement, in which the tibial condyles are flush with the femoral condyles. A grade III posterior drawer reflects > 10-mm posterior displacement. In a grade III posterior drawer, the tibial condyles are displaced posterior to the femoral condyles.

6. **What is the primary restraint to the 90° posterior drawer test?**
   The PCL provides 90% of the posterior restraint to the posterior drawer test at 90° of knee flexion. It contributes relatively little to varus, valgus, and internal and external rotation restraint.

7. **What is posterolateral rotatory instability?**
   Posterolateral rotatory instability is laxity or incompetence of the structures of the posterolateral corner of the knee, including the lateral collateral ligament and the arcuate ligament complex (arcuate ligament, popliteus tendon, fabellofibular ligament, and posterolateral capsule).
   Selective ligament-cutting experiments reveal that sectioning all of the structures of the posterolateral corner produces only small amounts of posterior translation of the knee. However, sectioning of the posterolateral ligaments results in markedly increased varus rotation and external tibial rotation with stress testing.

8. **What is the posterior sag test?**
   The posterior sag test is similar to the posterior drawer test. It essentially detects the amount of posterior displacement caused by gravity when the knee and hip are flexed to 90°. When compared with the opposite side, the PCL-injured knee reveals a posterior sag of the tibial condyles relative to the femoral condyles. A positive test reflects absence of the PCL.

9. **What is the quadriceps active test?**
   This test is also useful in evaluating PCL tear. The patient is placed in the same position as for a posterior drawer test. In the PCL-deficient knee, the tibia sags as in the posterior sag test. Quadriceps contraction at this position produces anterior translation of the tibia, verifying PCL injury.

10. **What is the natural history of the isolated PCL tear?**
    Most patients do not have symptomatic instability of the knee. Several studies have demonstrated that > 80% of patients return to preinjury sport level. Quadriceps rehabilitation to a level equal to that of the opposite side correlates with satisfactory activity level. Associated meniscus tears are uncommon.
    The PCL-deficient knee appears to be at risk for medial compartment and patellofemoral compartment arthritis. It is not clear whether the risk is related to activity level, but it does appear related to advancing time from injury. PCL-deficient cadaver knees have increased medial and patellofemoral compartment contact pressures, which may lead to articular surface degeneration.

11. What is the recommended treatment for isolated posterior tears?

Because most patients with isolated PCL tears function well, nonoperative treatment is generally recommended. Maximal quadriceps rehabilitation is required. It is unclear whether functional bracing affords any benefit.

The results of surgical reconstruction of the isolated PCL-deficient knee have not been shown to be better than conservative treatment. Further support for conservative treatment has recently been demonstrated in a biomechanical study in our laboratories. Multiple biomechanical and kinematic parameters were studied with high-speed video cinematography, computerized digital measurements, and force plate analysis. No significant difference could be detected when comparing the normal knee with the isolated PCL-deficient knee in young athletes.

12. If the PCL is avulsed from the tibia rather than torn in midsubstance, are the treatment recommendations any different?

Repair of the PCL bone avulsions from the tibia is generally advised. The ligament itself is intact. A simple posteromedial surgical approach affords easy reduction and fixation of the bone fragment. Results are uniformly good, in contrast to the midsubstance PCL tear described in question 11.

13. What are the principles of rehabilitation of the isolated PCL-deficient knee?

Nonoperative rehabilitation treatment emphasizes closed kinetic chain extension exercises, including squats, leg press, bicycling, and stair-stepper exercises. Open kinetic chain extension exercises, which are performed with the foot free, are avoided. Examples include seated or standing knee extension exercises.

In general, before beginning rehabilitation, the patient is evaluated by MRI. Any associated meniscus pathology is treated arthroscopically. Athletes commonly return to their sport within 3–6 weeks after injury. We generally prescribe a posterior cruciate functional brace for athletes involved in contact sports.

14. When should the isolated PCL-deficient knee be reconstructed?

Some clinicians believe that an acute knee injury with a grade III posterior drawer should be acutely reconstructed. Most, however, still recommend conservative treatment. If conservative treatment fails, resulting in persistent pain or functional instability, surgical reconstruction may still be performed.

15. What graft options are available for PCL reconstruction?
- Central one-third patella tendon autograft
- Patella tendon allograft
- Achilles tendon allograft
- Semitendinosus/gracilis autograft

Graft selection depends on the preference of surgeon and patient, availability of graft sources, and whether additional ligament reconstructions are required. Patella tendon autografts appear to result in better success rates (similar to ACL reconstructions). However, many knees undergoing PCL reconstruction have multiple ligament injuries. The morbidity of multiple autogenous graft harvests leads many surgeons to use allograft sources in such cases.

16. What is the best position for postoperative immobilization after PCL reconstruction?

If posterior capsule is intact, the best position is full extension. The posterior capsule limits gravity-induced posterior sag. If the posterior capsule has been injured or if other extraarticular repairs or reconstructions are performed, the position of postoperative immobilization depends more on those repairs than on the PCL.

17. In what position is the PCL graft tensioned and fixated?

Warren advises tensioning and fixation in full extension if the posterior capsule is intact. Paulos performs tensioning and fixation in 70° of knee flexion, which is the quadriceps neutral position.

18. What are the principal techniques involved in PCL reconstruction?

1. Reconstruction can be performed by either open or arthroscopic techniques, depending on degree of associated injury and the preference and skill of the surgeon.

2. Placement of the tibial guidepin should be directed by intraoperative radiographic evaluation. It is imperative that the tibial guidepin be in the central low position of the tibial attachment of the PCL.

3. A miniposterior incision should be used to allow digital evaluation of guidepin placement at the tibial attachment. This incision also allows better control of reamer penetration of the posterior tibial cortex during tunnel preparation.

4. The tendon of the graft must be at least 40 mm in length to allow the bone portions of the graft complex to be seated fully within the femoral and tibial tunnels.

5. Tibial tunnel orientation, placement, and graft fixation are possible through multiple methods. Some advocate beginning the tibial tunnel on the medial tibial metaphysis, whereas others begin the tibial tunnel on the lateral side. Some surgeons avoid the tibial tunnel altogether, preferring to fix the bone portion of the graft construct to the posterior tibial cortex at the site of PCL attachment.

6. Femoral tunnel placement should be 4 mm distal (shallow when viewed arthroscopically) to the femoral isometric attachment site. This position is still within the PCL femoral footprint.

19. Describe the clinical examination of the knee with combined PCL and posterolateral ligament instability.

The knee is markedly lax to posterior drawer at both 30° and 90°, usually with a grade III posterior drawer at 90°. The prone external rotation test and varus stress test at 30° are markedly positive. There may be varus opening in 90° of knee flexion. The patient may walk with a varus thrust gait.

20. What is the treatment of combined PCL/posterolateral rotatory instability injuries?

Surgical repair and reconstruction are required. Patients generally are markedly symptomatic, with both pain and instability, if untreated. The rate of medial compartment arthritis is significant.

If the patient has a varus knee or walks with a varus thrust gait, valgus high tibial osteotomy placing is performed first. Some patients are so dramatically improved by this procedure alone that later ligament reconstruction is not required. Most of the time, however, the PCL and posterolateral corner must be reconstructed. The PCL is reconstructed by one of the techniques described above. The posterolateral corner is reconstructed by either ligament advancement, biceps tenodesis, or anatomic reconstruction of the posterolateral corner. Posterolateral corner injuries and reconstruction are further described in the chapter on lateral ligament injury.

21. What is the treatment of an acute PCL tear combined with a medial side injury?

In a patient with an acute grade III medial collateral injury, open primary repair and approximation of the medial structures combined with acute PCL reconstruction is indicated. Patients with grade I or grade II MCL injuries may be treated nonoperatively if they are not athletes. The MCL and PCL injuries are both treated conservatively. Athletes with such an injury may be considered for subacute PCL reconstruction after allowing the partial MCL injury to heal.

22. In patients with knee dislocations or near knee dislocations with multiple ligament injuries, what surgical treatment should be considered?

If the PCL is avulsed, direct repair of the PCL combined with reconstruction of the ACL at the index procedure is an acceptable option. When both the ACL and PCL are torn in midsubstance and thus each requires reconstruction, the cruciates should be reconstructed in stages. At the initial surgery, PCL reconstruction combined with collateral and capsular repair is performed. Once the patient has satisfactorily recovered from the initial surgery, late ACL reconstruction is performed. Staged reconstruction is preferred because these individuals often develop postoperative knee stiffness after the operation if all structures are surgically repaired and reconstructed at the same time.

BIBLIOGRAPHY

1. Burks RT, Schaffer JJ: A simplified approach to the tibial attachment of the posterior cruciate ligament. Clin Orthop 254:216–219, 1990.
2. Clancy WG Jr, Shelbourne KD, Zoellner GB, et al: Treatment of knee joint instability secondary to rupture of the posterior cruciate ligament. Report of a new procedure. J Bone Joint Surg 65A:310–322, 1983.
3. Daniel DM, Stone ML, Barnett P, et al: Use of the quadriceps active test to diagnose posterior cruciate-ligament disruption and measure posterior laxity of the knee. J Bone Joint Surg 70A:386–391, 1988.
4. Fowler PJ, Messieh SS: Isolated posterior cruciate ligament injuries in athletes. Am J Sports Med 15:553–557, 1987.
5. Galloway MT, Grood ES, Mehalik MS, et al: Posterior cruciate ligament reconstruction. An in vitro study of femoral and tibial graft placement. Am J Sports Med 24:437–445, 1996.
6. Gollehon DL, Torzilli PA, Warren RF: The role of the posterolateral and cruciate ligaments in the stability of the human knee: A biomechanical study. J Bone Joint Surg 69A:233–242, 1987.
7. Miller RH: Knee injuries. In Canale ST (ed): Campbell's Operative Orthopaedics, 9th ed. St. Louis, Mosby, 1998, pp 1190–1195.
8. Parolie JM, Bergfeld JA: Long-term results of non-operative treatment of isolated posterior cruciate ligament injuries in the athlete. Am J Sports Med 14:35–38, 1986.
9. Skyhar MJ, Warren RF, Ortiz GJ, et al: The effects of sectioning of the posterior cruciate ligament and the posterolateral complex on the articular contact pressures within the knee. J Bone Joint Surg Am 74:594–699, 1993.
10. Torg JS, Barton TM, Pavlov H, et al: Natural history of the posterior cruciate ligament-deficient knee. Clin Orthop 246:208–216, 1989.
11. Velteri DM, Warren RF: Isolated and combined posterior cruciate ligament injuries. J Am Acad Orthop Surg 1:67, 1993.

72. MEDIAL COLLATERAL LIGAMENT INJURIES

Randall D. Neumann, M.D.

1. What is the medial collateral ligament?

The medial collateral ligament (MCL) complex is a supporting structure on the medial side of the knee. It is a sleeve of tissue extending from the midline anteriorly to the midline posteriorly.

2. What are the components of the MCL?

The important static structures are the superficial MCL, the posterior oblique ligament, and the middle third or deep capsular ligaments. The dynamic supporting structures include the semimembranosus complex and the vastus medialis.

3. What is the superficial MCL?

The superficial MCL, also called the tibia collateral ligament, attaches from the medial femoral epicondyle at the adductor tubercle and inserts distally 5–7 cm below the joint line under the pes anserinus.

4. What is the posterior oblique ligament?

The posterior oblique ligament is the thickened triangular capsular ligament originating posterior to the superficial MCL and inserting below the joint line. This ligament is important in maintaining medial stability and resists anterior medial tibial subluxation.

5. What is the deep capsular ligament?

The middle one-third of the capsular ligament or deep MCL is a short structure attached to the meniscus immediately beneath the superficial MCL. It is divided into meniscotibial and meniscofemoral fibers.

6. What is the function of the MCL?
The main function of the MCL is to resist valgus and external rotation forces of the tibia in relation to the femur.

7. Describe the clinical classification of MCL injuries.
Sprains of the MCL are classified as mild, moderate, or severe. Mild or grade I sprains have few torn fibers with no loss of ligamentous integrity. Moderate or grade II sprains are incomplete tears with no pathologic laxity; the fibers are still opposed. In severe or grade III sprains, the integrity of the ligament is completely disrupted.

8. What is the typical history obtained from a patient with an MCL injury?
Usually the patient discusses the mechanism. Lower-grade MCL injuries may occur with noncontact valgus and external rotation injuries, such as seen in skiing. Moderate-to-severe MCL injuries usually result from a lateral blow to the lower thigh or upper leg that causes valgus stress to be placed on the knee. This mechanism of injury commonly occurs in contact sports such as football, soccer, and rugby. Patients may or may not have the ability to ambulate. Some patients describe the sensation of a "pop" or a tearing of tissue. Usually no deformity exists.

9. Do most patients with a grade III sprain have severe hemarthrosis?
Because patients with a grade III sprain have complete tearing of the capsule, fluid from inside the joint may escape into the soft tissues. Therefore, patients may have only minimal joint space effusion.

10. Do patients with grade III injuries have severe pain and inability to walk?
Hughston et al. found that 50% of athletes with grade III injuries could walk into the office unaided by external support. They also found that some grade I and grade II sprains are actually more painful than grade III. Therefore, the absence of severe pain does not rule out a severe injury.

11. What other ligament is commonly injured along with the MCL?
The anterior cruciate ligament (ACL).

12. Describe the grading system for pathologic laxity of the MCL.
With abduction stress testing, joint opening may occur, displacing the tibia on the femur. Grade 0 is considered normal. Grade I has 1–4 mm of laxity; grade II, 5–9 mm of laxity; and grade III, 10–15 mm of laxity.

13. Where is maximal tenderness located in MCL injuries?
On physical examination palpation reveals that most patients have tenderness over the adductor tubercle. Such tenderness may signify that the posterior oblique ligament and deep fibers of the collateral ligament are torn. Other areas of tenderness occur over the joint line and distally over the insertion of the tibial collateral ligament.

14. What percentage of patients have injury to the extensor mechanism?
Approximately 10–20% of patients damage the extensor mechanism (usually the vastus medialis with patellar dislocation) in association with MCL injuries.

15. What tests on physical examination signify MCL injury?
1. The **abduction stress test** is done with the patient's knee flexed at 30°. It is best to have the thigh resting on the edge of the table, with the foot supported by the examiner. Abduction stress testing is done with a valgus load to open the medial compartment of the knee. The test should be done with the foot in the same degree of external rotation, because an extra grade of instability may be perceived if the examination allows the tibia to move externally. The test is considered positive when medial instability is present at 30° of flexion.

2. The **anterior drawer test** checks for anterior medial instability. With the foot in external rotation and the knee flexed at 90°, an anterior pull on the proximal calf is used to palpate laxity. It is best that the examiner sit on the patient's foot and relax the hamstrings before testing. Perceivable anterior rotational instability is seen if the MCL with its posterior oblique portion is torn. Both tests should be done when MCL injury is suspected.

3. The **Lachman test** should be done for evaluation of the ACL. Instability in full extension suggests that the posterior capsule is disrupted and possibly the posterior cruciate ligament (PCL). Some patients with patellar apprehension also have dislocated the patella.

16. What diagnostic tests are available for evaluation of MCL injuries?

1. **Stress radiography.** This test is done using abduction stress testing at 15–20°. Radiographs are then taken to assess the opening on the medial side of the joint.

2. **Magnetic resonance imaging (MRI).** MRI is helpful in assessing the location of the MCL tear and associated meniscal and cruciate pathology.

3. **Arthrograms.** Arthrograms are an invasive examination that may show meniscal pathology or contrast extravasation as evidence of capsular tearing; they also may be negative, because the capsule seals in 2–4 days. Arthrograms are generally not indicated at this time, because noninvasive tests are more accurate.

4. **Arthroscopy.** Examination under anesthesia and arthroscopy may be helpful in assessing meniscal pathology, ligamentous injury, and cruciate pathology. This invasive test is reserved for patients who are undergoing operative treatment.

17. What is a Pellegrini-Steida lesion?

The Pellegrini-Steida lesion is seen on the anteroposterior radiograph. Calcification adjacent to the adductor tubercle signifies an old collateral ligament injury of longer than 6 weeks.

18. Why are stress radiographs of the knee needed for adolescents?

Adolescents with open epiphyseal lines may have physeal injuries that are mistaken for medial instability because of the appearance of medial laxity. Physeal fractures generally require reduction and casting or internal fixation.

19. What are the treatments for grades I and II isolated MCL injuries?

Grades I and II isolated MCL injuries are treated conservatively. Icing is applied for 20 minutes 2–3 times/day. An elastic wrap may be used. Non–weight-bearing crutches are used. Isometric quadriceps contractures usually can be done within the first 2–3 days of injury. The knee is immobilized to block full extension for 7–10 days. Progressive ambulation and range-of-motion and strengthening exercises are done as the swelling subsides, pain diminishes, and the patient regains the ability to ambulate. Most patients can return to full activities and contact sports within 3–6 weeks.

20. How are isolated grade III MCL injuries treated?

Most patients are now treated nonoperatively. Historically, such patients underwent operative repair of the MCL. Multiple studies have shown that repair in an isolated MCL injury occurs without surgery. Treatment consists of crutches, cast, or bracing. Bracing can continue for 3–6 weeks, depending on healing.

CONTROVERSIES

21. Describe the treatment for ACL tears combined with MCL lesions.

Controversy exists about the approaches to MCL treatment in association with ACL treatment. Some authors believe that treatment of the MCL with protective weightbearing and bracing should restore full motion and stability before ACL ligament surgery is performed. At approximately 4–6 weeks, the ACL is reconstructed with patellar tendon graft, allograft, or hamstring tendons. If at that time instability continues, the posterior oblique and the superficial MCL are reconstructed. Other authors believe that the isolated MCL injuries should be treated surgically with open repair within 5–7 days after injury. The ACL is reconstructed at that time. Some evidence suggests that increased scarring and arthrofibrosis occur with a higher reoperation rate, when the surgery is done acutely during the first 7–10 days.

BIBLIOGRAPHY

1. Hughston JC, Andrews JR, Cross MJ, Moschi A: Classification of knee ligament instabilities: Part I. The medial compartment in cruciate ligaments. J Bone Joint Surg 58A:159–172, 1976.
2. Hughston JC, Barret GR: Acute anterior medial rotatory instability: Long term results of surgical repair. J Bone Joint Surg 65A:145–153, 1983.
3. Indelicato PA, Hermansdorfer J, Huegel M: The nonoperative management of complete tears of the medial collateral ligament of the knee in intercollegiate football players. Clin Orthop 256:174–177, 1990.
4. Linton RC, Indelicato PA: Medial ligament injuries. In DeLee JC, Drez D (eds): Orthopedic Sports Medicine: Principles and Practice, vol. 1. Philadelphia, W.B. Saunders, 1994, pp 1261–1274.
5. Neumann RD: Traumatic knee injuries. In Mellion MB (ed): Sports Medicine Secrets, 2nd ed. Philadelphia, Hanley & Belfus, 1999, pp 307–311.
6. O'Donoghue DH: Treatment of acute ligamentous injuries at the knee. Orthop Clin North Am 4:617–645, 1973.
7. Warren LF, Marshall JL: The supporting structures and layers of the medial side of the knee. An anatomical analysis. J Bone Joint Surg 61A:56–62, 1979.
8. Warren LF, Marshall JL, Girgis F: The primary static stabilizer of the medial side of the knee. J Bone Joint Surg 56A:665–674, 1974.

73. LATERAL LIGAMENT INJURIES

David E. Brown, M.D.

1. What is the incidence of isolated fibular collateral ligament tear?

The true incidence is unknown. However, an isolated ligament injury is quite uncommon. Many patients who are given a diagnosis of fibular collateral ligament (FCL) strain (often by inexperienced examiners) have anterior cruciate ligament (ACL) injuries.

2. What is the mechanism of an isolated FCL injury?

Such injuries are thought to result from either a contact or noncontact hyperextension varus stress. Perhaps the incidence is low because varus stress generally has to be applied from the medial side of the knee, a mechanism that is quite uncommon. Because the contralateral knee is likely to be "in the way," the injured knee is more likely to sustain a valgus stress to its lateral side.

3. Describe the examination of isolated FCL injuries.

Examination should show tenderness along the FCL, which is best palpated with the knee in a figure-four position with varus stress applied. There is generally little effusion, because the FCL is extraarticular. The presence of an effusion should arouse suspicion for a cruciate ligament tear. Selective ligament-cutting experiments in cadavers have demonstrated only **slight** varus laxity in knees with sectioned FCLs. **Moderate** varus laxity occurs only with additional sectioning of the posterolateral corner ligaments. **Severe** varus laxity should arouse suspicion of combined FCL, posterolateral corner, and cruciate ligament injuries.

4. What is the treatment of isolated FCL injuries?

Treatment includes elastic wrapping, ice application, functional bracing, and protection from repeat varus stress for a period of 4–6 weeks. Some authors advocate surgical repair of isolated FCL injuries. However, no study has scientifically evaluated the treatment of isolated FCL injuries.

5. Describe the anatomy of the posterolateral corner ligaments.

The principal structures of the posterolateral corner include:

- FCL
- Arcuate ligament
- Popliteus tendon
- Popliteofibular ligament
- Short lateral ligament
- Fabellofibular ligament
- Posterolateral deep capsule

Baker has described the arcuate ligament complex as the arcuate ligament, FCL, popliteus tendon, and lateral head of the gastrocnemius. Only the FCL and the popliteus tendon are invariable in all cadaver specimens; all other structures described above have a variable presence in knees. The fabellofibular ligament is present in approximately two-thirds of specimens. If the fabella is present, the fabellofibular ligament is present. If the fabellofibular ligament is not present, then the short lateral ligament is generally present. The popliteofibular ligament and the arcuate ligament are present in approximately 50% of specimens.

6. What is posterolateral rotatory instability?

Posterolateral rotatory instability is laxity or incompetence of the structures of the posterolateral corner of the knee, including the lateral collateral ligament and the posterolateral ligaments. Selective ligament-cutting experiments reveal that sectioning of all of the structures of the posterolateral corner produces only small amounts of posterior translation of the knee. However, sectioning the posterolateral ligaments resulted in markedly increased varus rotation and external tibial rotation with stress testing.

7. What is the mechanism of injury to the posterolateral corner?

- Posterolaterally directed blow to the medial part of the tibia
- Hyperextension and external rotation
- Pure hyperextension

8. What are the symptoms in patients with posterolateral instability of the knee?

The major symptom is pain in the posterolateral aspect of the knee. Up to 25% of patients may have dysesthesias and weakness of the foot and leg muscles due to associated injury of the peroneal nerve. Patients may complain of instability with the knee in full extension, thus leading to a gait pattern that emphasizes knee flexion to avoid instability. With greater laxity, the gait may demonstrate a varus thrust.

9. What is the external rotation recurvatum test?

The external rotation recurvatum test may reflect posterolateral rotatory instability. With the patient supine, the great toe is grasped and the foot is raised from the table. The test is positive if the knee falls into hyperextension, external rotation, and varus.

10. How does one test for varus instability of the knee? Why is such testing important?

With the patient relaxed and supine on the examination table, the distal femur is stabilized manually. The lower leg is grasped with the opposite hand, and varus stress is placed on the knee. The test should be performed at 0°, 30°, 60°, and 90° of knee flexion.

Isolated FCL injury causes minimal varus laxity. When combined with posterolateral corner injury, the varus laxity is moderate to severe. Large degrees of varus instability in full extension should arouse suspicion for combined injuries of the posterolateral corner and one of the cruciate ligaments. An isolated cruciate ligament injury does not affect varus or valgus stability. The presence of varus laxity in full extension is primarily indicative of a posterolateral corner injury.

11. How do you test for external rotation of the tibia? Why is such testing important?

The patient is placed prone on the examining table with the hips and knees resting on the table. The knees are flexed at 30°, and the feet are rotated externally. If external rotation on the injured side is 10° more than on the normal side, the test is considered positive. A positive test is usually consistent with a tear of the posterolateral corner.

12. Describe the clinical examination of the knee with combined posterior cruciate and posterolateral ligament instability.

The knee is markedly lax to posterior drawer at both 30° and 90°. At 90° there is usually a grade III posterior drawer. The prone external rotation test and varus stress test at 30° are markedly positive. Varus opening may be present in 90° of knee flexion. The patient may walk with a varus thrust gait.

13. What is the role of MRI in the evaluation of posterolateral corner injuries?

MRI accurately depicts the extent of injury to the posterolateral ligaments. A bone contusion on the anterior medial femoral condyle is invariably present with complete posterolateral ligament injuries.

14. What are the treatment options in patients with posterolateral rotatory instability?

If tears of the posterolateral corner are recognized acutely, primary repair of all injured structures is recommended. If there is insufficient tissue for primary repair, augmentation is indicated but depends on what healthy tissues remain in severe posterolateral corner injuries. For example, if the knee has been laterally dislocated, it is common for the iliotibial band and biceps tendon to be disrupted. If the biceps tendon and iliotibial band are intact, they can be used as augmentation sources.

Clancy advocates biceps tenodesis. The entire distal portion of the tendon is advanced and secured to the lateral femoral epicondyle with a soft-tissue screw and washer. This procedure augments the FCL and theoretically advances part of the posterolateral corner through intertendinous attachments between the biceps tendon and the posterolateral corner.

Warren has devised procedures to augment the popliteus tendon with central slips of either the biceps or iliotibial band.

Chronic posterolateral corner injuries also may be reconstructed with either the Clancy or Warren techniques. If the biceps tendon and iliotibial band are insufficient because of chronic stretching laxity or previous tear, Warren has described reconstruction of the popliteus and/or FCL with a bone-tendon-bone patellar ligament graft. The graft may be split on one end to allow reconstruction of both portions of the popliteus tendon.

BIBLIOGRAPHY

1. Baker CL Jr, Norwood LA, Hughston JC: Acute posterolateral rotatory instability of the knee. J Bone Joint Surg 65A:614–618, 1983.
2. Baker CL Jr, Norwood LA, Hughston JC: Acute combined posterior cruciate and posterolateral instability of the knee. Am J Sports Med 12:204–208, 1984.
3. Clancy WG Jr: Repair and reconstruction of the posterior cruciate ligament. In Chapman MW (ed): Operative Orthopedics, vol. 3. Philadelphia, J.B. Lippincott, 1988, pp 1651–1665.
4. DeLee JC, Riley MB, Rockwood CA: Acute straight lateral instability of the knee. Am J Sports Med 11:404, 1983.
5. Gollehon DL, Torzilli PA, Warren RF: The role of the posterolateral and cruciate ligaments in the stability of the human knee. A biomechanical study. J Bone Joint Surg 69A:233–242, 1992.
6. Ross G, Chapman AW, Newberg AR, et al: Magnetic resonance imaging for the evaluation of acute posterolateral complex injuries of the knee. Am J Sports Med 25:444–448, 1997.
7. Veltri DM, Warren RF: Posterolateral instability of the knee. J Bone Joint Surg 76A:460–472, 1994.
8. Wascher DC, Grauer JD, Markoff KL: Biceps tendon tenodesis for posterolateral instability of the knee: An in vitro study. Am J Sports Med 21:400–406, 1993.

74. PATELLOFEMORAL JOINT DISORDERS

Michele Helzer-Julin, PA.-C., M.S.

1. How common are disorders of the patellofemoral joint?

Problems related to the patellofemoral joint are likely to be the most common knee problems encountered in clinical practice. Routinely, they are not related to trauma but to overuse.

2. List some of the many general labels and specific clinical entities related to problems of the patellofemoral joint.

General Labels	Clinical Entities
Extensor mechanism malalignment (EMM)	Patellar tendinitis (jumpers' knee)
Patellofemoral pain syndrome	Quadriceps tendinitis
Runner's knee	Osgood-Schlatter disease
Chondromalacia	Plica
Patellar subluxation/dislocation	Fat pad impingement
	Bipartite patella

3. Is there a characteristic somatotype for the patient with patellofemoral problems?

No. Early discussion popularized the concept that patellar problems affect only chubby, knock-kneed, teenage girls—certainly not the vigorous male athlete. It is now clear that the patellofemoral joint is a major source of pain and dysfunction for both males and females in sedentary and athletic populations alike.

4. What anatomic predispositions contribute to patellofemoral disorders?

The many anatomic factors include both soft-tissue and bony abnormalities:

Bony Abnormalities	Soft-tissue Abnormalities
Patella alta	Vastus medialis obliquus dysplasia
Lateral tilting and subluxation of the patella	Tight lateral retinaculum
Shallow trochlear groove	Patellar hypermobility
Genu valgum	Generalized ligamentous laxity
External tibial torsion	Hamstring tightness
Femoral anteversion	Weak ankle dorsiflexors
Pes planus, pronation, forefoot supination	Increased lateral deviation of patellar tendon

5. Does the presence of any or all of the above predispositions guarantee that an individual will have problems?

No. Predispositions are merely that. Anatomic variations are widespread in the general population and may lie dormant, leaving affected individuals asymptomatic for years, decades, or even their entire life. Symptoms are usually provoked by overuse but also may be triggered by a single traumatic event that creates symptoms in a previously asymptomatic individual.

6. What are typical patellofemoral complaints?

Most symptoms and complaints relate to either pain, instability, or both:

1. **Anterior knee pain**, the most frequent complaint, may be aggravated by any physical activity, but most commonly by repetitive stair climbing or sitting with the knee flexed at 90° for a prolonged period (e.g., sitting in an airplane, car, or theater).

2. **Swelling** is not routine and, if present, is only minimal. Many patients have a general puffy appearance to their knees, although no effusion within the joint itself is detectable.

3. **Catching or slipping sensations** are common. Catching may occur when underlying inflamed tissue is caught on bony prominences, or it may be due to roughness on the patellar surface or inflamed plica. Even minor instability episodes may be interpreted by the patient as catching. Feelings of lateral patellar slipping range from a mild catching sensation to a feeling that the patella has completely left the trochlear groove, resulting in the knee giving way.

7. What activities typically aggravate the patellofemoral joint?

Activities that load the patellofemoral joint or create high compressive forces, such as ascending and descending stairs, squatting, and sitting with the knee flexed to 90° for prolonged periods of time, cause significant patellofemoral pain. Many patients also are bothered by running, jumping, cutting, and twisting activities.

8. Describe the typical physical findings.

The most common physical findings are the anatomic predispositions listed in question 4. In addition, there may be pain with compression of the patella, crepitation of the patellofemoral joint with knee range of motion, and apprehension with lateral displacement of the patella.

9. What radiographic techniques are useful?

For routine problems of the patellofemoral joint, radiographs may lend little additional information to a detailed history and physical examination. Routine anteroposterior and lateral views can rule out other pathologic processes. The lateral view assesses patellar height. The most significant view in dealing with the patellofemoral joint is the infrapatellar view, which assesses lateral tilting and subluxation of the patella. Because the patellofemoral joint is dynamically affected, static radiographs may appear normal in a patient with severe patellofemoral disability.

10. What are the current recommendations for initial treatment of patellofemoral problems?

Physical therapy with a rehabilitative exercise routine is the mainstay of treatment. Techniques, such as biofeedback, that emphasize patellar control rather than pure strength are essential. Flexibility is important. Knee extension exercises should be eliminated. External supports such as bracing and taping may be helpful. Nonsteroidal antiinflammatory drugs, modalities, activity modifications, and correction of forefoot abnormalities may be appropriate in select patients.

11. Do the above techniques cure the problem?

No. Anatomic predisposition is still present. The goal should be return to a normal, pain-free, and functional status. Nonsurgical means control symptoms in 80–90% of individuals. It is human nature to stop rehabilitative efforts once symptoms subside, despite the recurrent nature of patellofemoral problems. Therefore, patients must be made aware that this is a potentially life-long problem with which they need to cope. The patient should be reminded to reintroduce rehabilitative efforts if symptoms return.

12. What surgical options are available for patients in whom conservative treatment fails?

Various surgical options are designed to realign the patella. The simplest is an arthroscopic lateral release, which, unfortunately, does not help in all cases. A more extensive open procedure uses not only a lateral release, but also advancement of the vastus medialis obliquus and transfer of the patellar tendon medially and distally. Other less common surgical options include anterior advancement of the tibial tuberosity to decompress the patellofemoral joint, derotational osteotomy of the limb, and patellectomy.

13. At what point during conservative treatment should surgical options be considered?

No set length of time exists. Routinely, patients have tried conservative treatment and lifestyle modification for months to years. Surgical intervention should occur when the patient feels symptoms are at an unacceptable level and when the patient and surgeon agree that there is no trend toward improvement.

14. Can the patient expect a normal knee after surgery?

No. Although surgery may help considerably and allow for further improvement with post-operative physical therapy, the patient will still have anatomic variations that may continue to cause problems in the future.

15. How does treatment change when the patient sustains an acute lateral patellar dislocation?

The acute injury, of course, must be treated in and of itself, including the usual measures for control of swelling and possibly a brief period of immobilization. Current trends replace a strict 6 weeks of immobilization with modest immobilization for symptom control and early return to functional rehabilitation. As the acute phase resolves, treatment options are similar.

16. What findings prompt early surgical intervention after an acute patellar dislocation?

1. An osteochondral fracture of the patella, trochlea, or lateral femoral condyle may occur as the patella either leaves or reenters the femoral trochlea. Some large fractures can be reattached with internal fixation, whereas other smaller fractures need to be removed because of mechanical locking episodes.

2. If the vastus medialis obliquus has been ruptured at its insertion and a defect is palpable along the superior medial edge of the patella, early surgical repair is the best option.

BIBLIOGRAPHY

1. Bourne MH, Hazel WA, Scott SG, Sim FH: Anterior knee pain. Mayo Clin Proc 63:482–491, 1988.
2. Carson WG, James SL, Larson RL, et al: Patellofemoral disorders: Physical and radiographic evaluation. Part I. Physical examination. Clin Orthop 185:165–177, 1984.
3. Carson WG, James SL, Larson RL, et al: Patellofemoral disorders: Physical and radiographic evaluation. Part II. Radiographic examination. Clin Orthop 185:178–186, 1984.
4. DeLee JC, Drez D (eds): Orthopedic Sports Medicine: Principles and Practice. Philadelphia, W.B. Saunders, 1994, pp 1163–1248.
5. Dugdale TW, Barnett PR: Historical background: Patellofemoral pain in young people. Orthop Clin North Am 17:211–219, 1986.
6. Dutkowsky JP: Miscellaneous nontraumatic disorders. In Canale ST (ed): Campbell's Operative Orthopaedics, 9th ed. St. Louis, Mosby, 1998, pp 787–855.
7. Fisher RL: Conservative treatment of patellofemoral pain. Orthop Clin North Am 17:269–272, 1986.
8. Franz WB III: Overuse syndromes in runners. In Mellion MB, Walsh WM, Shelton GL (eds): Sports Injuries and Athletic Problems. Philadelphia, Hanley & Belfus, 1990, pp 289–309.
9. Galland O, Walch G, Dejour H, Carret JP: An anatomical and radiological study of the femoropatellar articulation. Surg Radiol Anat 12:119–125, 1990.
10. Henry JH: Conservative treatment of patellofemoral subluxation. Clin Sports Med 8:261–278, 1989.
11. Hughston JC: Knee Ligaments. Injury and Repair. St. Louis, Mosby, 1993.
12. Hughston JC: Patellar subluxation: A recent history. Clin Sports Med 8:153–162, 1989.
13. Hughston JC, Flandry F, Brinuer MR, et al: Surgical correction of medial subluxation of the patella. Am J Sports Med 24:486–491, 1996.
14. Hughston JC, Walsh WM, Puddu G: Patellar Subluxation and Dislocation. Philadelphia, W.B. Saunders, 1984.
15. Maenpaa H, Lehto Mu: Patellar dislocation: The long-term results of nonoperative management in 100 patients. Am J Sports Med 25:213–217, 1997.
16. McConnell J: The management of chondromalacia patellae: A long term solution. Aust J Physiother 2:215–223, 1986.
17. Minkoff J, Fein L: The role of radiography in the evaluation and treatment of common anarthrotic disorders of the patellofemoral joint. Clin Sports Med 8:203–260, 1989.
18. Reider B, Marshall JL, Warren RF: Clinical characteristics of patellar disorders in young athletes. Am J Sports Med 9:270–274, 1981.
19. Shelton GL, Thigpen LK: Rehabilitation of patellofemoral dysfunction: A review of literature. J Orthop Sports Phys Ther 14:243–249, 1991.
20. Walsh WM, Helzer-Julin MJ: Patellar tracking problems in athletes. Prim Care 19:303–330, 1992.

75. SURGICAL TREATMENT OF PATELLOFEMORAL DISEASE

W. Michael Walsh, M.D.

1. How often is surgical treatment needed for patellofemoral disorders?

Compared with other orthopedic problems, not frequently. Although the number of patients with patellofemoral disease is high, most can be handled with nonsurgical means. Currently, 10–20% of our patients with a patellofemoral disorder need surgical intervention.

2. What surgical procedures are generally used?

As a general concept, surgery should alter the forces working on the patella and attempt to make patellofemoral tracking as normal as possible. The most commonly used procedures are isolated lateral retinacular release (LRR), done as either an arthroscopic or open procedure, and open reconstruction of the extensor mechanism.

3. How does the LRR procedure work?

With respect to the abnormal forces at work on the patella, a predominance of laterally directed forces is usually quite significant. Such lateral forces may come from both the static structures (lateral retinaculum, lateral patellofemoral ligament, lateral patellotibial ligament) and dynamic structures (oblique portion of the vastus lateralis muscle). An LRR attempts to decrease the lateral forces by dividing the lateral retinaculum and a small portion of the vastus lateralis. Theoretically the patient may be able to control patellar tracking better through rehabilitation of the vastus medialis obliquus. LRR can be done through arthroscopic techniques or a small open incision.

4. Which patients should have an LRR?

In the past, LRR has had a somewhat poor reputation because of its unpredictable results and high complication rate. Therefore, it should not be done unless proved absolutely necessary after failure of nonsurgical treatment, including extensive rehabilitative exercise techniques, external support, and activity modification. If the patient continues to have significant disability (pain, swelling, limitation of function), LRR may be considered. Usually nonsurgical treatment is carried out for at least several months. The surgeon then looks for the specific anatomic finding, either on preoperative computed tomographic (CT) scan or by arthroscopic examination of the patellofemoral joint, that indicate the appropriateness of LR. Such findings include tightness in the lateral retinaculum and lateral tilting of the patella, with or without lateral malposition.

5. Since LRR is an arthroscopic procedure, is it simple to do and followed by quick recovery?

In many instances, no. In addition to possible complications that slow recovery, patients still need to rehabilitate the quadriceps and perhaps to use other forms of nonsurgical treatment (e.g., bracing, orthotics) before returning to normal activity. Routinely 3–6 months may be required for full return of function. This time frame should be emphasized to the patient preoperatively as well as the fact that the surgery is not a total substitute for continued nonsurgical efforts in the future.

6. What complications are seen with LRR?

In studies carried out by the Arthroscopy Association of North America, arthroscopic LRR was the procedure most commonly associated with significant complications, the majority of which involved postoperative development of hemarthrosis. Occasionally, this complication requires return to the operating room for drainage and coagulation of bleeding points. For this reason some surgeons prefer to do LRR as a small open procedure rather than arthroscopically. The open procedure allows identification and coagulation of the large vessels at the time the release is done. Other complications include profound quadriceps disability and medial subluxation of the patella, both of which come from overreleasing the vastus lateralis, and rupture of the quadriceps tendon, which results from releasing too far around the superior edge of the patella.

7. How does an open reconstruction of the extensor mechanism work?

There are three basic components: lateral release, medial advancement or stabilization, and transposition of the patellar tendon insertion. Lateral release is done as described above for the isolated LRR. Various authors have described different techniques for medial advancement or stabilization. The important structure to advance or stabilize is the vastus medialis obliquus muscle. In the past, the routine procedure was to advance the muscles' insertion onto the superomedial patella. Recently, we have found it more satisfying in many cases to restabilize the origin of the vastus medialis obliquus in the region of the adductor tubercle. The distal part of the reconstruction is a transfer of the patellar tendon insertion on the tibial tuberosity to a more medial and distal position. The goal is to correct an excessive Q angle as well as excessive patella alta. Many variations on this basic theme have been described over the years, but most still include the same three elements.

8. Which patients should have an extensor mechanism reconstruction?

In general, the decision to proceed with surgery follows the same line of reasoning mentioned above for LRR. Most patients want to try the arthroscopic procedure first because it is simpler. Isolated lateral release may work in 75% or more of patients. The remaining 25% have the option of trying an open reconstruction. Some may decide that they do not wish to try further surgery. On the other hand, certain patients want the greatest correction that can be attempted with their first trip to the operating room. For these patients, it may be decided to skip the arthroscopic LRR and to proceed directly with an open reconstruction of the extensor mechanism. An initial recommendation of open reconstruction also may be prudent in patients with greater degrees of malalignment or in patients with recurrent dislocation rather than pain syndromes. For some authors, the presence of lateral malposition of the patella rather than simple lateral tilt indicates the need for open reconstruction rather than lateral release. No well-done long-term studies substantiate one viewpoint over the other.

9. What is involved in recovery from an extensor mechanism reconstruction?

When the patellar tendon insertion is repositioned, some internal fixation with hardware is usually necessary. Traditionally internal fixation has led to a period of immobilization after reconstruction. Most surgeons limit the period of absolute immobilization to 3 or 4 weeks. At that point protected motion can be started with an adjustable hinge brace. Part-time immobilization may be continued for 6 weeks. Crutches are used until ambulation is normal. Extensive quadriceps rehabilitation is necessary postoperatively. Overall functional recovery may easily take 6–9 months after surgery.

10. What specific complications may occur after open reconstruction of the extensor mechanism?

The most frequent complications are related to overzealous repositioning of the patella. If an excessive release is done laterally, along with excessive advancement of the medial structures, medial subluxation or even dislocation may be created. Extreme distal positioning of the patella by excessive transfer of the patellar tendon insertion creates a pathologically low-lying patella, often with abutment of the patella against the proximal tibia. This complication is terribly painful.

11. Do the above surgical procedures cure the problem?

No surgical procedure completely cures patellofemoral disorders. The predisposition is anatomic. The factors are many and varied. Even after surgery, patients must continue with rehabilitative efforts and other adjunctive means, such as bracing and foot orthotics. In the best of cases, patients often have residual symptoms during such high patellar stress activities as walking stairs. These points should be absolutely clear to patients before they undergo surgery.

12. Can other surgical procedures be done?

Yes. Many other surgical procedures have been applied to the patellofemoral joint. Some are now of historical interest only. Simpler procedures that may still be appropriate include excision of areas of chondromalacia (although not as an isolated procedure), removal of osteochondral fractures, synovectomy for pathologic synovial plica, and excision of painful accessory ossification centers of the patella. More complicated as well as controversial is the concept of anteriorization of the tibial tuberosity to decompress the patellofemoral joint. This procedure has enjoyed mixed reviews and somewhat unpredictable results in the past. It should probably be viewed as a salvage procedure. Patellectomy likewise may be used as a salvage procedure when marked deterioration of the patellar articular surface has occurred. In patients who have a severe rotational component to limb malalignment, derotational osteotomies of the femur and tibia may be appealing. However, the sheer magnitude of the undertaking has prevented practical application.

13. Should early surgery be done for an acute patellar dislocation?

It seems sensible that an acute patellar dislocation should be treated like other acute disruptions of soft tissue (e.g., torn ligaments). If this analogy were to hold true, then early, direct suture repair may hold promise of decreasing the incidence of recurrent dislocation. This concept has been promoted by some researchers in the past and may be gaining in popularity. Studies have shown the particular importance of the medial patellofemoral ligament. An acute dislocation rupture of this ligament may be demonstrated by MRI. If documented, early repair would make perfect sense. However, considering the facts that one-half of patients with patellar dislocation may not experience recurrence and that reconstructive techniques work reasonably well, early surgical intervention is not used by most orthopedists.

BIBLIOGRAPHY

1. Canale ST (ed): Campbell's Operative Orthopaedics, 9th ed. St. Louis, Mosby, 1998.
2. Evans IK, Paulos LE: Complications of patellofemoral joint surgery. Orthop Clin 23:697–710, 1992.
3. Flandry F, Hughston JC: Complications of extensor mechanism surgery for patellar malalignment. Am J Orthop 24:534–543, 1995.
4. Fox JM: The Patellofemoral Joint. New York, McGraw-Hill, 1993.
5. Fulkerson JP (ed): Disorders of the Patellofemoral Joint, 3rd ed. Baltimore, Williams & Wilkins, 1996.
6. Fulkerson JP: Patellofemoral pain disorders: Evaluation and management. J Am Acad Orthop Surg 2:124–132, 1994.
7. Sallay PI, Poggi J, Speer KP, Garrett WE: Acute dislocation of the patella. Am J Sports Med 24:52–60, 1996.
8. Walsh WM: Patellofemoral joint. In DeLee JC, Drez D Jr (eds): Orthopaedic Sports Medicine: Principles and Practice. Philadelphia, W.B. Saunders, 1994, pp 1163–1260.

76. KNEE ARTHRITIS

Randall D. Neumann, M.D.

1. What are the three compartments of the knee?

Patellofemoral, medial, and lateral.

2. Which compartments are generally affected in degenerative osteoarthritis of the knee?

The medial compartment is the most commonly affected, followed by the lateral compartment and then the patellofemoral compartment.

3. What is the mechanical axis of the lower extremity?

The mechanical axis goes directly through the femoral head, through the intercondylar notch of the knee to the midportion of the ankle.

4. What is a varus deformity?

In patients with osteoarthritis who have primarily medial compartment disease, collapse of the medial joint space causes medial angulation of the tibia. The clinical appearance is bow-leggedness, which causes the mechanical axis to go through or inside the medial compartment of the knee. This condition is considered varus of the knee.

5. What is valgus of the knee?

When lateral compartment arthritis predominates, joint space collapse occurs in the lateral compartment and causes the weight-bearing axis to fall outside the lateral compartment of the knee. The patient appears knock-kneed. This condition represents a valgus deformity of the knee.

6. What is a flexion contracture?

Patients with degenerative arthritis of the knee commonly have a flexion contracture. Minimal flexion contracture may be 1–2°, whereas other contractures may be as high as 45°. Flexion contracture is commonly caused by posterior osteophytes on the femur, tibial plateau deformities, fracture, or loose bodies. Contractures of the ligaments may occur, especially with the posterior cruciate and posterior capsule.

7. What is the most common symptom in patients with osteoarthritis of the knee?

Pain.

8. Describe the clinical history of patients with degenerative arthritis of the knee.

Most patients report an insidious onset, perhaps with a history of trauma or repetitive trauma that patients may describe as minor or major. The pain is usually described as aching to sharp and is likely to present after excessive activity. With severe stages of arthritis, night pain may occur. Patients describe stiffness on waking in the morning, which gradually diminishes with activity. If the patient is sitting or riding in a car, pain and stiffness occur upon standing or walking. Pain is located at the site of the most affected compartment of the knee. The patient has diminished function, including inability to climb stairs, especially without the help of a railing. Walking may be limited to several blocks or several miles. Some patients lose the ability to do their own grocery shopping or must use the shopping cart as a mandatory aid. Patients commonly notice deformity with swelling, osteophyte function, and varus or valgus deformity.

9. Describe the physical findings in osteoarthritis of the knee.

Patients generally lack some degree of motion. Commonly they will lack 5–10° of full extension and will not be able to lay the leg with the knee flat. Most patients lose flexion because of posterior osteophytes and contracture of the posterior capsule. Tenderness is palpable along the joint line. Effusion may be mild to moderate. Crepitation is generally felt in the affected compartment. Clinical varus or valgus may be present.

10. What other joints should be examined in elderly patients complaining of knee pain?

Elderly patients commonly have degenerative changes in other joints. Patients with spinal stenosis may have referred pain to the knee that increases with walking and is relieved with rest. The referred pain may be due to spinal claudication rather than knee arthritis. Patients with degenerative arthritis of the hip have referred pain through the obturator nerve to the medial side of the knee. It is not uncommon for patients to present with complaints of knee arthritis when the pathology is related to the hip joint.

11. What are the radiographic findings in patients with osteoarthritis of the knee?

Patients have narrowing of the joint space in either the medial, lateral, or patellofemoral compartment. Axial alignment may show varus or valgus deformity on weight-bearing views. Osteophytes are commonly seen in the intercondylar notch area and along the most severely affected joints. Loose bodies from fragmentation of articular cartilage may be seen along the posterior femoral condyles. Destruction of the posterior condyles or posterior portions of the medial and lateral tibia plateau may be seen. On the sunrise view, subluxation of the patella or frank dislocation is noted. Lateral subluxation of the tibial plateau on the femur may be seen on the anterior radiographs.

12. Which disease processes with arthritis may have loose bodies in the knee?
- Osteochondritis dissecans
- Osteonecrosis
- Chondromalacia of the patella
- Degenerative arthritis
- Neuropathic joints

13. Discuss the synovial fluid analysis in patients with degenerative arthritis.
The white blood cell count is generally < 2,000 mm³, with < 50% neutrophils. Cultures are negative. No crystals are seen on light microscopy.

14. What other disease entities should be ruled out before treatment for knee arthritis?
- Spinal stenosis
- Degenerative changes in the hips
- Tumors
- Neuropathy
- Vascular insufficiency
- Diabetes and metabolic disorders
- Systemic arthritis, such as rheumatoid arthritis
- Osteonecrosis

15. What conservative treatments should be tried in patients with osteoarthritis of the knee?
Patients should be placed on a trial of nonsteroidal antiinflammatory medication. Appropriate counseling should be given. Patients may respond to icing of an overly inflamed joint. Protective weightbearing, such as occasional use of crutches or cane, may be beneficial. Generalized exercise may include walking, swimming, or bicycling. Range-of-motion exercises should be done on a daily basis. Knee braces or neoprene sleeves may be used for comfort and control of swelling. The occasional and cautious use of intraarticular steroids is permitted; overuse of corticosteroids has been known to lead to progression of disease.

16. What arthroscopic treatment can be used for degenerative arthritis?
Some success has been gained with arthroscopic debridement. Candidates include patients without contracture or subluxation and patients with mechanical symptoms, including catching or locking, and localized disease. Arthroscopic treatment includes removal of spurs in the intercondylar notch along the anterior cruciate, medial, and lateral gutters. The articular cartilage can be shaved. Loose bodies are removed, commonly from behind the medial and lateral condyles posteriorly, the intercondylar notch area, and beneath the medial and lateral menisci posteriorly.

17. What is abrasion arthroplasty?
Abrasion arthroplasty is an arthroscopic technique that uses a high-speed burr to remove the subchondral bone down to bleeding bone, usually a depth of 2–3 mm. Patients are protected on crutches for various periods of time—from 6 weeks to 3 months. Abrasion arthroplasty may be indicated for patients with localized lesions when the cartilage surrounding the defect is normal and when the alignment of the extremity is normal. In patients with generalized arthritis throughout the joint, the procedure is much less reliable. Most surgeons have lost interest in this procedure, because it is highly unpredictable.

18. Describe the synovial fluid analysis in patients with inflammatory arthritis such as rheumatoid arthritis.
The inflammatory fluid is usually translucid or opaque. Newspaper cannot be read through the tube. The color ranges from yellowish to yellow-green. The white blood cell count is generally much less than 50,000 mm³. Gram stain and cultures are negative. White blood cells may be 50% neutrophils.

19. Describe the radiologic findings of rheumatoid arthritis of the knee.

Soft-tissue swelling due to joint effusion synovitis and periarticular edema is usually easily detectable, along with uniform narrowing of the patellofemoral, medial, and lateral compartments. Juxtaarticular osteoporosis is evident. Erosions, if present, are usually sharply marginated. Severe bone destruction may be seen in the advanced stage with considerable angulation, resulting in a varus or valgus knee. Marginal osteophytes and sclerosis are generally lacking.

20. What treatments are available for rheumatoid arthritis of the knee?

Conservative treatment should include nonsteroidal antiinflammatory drugs, interarticular steroids, and aspiration. Joint splinting may be helpful in patients who have tense effusions and synovitis. If synovitis persists, arthroscopic synovectomy may temporarily arrest the disease. Open synovectomy also helps to alleviate symptoms. In late stages, patients may require joint replacement or knee fusion.

21. Describe the hallmark of calcium pyrophosphate dihydrate deposition (CPPD) disease.

The hallmark of CPPD is calcium deposition on fibrocartilage, particularly the menisci of the knee, which is readily seen on radiographs. Cysts, which may be quite large, are generally found next to the joint margin and may mimic a neuropathic joint.

22. What tests should be done on the synovial fluid in crystalline arthropathies?

Routine microscopy and polarization should be done. The calcium pyrophosphate dihydrate crystals are seen on nonpolarized light microscopy and the uric acid crystals on polarized light microscopy.

23. What are the radiographic findings in patients with hemophilic arthropathy of the knee?

Overgrowth of the distal femur and tibial epiphysis may result in metaphyses that fit the diaphyses poorly. The intercondylar notch of the femur is commonly widened. Squaring of the inferior pole of the patella has been recognized by many investigators. Because flexion contractures are common, patients may have posterior lateral displacement of the tibia on the femur. The patella may be dislocated.

24. Describe the arthritis in neuropathic joint disease.

Neuropathic joints are commonly seen in diabetes mellitus, tabes dorsalis, and meningomyelocele. The earliest manifestations are soft-tissue swelling that may be massive. Generally pain is minimal despite the massive joint destruction. Typically the joint shows gross disorganization. Subluxation of the tibia on the femur is common, along with complete laxity of the entire joint and dislocation of the patella. Intraarticular fractures and loose bodies are also common. Calcification and bone fragments are seen within the soft tissues adjacent to the joint. The arthropathy is progressive, and severe destruction may take place over several months.

25. What is the differential diagnosis of a neuropathic joint?

- Diabetes mellitus
- Syphilis
- Syringomyelia
- Leprosy
- Amyloidosis
- Charcot-Marie-Tooth disease
- Multiple sclerosis
- Gigantism
- Alcoholism
- Chronic demyelinating polyradiculopathy

26. What is the differential diagnosis for hemarthrosis found on synovial fluid aspiration?

- Trauma with injury to the anterior cruciate ligament
- Peripheral meniscal tears
- Medial or collateral ligament injuries
- Osteochondral fractures
- Hemophilia
- Pigmented villonodular synovitis
- Sickle-cell disease
- Degenerative arthritis
- Other bleeding disorders

BIBLIOGRAPHY

1. Alpert SW, Koval KJ, Zuckerman JD: Neuropathic arthropathy: Review of current knowledge. J Am Acad
   Orthop Surg 4:100–108, 1996.
2. McCarty DJ: Synovial fluid. In McCarty DJ, Koopman WJ (eds): Arthritis and Allied Conditions.
   Philadelphia, Lea & Febiger, 1993.
3. Resnick DA: Degenerative diseases of extra spinal location. In Resnick D (ed): Diagnosis of Bone and
   Joint Disorders. Philadelphia, W.B. Saunders, 1991, pp 1270–1368.
4. Silver RM (ed): Primer on the Rheumatic Diseases, 11th ed. Atlanta, Arthritis Foundation, 1997.

77. OSTEOCHONDRITIS DISSECANS AND OSTEONECROSIS

Randall D. Neumann, M.D.

1. What is osteochondritis dissecans?

Osteochondritis dissecans (OCD) is a disorder of one or more ossification centers with sequential degeneration and/or aseptic necrosis and recalcification.

2. List the common sites of OCD in the body.

1. Medial femoral condyle of the knee
2. Capitellum of the distal humerus
3. Talus

3. Describe the theories of the etiology for OCD.

1. **Exogenous trauma.** Significant knee trauma is found in approximately 50% of patients with OCD. The trauma may be minor or include falls and twisting injuries.

2. **Endogenous trauma.** Patellar dislocations, mensical tears, and instability syndromes have been associated with OCD.

3. **Ischemia.** The obstruction of blood supply to the femoral condyle at the site of involvement has been theorized to precipitate cartilage and bone separation.

4. **Abnormal ossification within the epiphysis.** Accessory centers of ossification are known to occur. In children this process often is exhibited by a rough or irregular epiphyseal outline. It has been suggested that this accessory bony nucleus separates in childhood and partially reattaches with time.

5. **Multiple epiphyseal dysplasia** must be considered in patients with OCD.

4. Where does OCD occur in the knee?

Approximately 85% are found on the medial femoral condyle, with 15% on the lateral condyle. The classic presentation is immediately adjacent to the intercondylar notch. Affected areas may extend over the weight-bearing surface. On the lateral condyle, they are generally on the weight-bearing surface but may occur anteriorly. Such lesions are usually from 2–2.5 cm in diameter on the medial side of the joint and have a reasonably thick bony backing. Lateral lesions tend to be large (3–4 cm in diameter) and usually have a slim underpinning of bone that makes them more prone to fragmentation. As a result, multiple small fragments may exist.

5. What is the natural history of OCD?

The majority of juvenile patients (< 15 years of age or still skeletally immature) proceed to spontaneous healing. Young adults have more progressive forms. Patients with intact articular cartilage may have only intermittent symptoms, especially when they are vigorously active. Once the articular cartilage fractures, symptoms increase and swelling ensues. Patients who have sloughed the articular cartilage and bone have symptoms due to loose bodies, including catching, locking, and pain. With the larger defect more readily identified, arthritic symptoms may appear, along with radiographic evidence of degenerative changes.

6. What is the typical history in patients with OCD?
Symptoms usually associated with OCD are often vague and poorly localized. Symptoms include pain, stiffness, and swelling. With progression of joint incongruity, sensations of locking, catching, or giving way develop. Pain may be severe if the defect is large.

7. Describe the physical findings in the patient with OCD.
Most patients are extremely comfortable. The range of motion is usually within normal limits. Some patients have a small lack of extension, slight quadriceps atrophy, and weakness. Patients with articular surface defects may have recurrent episodes of swelling, and effusion is likely. Tenderness may be present along the medial or lateral joint lines. Loose bodies may be identified, and some patients are able to move them around in their knees. Wilson's sign is elicited by flexing the knee to 90°, internally rotating the tibia, and extending the knee slowly. Pain at approximately 30° of flexion is a positive sign that signifies impingement of the tibial spine on the medial femoral condyle OCD.

8. What radiographic studies are done to determine if OCD is present?
The standard films are the anteroposterior, lateral, tunnel, and sunrise views. The most useful view is the tunnel view. Lesions on the posterior portion of the medial femoral condyle are commonly missed on standard anteroposterior views. Therefore, when OCD is suspected, an intercondylar notch or tunnel view is mandatory.

9. What is the classic radiographic appearance of OCD?
The classic radiographic appearance is a well-circumscribed area of subchondral bone, separated from the remaining femoral condyle by a crescent-shaped radiolucent line. OCD is located on the posterior lateral aspect of the medial femoral condyle or the central portion of the lateral femoral condyle. The typical position is seen on the lateral photograph. A line drawn distally from the posterior margin of the femoral shaft and intersecting a line along the intercondylar notch shows the location of approximately 75% of cases of OCD involving the medial femoral condyle. The lateral femoral condyle lesions are seen on the lateral radiograph and are located posterior to the line drawn distally from the posterior femoral cortex.

10. What other radiographic techniques are used for evaluating OCD?
CT and MRI have been found to be more frequently helpful in the evaluation of OCD. MRI is capable of detecting focal defects in articular cartilage as small as 2 mm. MRI can differentiate in situ versus unstable fragments.

11. Is bone scan helpful in the diagnosis of OCD?
Bone scan is used for diagnostic purposes and for following the healing and pathologic processes. Some studies suggest that bone scans may be more sensitive and more specific in determining the mechanical stability of the lesions.

12. What invasive diagnostic test is used in patients with OCD?
Arthroscopy directly visualizes the involved area and allows the examiner to probe the zone of involvement and to determine the degree of articular cartilage separation. Loose bodies are also removed during arthroscopy if it is indeed determined that they are loose. After surgical procedures, arthroscopy can be used to assess the articular surface for healing, degeneration, and mechanical stability.

13. Describe the two types of OCD that are found clinically.

The first distinct clinical picture is found in children or young adolescents from 5–15 years of age with open epiphyses. The second type is found in skeletally mature adults from ages 15–50 years. The two types are separated by their distinctly different natural histories.

14. What is the treatment for patients with juvenile OCD?

Juvenile OCD differs from the adult form in that the majority of the lesions heal spontaneously. Lesions should be monitored with radiographs or bone scans for healing in 6–12 months. Symptomatic treatment with rest for 3–6 months usually suffices. Long-leg cast may be used in the initial stages if pain is excessive. If the lesions continue to be symptomatic, arthroscopic drilling and pinning are necessary. Treatment depends on the stage of the lesion. Patients who have minor abnormalities with the articular surface still intact may be treated symptomatically.

Patients with fracture and disengagement may be treated arthroscopically. A bony peg fixation after debridement of the defect and replacement of the bone fragment can be used. Pin fixation with a Kirchner wire or a resorbable pin may also be used. Herbert compression screw fixation has been used for large defects and has the advantage of firm fixation and the ability to countersink the screw. In patients with complete fragmentation, arthroscopy with loose body removal is performed. The remaining crater area is grafted with bone or osteochondral allografts. Patients with unsalvageable fragments and significant degenerative changes may be candidates for total knee arthroplasty.

15. What is the incidence of osteoarthritis among adult patients with OCD?

Degenerative changes usually begin at age 40 years, with highly progressive deterioration. Approximately 70% of patients at age 50 and 80% at age 60 have osteoarthritis.

16. What are the five stages of OCD as described by Kahill and Berg?

Stage 0 has normal bone scan and plain films. Stages 1–4 have abnormal radiographic findings characteristic for OCD, but the bone scans are different for each stage. Stage 1 shows no activity on bone scan. Stage 2 has focal activity at the site of the OCD defect. Stage 3 has focal activity at the OCD defect and increased activity in the femoral condyle supporting the OCD lesion; stage 4 is similar to stage 3 with activity on the tibia plateau. With regard to healing, Kahill and Berg observed that the OCD with a stage 2 or greater scan has the highest probability of healing. This level of activity indicates potential for repair. Because stage 1 lesions have a poor potential for handling by conservative therapy, surgical intervention may be necessary.

17. Should the loose articular portion be removed arthroscopically with no other treatment?

Results of excision of adult or juvenile defects are poor. Therefore, attempts should be made to retain the full-thickness osteochondral defect. If this is not possible, bone grafting or allograft should be used.

18. How should the OCD lesion be prepared for arthroscopic treatment?

Arthroscopy includes the removal of the fibrous membrane, curretting of the necrotic base, and retrograde or antegrade drilling to allow ingrowth of vascular tissue and bone grafting. Fixation of the fragment is mandatory.

19. What new treatments are available for articular cartilage defects?

Fresh frozen osteochondral allografts are prepared by removing the diseased area with a section of bone. A fresh frozen allograft is then matched for size, depth, and radii and held in position by screws.

A **mosaic graft** is also an allograft. Osteochondral plugs are taken from the peripheral area of the anteromedial or anterolateral femoral epicondyle. Corresponding holes that match the size and depth of the plugs are drilled, which are then inserted into the defect. Differing plug size creates a "mosaic" look.

Chondrocyte transplantation. Articular cartilage is harvested via arthroscopy from the knee. Chondrocytes are cultured and then placed in a defect. With the cells present, a periosteal flap is then sutured over the defect. Weightbearing is not allowed for 3 months.

OSTEONECROSIS

20. What is osteonecrosis?

Osteonecrosis is a clinical syndrome in which a segment of bone in the weight-bearing portion of the femoral condyle loses its blood supply; later it is associated with subchondral fracture collapse and degenerative arthritis.

21. What is the etiology of osteonecrosis?

An occlusion in the blood supply to the femoral condyle interferes with microcirculation in the bone. The diminished microcirculation produces edema in a nonexpandable compartment and leads to increased pressure in the bone marrow, further diminishing the blood supply and resulting in osseous ischemia.

22. In what disease processes is osteonecrosis of the knee seen?

Steroid therapy	Hemoglobinopathies
Renal transplantation	Caisson's disease
Gaucher's disease	Systemic lupus erythematosus
	Idiopathic spontaneous osteonecrosis

23. Describe the clinical presentation of patients with osteonecrosis of the femoral condyle.

The typical patient is a woman over 60 years of age who has sudden onset of severe pain on the medial side of the knee that may or may not be associated with trauma. Women are affected approximately three times more commonly than men. The pain is present frequently at night. It may be severe for 6–8 weeks and then gradually subsides.

24. Can osteonecrosis occur in the tibia?

Osteonecrosis of the tibia usually occurs in the medial compartment. It is not nearly as common as its counterpart on the femoral side.

25. Describe the physical findings in patients with osteonecrosis.

Depending on the stage, examination may reveal minimal clinical signs. Mild synovitis and effusion are commonly present. Stability and overall range of motion are generally not affected. Tenderness is localized over the compartment with the disease process and ranges from mild to severe. Loss of range of motion is common when significant degenerative changes occur.

26. Describe the radiographic classification of osteonecrosis of the knee.

In stage I the radiographic appearance is normal. Stage 2 is characterized by slight flattening of the convexity of the condyle, which may be subtle and is easily missed. In stage 3 the typical lesion of osteonecrosis is evident. A radiolucent area of variable size surrounds a sclerotic area in the subchondral bone. In stage 4 the radiolucency is surrounded by a definitive sclerotic halo. In stage 5 secondary changes develop, including narrowing of the joint space, sclerosis, formation of osteophytes, and destructive changes on the tibial side of the joint.

27. What other radiographic abnormalities are seen with osteonecrosis?

Technetium 99-m is the scanning agent of choice. An osteonecrotic lesion appears as a focally intense area of uptake over the affected condyle. If uptake is increased on both sides of the joint, concomitant arthritis may be present. Magnetic resonance imaging shows an area of low signal intensity in the central lesion on T2-weighted image, with a high-intensity signal about the margin.

28. Which is better for diagnosing osteonecrosis: arthroscopy or MRI?

MRI is better. Arthroscopy cannot visualize the bone changes of necrosis, because the articular cartilage overlying the lesion is usually normal. MRI identifies the area and extent of the lesion.

29. What laboratory studies are significant in osteonecrosis?

Routine laboratory studies are not helpful. The sedimentation rate may be mildly elevated. All other laboratory tests are within normal limits, except those associated with other medical problems.

30. What risk factors affect the clinical course and prognosis in osteonecrosis?

Patients who are in stage 1 or who have a small lesion that is < 45% of the condylar width have a favorable prognosis. Patients who have a large lesion (> 50% of the width of the condyle) generally become disabled with increasing pain, deformity, and eventually secondary joint destruction. Patients with stage 1 or small lesions generally have intense symptoms initially, but they slowly resolve over a period of 9–15 months. Pain may resolve completely.

31. What is the treatment for osteonecrosis?

Conservative treatment consists of nonsteroidal antiinflammatory medications, analgesics for night pain, and protected weight bearing. Most small lesions heal without surgical treatment.

32. What surgical treatments are available for patients with osteonecrosis?

1. **Proximal tibial osteotomy** may be beneficial in association with bone grafting by preventing collapse of the lesion and encouraging healing.

2. **Drilling or burring of the lesion** involves drilling into the subchondral bone to stimulate new vascularity. This treatment has not been very successful.

3. **Allograft bone** involves removal of diseased bone and replacement with matched femoral allograft.

4. **Joint replacement.** In reality, patients with osteonecrosis are usually elderly and prosthetic replacement should be considered for most patients who need surgical intervention.

BIBLIOGRAPHY

1. Cahill BR: Osteochondritis dissecans of the knee: Treatment of juvenile and adult forms. J Am Acad Orthop Surg 3:237–247, 1995.
2. Canale ST (ed): Campbell's Operative Orthopedics, 9th ed. St. Louis, Mosby, 1998.
3. Ecker ML, Lotke PA: Spontaneous osteonecrosis of the knee. J Am Acad Orthop Surg 2:173–178, 1994.
4. Federico DJ, Lynch JK, Jokl P: Osteochondritis dissecans of the knee: A historical review of etiology and treatment. Arthroscopy 6:190–197, 1990.
5. Garret JC: Osteochondritis dissecans. Clin Orthop Sports Med 10:569–593, 1991.
6. Kahill B, Berg B: 99-M Technetium phosphate compound joint scintigraphy in the management of juvenile osteochondritis dissecans of the femoral condyle. Am J Sports Med 11:329–335, 1983.
7. Lotke PA, Ecker ML: Current concepts review: Osteonecrosis of the knee. J Bone Joint Surg 70A:470–473, 1988.
8. Sebast, Denelli WJ: Osteochondrosis. In DeLee JC, Drez D (eds): Orthopedic Sports Medicine: Principles and Practice, vol. 1. Philadelphia, W.B. Saunders, 1994.

78. TOTAL KNEE ARTHROPLASTY

Adolph V. Lombardi, Jr., M.D., FACS

1. What are the major indications for total knee arthroplasty (TKA)?

TKA is indicated for end-stage degenerative joint disease of the knee, which may result from primary or secondary osteoarthritis, avascular necrosis, and inflammatory arthropathies, such as rheumatoid arthritis.

2. What are the nonoperative treatment modalities of degenerative joint disease of the knee?

1. Limited periods of rest
2. Orthoses, such as elastic knee supports, or valgus unloading braces
3. Nonsteroidal antiinflammatory agents (NSAIDs)
4. Corticosteroid injections
5. Viscosupplementation
6. Ambulatory aids, such as a cane, crutches, or walker

3. What is viscosupplementation?

Viscosupplementation is the use of an injectable viscoelastic preparation containing hyaluron or hylan (crosslinked hyaluron), which has been reported to provide extra joint protection. The preparations are available in various molecular weights. Treatment consists of a series of injections, which may be repeated at 6 month intervals. Since hyaluronic acid is a naturally occurring material, the body absorbs it over a 4-week period. Despite the absorption of the preparation, it has been reported to work for periods ranging from 6 months to 2 years.

4. Describe the ideal candidate for a valgus unloading brace.

A valgus unloading brace is a brace that induces a valgus thrust and therefore decompresses the medial compartment. A patient presenting with moderate degenerative joint disease involving the medial compartment is an acceptable candidate for a valgus unloading brace. These braces are typically used in members of the younger patient population who wish to maintain a high-activity lifestyle. The use of valgus unloading braces has been justified in several reports to date.

5. What are the operative treatments of degenerative joint disease of the knee?

1. Arthroscopic debridement
2. Osteotomy
   High tibial osteotomy for treatment of varus deformity
   Distal femoral osteotomy for treatment of valgus deformity
3. Unicompartmental knee arthroplasty
   Medial
   Lateral
4. Patellofemoral arthroplasty
5. Total knee arthroplasty

6. Describe the ideal candidate for arthroscopic treatment of osteoarthritis of the knee.

- Symptoms of < 1 year duration
- Nontraumatic etiology
- Normal limb alignment
- Mechanical symptoms, such as clicking and catching
- No history of previous knee surgery

7. What are the major indications for high tibial osteotomy in the treatment of degenerative joint disease of the knee?
1. Isolated medial compartment arthritis demonstrated by history, physical examination, and radiograph
2. Young, active patients with a strong desire to continue a vigorous lifestyle
3. Overweight patients
4. Patients with a range of motion > 90° and < 15° of flexion contracture
5. Varus deformity < 15°

8. What are the major indications for distal femoral osteotomy in the treatment of degenerative joint disease of the knee?
The indications for distal femoral osteotomy in treatment of degenerative joint disease of the knee are the same as the above indications for high tibial osteotomy with the following exceptions:
1. Isolated lateral compartment arthritis (rather than medial compartment arthritis)
2. Valgus deformity < 15°

9. Describe the ideal candidate for unicompartmental knee arthroplasty.
- Physiologic age > 60 years
- Relatively sedentary lifestyle
- Primary diagnosis of osteoarthritis
- Preoperative range of motion ≥ 90°
- < 10° of flexion contracture
- Angular deformity < 15° that is correctable to neutral

10. What are the absolute contraindications to unicompartmental knee arthroplasty?
Inflammatory arthropathy and infection.

11. What is the difference between unicompartmental knee arthroplasty and TKA?
Unicompartmental knee arthroplasty involves replacement of a singular compartment of the knee, either medial or lateral, whereas TKA involves replacement of all three compartments of the knee: the medial and lateral compartments and most of the patellofemoral compartment.

12. Describe the ideal candidate for patellofemoral arthroplasty.
No ideal candidate can be described; results of this procedure have been less than ideal. The nonsurgical, conservative modalities of treatment for patellofemoral arthrosis include physical therapy, NSAIDs, and intraarticular injections of hyaluronic acids or corticosteroids. Surgical treatments include arthroscopic debridement with or without a lateral retinacular release, Maquet osteotomy (elevation of the tibial tubercle to facilitate a reduction in patellofemoral contact stresses), and, in the case of the elderly patient, TKA.

13. What are the primary goals of TKA?
- Relief of pain
- Restoration of function
- Achievement of intrinsic stability
- Creation of a durable reconstruction

14. What are the major contraindications to TKA?
Infection represents the major contraindication to TKA. Relative contraindications include young age; active, physical lifestyle; and obesity.

15. Should the patella always be resurfaced in TKA?
The answer to this question is twofold. For the treatment of inflammatory arthritis, it is universally agreed that the patella should be resurfaced. Resurfacing of the patella in patients with

osteoarthritis, however, is controversial. Close review of the literature reveals that patients with-out patellofemoral resurfacing experience discomfort during activities associated with patello-femoral compression, such as ascending and descending stairs and rising from a chair.

16. What is the standard surgical approach to TKA? What is the rationale for its use?

The standard surgical approach for TKA involves a straight midline incision followed by a standard medial parapatellar capsular arthrotomy. Despite the fact that a standard medial para-patellar skin incision follows more adequately the lines of Langers, a straight midline skin inci-sion is used with a subsequent medial parapatellar arthrotomy so that the skin and subcutaneous incision are not directly over the capsular incision. This slight mismatch of the capsular and skin incision provides an overlap that allows a better seal and therefore effectively reduces postopera-tive drainage and subsequent possibility of related infection.

17. Have any approaches other than the straight midline skin incision and the medial para-patellar capsular arthrotomy been popularized?

The midline skin incision remains the standard approach. However, several alternative cap-sular arthrotomies have been described: the subvastus approach, the vastus medialis splitting ap-proach, the trivector approach, and lateral parapatellar approach.

18. What is the advantage of the subvastus, or southern, approach?

The subvastus approach spares the quadriceps tendon. From proximal to distal aspect, it in-volves elevation of the vastus medialis obliquus with a medial capsular arthrotomy that begins at the superior medial pole of the patella. Therefore, no incision is made into the quadriceps tendon. Advocates of this approach have noted a quicker return of quadriceps function, but no long-term advantages are seen over the more popular medial parapatellar arthrotomy. Limiting this ap-proach to primary TKA in thin patients is advised.

19. Describe the vastus medialis splitting approach.

The vastus medialis splitting approach begins with a division of the vastus medialis along its fibers at the proximal two-thirds and distal one-third junction. The muscle division ends at the su-perior medial pole of the patella and the capsular arthrotomy is then carried distally along the medial aspect of the patella. It was initially reported that this approach yielded a diminution in the number of lateral retinacular releases. However, when the study was repeated in a random-ized fashion, no difference in lateral retinacular release rates was noted between the medial para-patellar arthrotomy and vastus medialis splitting approach.

20. Describe the trivector approach.

The trivector approach involves an incision of the body of the vastus medialis obliquus, which begins approximately 5 cm proximal to the superior pole of the patella and extends distally along the medial aspect of the patella. Instead of splitting the quadriceps tendon, the muscle belly is divided. The term *trivector* arose as a result of the description of three vectors of pull on the patella: the vastus lateralis, the rectus femoris, and the vastus medialis obliquus. Proponents report that all three vectors are maintained with this approach. Original literature described early benefit with respect to the diminution of the number of lateral retinacular releases and an earlier recovery of the quadriceps function. However, a recent prospective study shows no difference be-tween a standard medial parapatellar arthrotomy and the trivector approach.

21. What is the indication for use of the lateral parapatellar approach?

A straight midline skin incision followed by the lateral parapatellar arthrotomy has become the exposure of choice for the severe valgus deformity. Patients with a valgus deformity often have an associated lateral subluxation of the patella and require a lateral retinacular release at the time of surgical intervention. When a surgeon performs a medial parapatellar arthrotomy and a subsequent lateral retinacular release for a valgus knee deformity, the vasculature to the patella may be somewhat compromised. In an effort to reduce compromise of the patellar vasculature, some surgeons advocate the performance of a lateral parapatellar arthrotomy.

22. If the surgeon experiences difficulty in everting the patella during the standard medial parapatellar approach, what maneuvers can be performed to facilitate eversion?
1. Extending the incision proximally into the quadriceps tendon
2. Releasing adhesions in the lateral retinaculum and patellofemoral ligament
3. Removing the peripheral osteophytes about the patella
4. Tethering the medial portion of the insertion of the patellar ligament
5. Performing a lateral retinacular release

23. Define the mechanical axis of the knee.
   The mechanical axis is defined as a line that intersects the center of the femoral head, the center of the knee, and the ankle. The goal of TKA is to reconstruct the mechanical axis with appropriate resection of the tibia and distal femur while carefully balancing the ligamentous structures.

24. What is the normal alignment of the distal femoral condyles with respect to the femoral axis and of the tibial plateau with respect to the tibial axis?
   The normal alignment of the distal femoral condyles with respect to the femoral axis is approximately 9° of valgus, whereas the normal alignment of the tibial plateau with respect to the tibial axis is approximately 3° of varus. Therefore, a resultant 6° of valgus facilitates creation of the mechanical axis.

25. How should the proximal tibia be cut with respect to the tibial axis?
   This question has a twofold response. Surgeons who follow the teaching of Insall et al. believe that the tibial resection should be created at 90° to the tibial axis in the coronal plane. They stress that varus malalignment leads to early failure. To reconstruct the mechanical axis, the distal femur must be resected at 6° of valgus. Hungerford et al., however, proposed that the proximal tibia be cut in 3° of varus and the distal femur in 9° of valgus. Hungerford argues that such resections place the joint line in the coronal plane parallel to the ground during gait. The majority of physicians, however, continue to resect the proximal tibia at 90° to the axis. As noted above, when the surgeon aims for 3° of varus, the margin is within several degrees; thus a 5° or 6° varus resection may inadvertently be performed. Because such varus malalignment is associated with accelerated loosening, it is safer to aim for a 90° resection and to accept a 2–3° variance in either varus or valgus.

26. What is the normal alignment of the proximal tibia in the sagittal plane?
   In the sagittal plane the proximal tibia generally has a posterior slope of approximately 7–10°. Therefore, in resecting the proximal tibia two options exist: (1) resection perpendicular to the axis, in which case the implant should have posterior slope built into the articulation, and (2) resection of the proximal tibia with 5–7° of posterior slope. Reconstruction of the posterior slope is especially important in cruciate-retaining total knee arthroplasty.

27. What are the palpable landmarks used to assist the placement of the extramedullary tibial alignment jigs?
   The palpable landmarks used to place the extramedullary tibial alignment jigs are the tibial tubercle, tibial spine, and medial and lateral malleolus. The jigs should be positioned over the tibial tubercle and aligned parallel with the tibial spine while intersecting the medial and middle thirds of the intermalleolar distance; thus, the jigs line up between the first and second ray.

28. Should intramedullary or extramedullary alignment jigs be used in performing the distal femoral and proximal tibial resections?
   The literature with respect to distal femoral resection is quite convincing. Intramedullary alignment jigs offer a more reliable, accurate, and reproducible distal femoral resection. The

literature with respect to the tibial resection, however, is controversial. The palpability of the landmarks identified above allows accurate placement of extramedullary alignment jigs and, therefore, reproducible resections. Furthermore, there is debate with respect to bowing of the tibia, which may make it difficult to appropriately place an intramedullary guide and may result in a slight valgus or varus malalignment.

29. Describe the anatomic considerations of the distal femur and proximal tibia that assist in determining rotation of the femoral component.

Rotation of the femoral component is determined by evaluating four distinct anatomic features of the distal femur and proximal tibia: (1) The transepicondylar axis, which intersects the medial and lateral epicondyle, represents the true axis of rotation of the distal femur: (2) the anterior/posterior axis of the femur has been described as a line from the center of the trochlear groove to the center of the intercondylar notch. This axis is reported to be 90° to the transepicondylar axis; (3) the posterior femoral condyles have been identified to be 3° internally rotated to the transepicondylar axis. Therefore, by using a guide that references the posterior condyles with 3° of external rotation the femoral component will be placed in line with the neutral transepicondylar axis; finally (4) the tibial shaft axis has been identified as being 90° to the transepicondylar axis. Therefore, at the time of surgical intervention, the surgeon may incorporate all four of the above anatomic references to assist in determining rotation of the femoral component.

30. What surgical maneuvers can be performed to facilitate patellofemoral tracking?

1. Appropriate resection and resurfacing of the patella to restore preoperative thickness
2. Slight medial displacement of the patellar component
3. Placement of the femoral component in neutral rotation or slight external rotation
4. Lateral deviation of the femoral component
5. Appropriate rotation of the tibial component
6. Release of the patellofemoral ligament and any adhesions within the lateral retinaculum
7. Lateral retinacular release with preservation of the superior geniculate vessel
8. Advancement and reefing of the vastus medialis obliquus

31. Outline the steps for correction of varus malalignment at the time of TKA.

In the varus arthritis knee, the medial ligamentous structures are contracted. The object of TKA is to restore alignment and to reestablish the mechanical axis. In addition to the appropriate bony resections, release of the contracted soft tissues with proper ligamentous balance must be performed. The first step in correction of the contracture is removal of peripheral osteophytes from the distal femur and proximal tibia. Next, the deep medial collateral and capsular attachment to the proximal tibia are released. If correction is not afforded at this time, subsequent release of the superficial medial collateral ligament should be performed, followed by release of the pes anserinus. These releases are performed off the proximal tibia and should create a continuous sleeve of soft tissues.

32. Which bony landmarks on the distal femur represent the most reproducible guides in determining the rotation of the femoral component?

Rotation of the femoral component is best determined by locating the transepicondylar axis, which intersects the medial and lateral epicondyles. The axis of the posterior condyles is internally rotated with respect to the transepicondylar axis and, therefore, should not be used as a guide to determine rotation.

33. Describe the steps in correction of a valgus deformity.

The valgus arthritic knee presents with contractures of the lateral soft-tissue structures. The goal of TKA is to restore the mechanical axis with proper soft-tissue balance. Therefore, in addition to the bony resections in the valgus knee, the lateral contracted soft-tissue structures must be released. All authorities agree that peripheral osteophytes should be removed first. The sequence and technique of releasing the various lateral structures, however, is debatable. Contracture of the iliotibial band is generally noted with the knee in full extension. The iliotibial band can be released using a variety of techniques: (1) release from Gerdy's tubercle versus; (2) fractional lengthening with multiple stab wounds; or (3) transection of the iliotibial band at the joint line. The posterior lateral capsule/arcuate complex can be transected with the knee in full extension, taking care to avoid the neurovascular structures. Alternatively, the posterior lateral capsule/arcuate complex can be released from the distal femur with the knee in flexion with a curved osteotome. If the knee remains unbalanced and further release is deemed necessary, gradual release of the popliteus tendon and the lateral collateral ligament from the distal femur is required. The release of these structures should be performed only to the degree deemed necessary, since partial attachment of such structures will allow for the use of a nonconstrained posterior cruciate retaining or posterior stabilized device. However, if full release of the popliteus tendon and lateral collateral ligament is required, a posterior stabilized constrained device is advised to achieve stability. Note that rarely the biceps femoris may require release. Also note that a lateral retinacular release is frequently required in a valgus knee to facilitate tracking of the patellofemoral articulation.

34. What are the steps in release of flexion contracture in TKA?

The type of implant that should be used in patients with degenerative disease and associated flexion contracture is controversial. The literature supports posterior-stabilized arthroplasty in this group of patients, because the posterior cruciate ligament is part of the deforming force and, therefore, must be released at the time of surgical intervention to correct the flexion contracture. Proponents of posterior cruciate-retaining arthroplasty advise that posterior cruciate-retaining devices can be used with special attention to the tension within the posterior cruciate ligament. They suggest that controlled release of the ligament should be performed as opposed to total excision and substitution of a posterior-stabilized device.

Whichever type of implant is selected, it is imperative to remove all of the posterior condylar osteophytes to assist in reconstruction of the posterior process. In posterior-stabilized arthroplasty, contracture of the posterior cruciate ligament can be dealt with by excision and use of an implant that substitutes for the posterior cruciate ligament. When a posterior cruciate-retaining system is used, the ligament may need to be tethered from its insertion either in the proximal tibia or distal femur. When the flexion contracture is excessive, the capsule should be released from the posterior femur; ultimately, the medial and lateral heads of the gastrocnemius also may need to be released to enhance extension. Increased distal femoral resection increases the extension space and therefore facilitates correction of the flexion contracture; this resection, however, also elevates the joint line. This effect is not as significant in a posterior-stabilized system. However, in posterior cruciate-retaining arthroplasty, retention of the joint line is crucial to function of the posterior cruciate ligament.

BIBLIOGRAPHY

 1. Engh GA, Parks NL, Ammeen DJ: Influence of surgical approach on lateral retinacular releases in total knee arthroplasty. Clin Orthop 331:56–63, 1996.
 2. Fisher DA, Trimble SM, Breedlove K: The medial trivector approach in total knee arthroplasty. Orthopedics 21:53–56, 1998.
 3. Fu FH (ed): Surgery of the Knee. Baltimore, Williams & Wilkins, 1994.
 4. Hewett TE, Noyes FR, Barber-Westin SD, Heckman TP: Decrease in knee joint pain and increase in function in patients with medial compartment arthrosis: A prospective analysis of valgus bracing. Orthopedics 21:131–138, 1998.
 5. Insall JN, Windsor RE, Scott WN, et al (eds): Surgery of the Knee, 2nd ed. New York, Churchill Livingstone, 1993.
 6. Krackow KA (ed): The Technique of Total Knee Arthroplasty. St. Louis, Mosby, 1990.
 7. Lombardi AV Jr, Mallory TH, Eberle RW: Constrained knee arthroplasty. In Scott WN (ed): The Knee. St. Louis, Mosby, 1993, pp 1305–1323.
 8. Miyaska KC, Ranawat CS, Mullaji A: 10 to 20-Year follow-up of total knee arthroplasty for valgus deformities. Clin Orthop 345:29–37, 1997.
 9. Rand JA (ed): Total Knee Arthroplasty. New York, Raven Press, 1993.
10. Scott WN (ed): The Knee (Vol. 1 and 2). St. Louis, Mosby, 1994.

79. COMPLICATIONS IN TOTAL KNEE ARTHROPLASTY

Adolph V. Lombardi, Jr., M.D., FACS

1. What is the most frequent complication following total knee arthroplasty (TKA)?

Complications with respect to the extensor mechanism represent the most frequently reported complications of TKA, with some centers reporting as high as 1.5–12% patellofemoral complications.

2. When minimal patellar resections are performed and a standard patellar component of approximately 8–9 mm is placed, "overstuffing" of the patellofemoral articulation may occur. What are the potential complications from overstuffing of the patellofemoral articulation?

Overstuffing of the patellofemoral articulation has both mechanical and functional implications. Increases in the contact stresses, as well as the shear stresses, that may be applied to the patellar implant may cause early loosening. A caliper should be used at the time of patellar resection to measure the anterior-posterior dimension of the patella (average thickness 23–25 mm); the appropriate amount of the patella should be resected, followed by proper reconstruction of patellofemoral articulation. Caution to avoid over-resection of the patella is also advised, because over-resection may lead to patellar fracture. A minimal postresection patellar thickness of 12–15 mm is required to avoid this complication. The postsurgical patellar composite should equal the presurgical patellar thickness.

3. What is lateral subluxation of the patella and how is it best treated?

Obtaining satisfactory tracking of the patellofemoral articulation is a difficult and multivariant task. It involves proper positioning of the femoral, tibial, and patellar components. To determine the appropriate surgical intervention requires addressing the cause for the subluxation. Radiographic evaluation of the implant may assist in determining proper alignment of the components but is not conclusive. Intraoperative inspection of all three components is required to rule out implant malalignment as the causative factor. Improper positioning of the components would necessitate revision of the implant. If it is determined that all components are in proper alignment, correction may be achieved with a lateral retinacular release, and in some cases a distal and lateral advancement of the vastus medialis obliquus.

4. If the femoral component rotation in the sagittal plane is placed along the axis of the posterior femoral condyles, what error and subsequent complication may result?

If the surgeon places the femoral component in line with the posterior femoral condylar axis, the femoral component will be placed in internal rotation with respect to the transepicondylar axis or true axis of the femur. This placement not only causes ligamentous imbalance but also increases the stresses across the patellofemoral articulation and leads to subluxation and perhaps dislocation of the patella.

5. What is the potential complication from intramedullary jigging of the femur and tibia for TKA?

The potential complication from intramedullary (IM) jigging of the femur and tibia is the generation of fat emboli. Literature stresses that the IM rod should be approximately 8 mm in diameter and should be fluted to allow drainage of fat from the femoral and tibial canals. In addition, the pilot holes should be 12 mm in diameter or approximately 4 mm larger than the intramedullary rod.

6. Describe the preoperative deformity more commonly associated with a postoperative peroneal palsy.

Postoperative peroneal palsy is a rare occurrence with TKA. However, it is more commonly seen in knees that present with significant combined valgus and flexion contracture deformities. Correction of such deformities may cause a stretching type injury to the peroneal nerve resulting in a postoperative neuropraxia. If this is identified in the early postoperative period, all dressings should be removed and the knee should be flexed. Some authors advocate exploration of the peroneal nerve.

7. Describe the patellar clunk syndrome and its treatment.

The patellar clunk syndrome has been described as an audible sound in conjunction with a visual displacement of the patella as the knee moves from a flexed position to an extended position. The clunk is caused by a fibrous nodule that is formed at the superior pole of the patella. Its definitive pathogenesis is debatable; however, it has been identified when there is superior overhand of the patellar component. Treatment generally requires surgical excision of the fibrous nodule and correction of the overhand of the patellar component.

8. What potential complication may result from notching of the anterior femoral cortex in TKA?

Although the significance of notching of the anterior femoral cortex in TKA is somewhat controversial, most of the literature suggests that notching should be avoided, because it may represent an etiologic mechanism for supracondylar fracture. Notching of the anterior femoral cortex is currently avoided by use of sophisticated instrumentation with appropriate sizing guides. Despite this sophisticated instrumentation, however, the surgeon must clear the suprapatellar fat and synovium and carefully monitor the anterior femoral resection.

9. Describe the etiology of an intercondylar distal femoral fracture in posterior stabilized TKA. What can be done to prevent it?

Intercondylar distal femoral fracture is a rare occurrence, exclusive to posterior stabilized arthroplasty (e.g., an intercondylar distal femoral resection for posterior stabilized arthroplasty). This complication occurs when the intercondylar femoral resection is slightly narrower than the intercondylar box of the femoral component or when the femoral component is inserted or extracted in slight varus or valgus malalignment. It may be avoided by accurate intercondylar resection. An intercondylar sizing guide should be used for measuring the intercondylar resection, and great care should be taken in inserting and extracting the trial and final components.

10. Describe the types of intercondylar distal femoral bone fractures that may occur in TKA and the appropriate management of each.

Two types of intercondylar distal femoral fractures may occur in posterior stabilized TKA: nondisplaced and displaced. Nondisplaced fractures are generally recognized on postoperative roentgenographs and require no further treatment. Patients should be placed in a routine physical therapy and rehabilitation program. A displaced intercondylar distal femoral fracture, however, is noted at the time of the surgical intervention and should be stabilized with screws and/or stemmed components. After stabilization of the fracture, no change in the postoperative physical therapy and rehabilitation routine is required.

11. What neurologic complication may arise in correction of the arthritic knee with a valgus malalignment and an associated flexion contracture?

Correction of the arthritic knee with a valgus deformity and associated flexion contracture sometimes leads to peroneal palsy, which is attributed to stretching of the peroneal nerve. If this complication is noted postoperatively, all compressive dressings should be removed immediately and the knee should be flexed. Surgical decompression of the peroneal nerve remains controversial, but recent literature cites the benefit of decompression if nerve function does not spontaneously recover.

12. Describe the major factors in proximal tibial resection that may lead to failure of TKA.

Critical to successful TKA is the technique of proximal tibial resection. The first and foremost factor is the level of proximal tibial resection. Overresection of the proximal tibia should be avoided, because the strength of the proximal tibia decreases with the level of resection. Underresection of the proximal tibia, however, also may be detrimental, because the joint line is elevated. An accurate level of resection is especially critical in a posterior cruciate-retaining arthroplasty. As a rule of thumb, the level of the proximal tibial resection should be approximately 8–10 mm from the lateral tibial plateau with a corresponding resection 3–5 mm from the medial plateau. The proximal tibia normally has approximately $7–10°$ of posterior slope; thus, resection of the proximal tibia to neutral or reverse angulation affects the flexion gap and may subsequently alter range of motion. This rule must be noted when using a posterior cruciate-retaining knee in which the articulating mechanism does not incorporate posterior slope.

13. What potential error may occur if the intramedullary guide, used for distal femoral preparation, is placed in the center of the intercondylar notch?

Anatomic studies have demonstrated that the femoral axis exits the distal femur at the lateral border of the medial femoral condyle. Therefore, if the intermedullary guide is inserted into the center of the intercondylar notch, it is placed in a slight valgus orientation of approximately $2°$; therefore, if one is aiming for $6°$ valgus resection, the guide should be placed at $4°$ of valgus.

14. What are the advantages and disadvantages of screw fixation in cementless TKA?

The literature recommends the use of 4 screws to augment fixation of the cementless tibial component. Screws have been shown to enhance stability, to decrease micromotion, and, therefore, to potentiate osseous integration into the tibial component. Several recent articles, however, have revealed osteolytic lesions about the screws; thus the term "screw osteolysis" has been coined. It is postulated that polyethylene debris invades the screw holes and tracks along the body of the screw. Removal of the screws and replacement with morsellized bone grafting has been shown to be an effective treatment of osteolytic lesions.

BIBLIOGRAPHY

1. Fu FH (ed): Surgery of the Knee. Baltimore, Williams & Wilkins, 1994.
2. Guyton JL: Arthroplasty of ankle and knee. In Canale ST (ed): Campbell's Operative Orthopaedics, 9th ed. St. Louis, Mosby, 1998, pp 232–295.
3. Hozack WJ, Rothman RH, Booth RE Jr, Balderston RA: The patellar clunk syndrome: A complication of posterior stabilized total knee arthroplasty. Clin Orthop 241:203–208, 1989.
4. Insall JN, Windsor RE, Scott WN, et al (eds): Surgery of the Knee, 2nd ed. New York, Churchill Livingstone, 1993.
5. Krackow KA (ed): The Technique of Total Knee Arthroplasty. St. Louis, Mosby, 1990.
6. Lombardi AV Jr, Mallory TH, Eberle RW: Constrained knee arthroplasty. In Scott WN (ed): The Knee. St. Louis, Mosby, 1993, pp 1305–1323.
7. Rand JA (ed): Total Knee Arthroplasty. New York, Raven Press, 1993.

80. ALTERNATIVES TO TOTAL KNEE ARTHROPLASTY: OSTEOTOMY AND FUSION

Daniel P. Hoeffel, M.D., and Randall D. Neumann, M.D.

OSTEOTOMY

1. Describe the mechanical axis of the lower limb.
The mechanical axis is a straight line originating from the center of the femoral head to the center of the tibiotalar (ankle) joint.

2. Define the tibiofemoral angle.
This angle is created by the intersection of lines along the long axes of the femur and tibia.

3. What are normal values for the mechanical axis and tibiofemoral angle?
The normal mechanical axis is zero because it is a straight line. The normal tibiofemoral angle is ~ 5–7° of valgus angulation.

4. What is the load distribution across the normal knee?
Approximately 60% of the load is borne by the medial compartment, and 40% is borne by the lateral compartment.

5. Describe the load distribution across a varus knee and a valgus knee.
A **varus deformity** often results from medial compartment degenerative changes with collapse of the medial tibial plateau. As the knee progresses into varus, the mechanical axis crosses the knee joint as a point more medial than normal, which results in greater relative loading of the medial compartment.

A **valgus deformity** results from lateral compartment degenerative changes with collapse of the lateral femoral condyle. The mechanical axis moves laterally. Relatively more weight is transmitted through the lateral compartment.

6. What are the goals of knee osteotomy?
1. To transfer load from the degenerative compartment to the less diseased compartment, thus preserving articular surface and relieving pain.
2. To alter the bony alignment at the point at which the mechanical axis crosses the knee joint, thereby altering load distribution across the knee.

7. What is the usual osteotomy for medial compartment degeneration?
A proximal tibial valgus osteotomy to correct the accompanying varus deformity is usually performed.

8. Which type of osteotomy is done for lateral compartment degeneration?
A distal femoral varus osteotomy corrects the accompanying valgus deformity.

9. List the indications for proximal tibial valgus osteotomy about the knee.
1. Absence of lateral compartment and patellofemoral degenerative arthritis
2. Younger patient (< 60–65 years)
3. Good bone stock (minimal osteoporotic change)
4. Minimum flexion arc (> 90°)
5. < 15° of fixed varus

10. What are the contraindications for proximal tibial valgus osteotomy?
- Lateral subluxation of the tibia on the femur > 1 cm
- Tibial subchondral bone loss
- Flexion contracture > 15°
- < 90° range of motion
- Peripheral vascular disease
- Lateral thrust of the knee during gait
- Rheumatoid or other systemic arthritides

11. List the indications for varus osteotomies of the femur.
1. Valgus deformities > 12° and > 10° deviation of the knee joint from the horizontal
2. No flexion contracture > 15°
3. ≥ 90° range of motion
4. No knee instability

12. What preoperative planning is necessary when considering a tibial osteotomy?
Full-length, weight-bearing radiographs are used to determine the desired amount of correction and the size of the bone wedge to be removed. To unload the arthritic medial compartment, the angle between the tibia and the femur should be 8–10° of valgus. Slight overcorrection provides the best long-term results.

13. What types of fixation have been used to stabilize tibial valgus osteotomy?
- Plates and screws
- Staples
- External fixators

14. What are the long-term results of proximal tibial valgus osteotomy?
At 5-year follow-up 88% of patients have satisfactory results; at 10-year follow-up the number drops to 63%. Adequate angular correction has a strong correlation with good outcome.

15. List the complications associated with proximal tibial osteotomies.
- Inadequate correction (most common)
- Overcorrection
- Violation of tibial articular surface
- Avascular necrosis of the tibial plateau
- Patella baja (low-riding patella)
- Anterior compartment syndrome
- Peroneal nerve syndrome
- Delayed union/nonunion (3–5%)
- Infection
- Vascular injuries to the popliteal vessels

16. How successful is total knee arthroplasty (TKA) after tibial osteotomy?
Results are less satisfactory than for primary TKA. Patella baja is not uncommon after tibial osteotomy, which makes adequate exposure for TKA more difficult. One study showed 81% good-to-excellent results for TKA after tibial osteotomy, whereas primary TKA had 100% good-to-excellent results.

17. Describe the usual bony deformity in the valgus arthritic knee.
Lateral compartment arthritis is usually associated with lateral femoral condyle bone deficiency. Thus, a medial closing wedge osteotomy of the tibia may cause significant obliquity of the knee joint and subluxation of the femur on the tibia. A femoral osteotomy avoids this complication.

18. What preoperative planning should be done before distal femoral varus osteotomy?
Full-length, weight-bearing radiographs are used to determine the desired amount of correction and the size of the bone wedge to be removed. The tibiofemoral angle should be corrected to 0°.

19. What types of fixation are used to stabilize femoral osteotomies?
The standard device is a 95 degree-blade plate with screws.

20. What are the follow-up results of distal femoral osteotomy?

Five to 10-year follow-up shows 70–80% good-to-excellent results that do not appear to decrease over time.

KNEE ARTHRODESIS

21. What is knee arthrodesis?

A knee arthrodesis is a surgical procedure designed to produce a bony ankylosis (fusion) of the knee joint.

22. What are the goals of a knee arthrodesis?

To create a stable, pain-free platform on which to ambulate or transfer.

23. List the disadvantages of a knee fusion.

1. Joints above and below the knee will transmit greater loads and may become stiff or undergo degenerative changes.

2. Loss of knee range of motion, which decreases gait efficiency (20% increased energy requirement)

3. Activities of daily living may be more difficult (e.g., rising from a seated position, dressing)

24. What are the indications for knee arthrodesis?

- A salvage procedure for severe unilateral knee afflictions
- Infected TKA that makes revision surgery unsuitable
- Posttraumatic arthritis in high-demand patients (i.e., manual laborers)
- Tumors requiring significant bony resection
- Severe infectious arthritis (resistant bacteria, fungal, TB)
- Paralytic conditions (especially with genu recurvatum)
- Congenital knee anomalies

25. What types of techniques are available for arthrodesis?

- Intramedullary (IM) rodding
- Compression plating
- External fixation

26. List the disadvantages of plating, IM rodding, and external fixation.

Plating
  May require placing metal in previously or currently infected site
  Large bulk of components
IM rodding
  Rod migration
  Difficult to obtain correct alignment
  Difficult to remove
External fixation
  Pin tract drainage/infection
  Muscle and soft tissue scarring at pin sites
  Long treatment course (6 months)

27. What is the ideal position for a knee fusion?

0–5° of valgus
10–15° of flexion
Slight external rotation

28. What is the reported success rate of arthrodesis with an IM nail?

Eighty-five percent of patients gain functional stability and overall union.

29. Does the type of knee arthroplasty originally performed affect the rate of fusion?
Yes. A hinged prosthesis adversely affects the fusion rate (56%). Nonhinged prostheses have a ~ 90% fusion rate.

30. What are the potential complications of knee fusion?
- Pseudarthrosis (failure to fuse)
- Recurrent infection
- Knee pain
- Back pain
- Pin tract infection
- Fracture of bone at pin site (external fixation)
- Nail breakage
- Tibia fracture (IM rod)

BIBLIOGRAPHY

1. Arroyo JS, Garvin KL, Neff JR: Arthrodesis of the knee with a modular titanium intramedullary nail. J Bone Joint Surg Am 79:26–35, 1997.
2. Christian CA, Donley BG: Arthrodesis of the ankle, knee, and hip. In Canale ST (ed): Campbell's Operative Orthopaedics, 9th ed. St. Louis, Mosby, 1998, pp 145–187.
3. Coventry MB, Ilstrup DM, Wallrichs SL: Proximal tibial osteotomy: A critical long-term study of 87 cases. J Bone Joint Surg 75A:196–201, 1993.
4. Edgerton BC. Mariani EM, Morrey BF: Distal femoral varus osteotomy for painful genu valgum. A five-to-11-year follow-up study. Clin Orthop 288:263–269, 1993.
5. Insall JN: Osteotomy. In Insall JN (ed): Surgery of the Knee, 2nd ed. New York, Churchill Livingstone, 1993, pp 635–677.
6. Jakob RP, Murphy SB: Tibial osteotomy for varus arthrosis: Indication, planning, and operative technique. Instr Course Lect 41:87–93, 1992.
7. Kelly MA: Nonprosthetic management of the arthritic knee. In Callaghan JJ (ed): Orthopaedic Knowledge Update Hip and Knee Reconstruction. Rosemont, IL, American Academy of Orthopaedic Surgeons, 1995, pp 245–251.
8. Mont MA, Alexander N, Krackow KA, Hungerford DS: Total knee arthroplasty after failed high tibial osteotomy. Orthop Clin North Am 25:515–525, 1994.
9. Pritchett JW, Mall BA: Knee arthrodesis with a tension band plate. J Bone Joint Surg 70A:285–288, 1988.

81. FRACTURES ABOUT THE KNEE

Randall D. Neumann, M.D.

1. What is a tibial plateau fracture?
A tibial plateau fracture involves the proximal 10–12 cm of the tibia, which consist largely of cancellous bone.

2. Describe the types of tibial plateau fractures.
Numerous classifications have been introduced over the years. The categories encompass many fracture configurations but are so broad that comparisons of treatment results are meaningless. Fractures can be described as minor or major and undisplaced or displaced. Compression may occur in either the medial or lateral compartment. Fractures may involve compression of one small fragment or a major fragment. Hohl's classification depicts many of these fractures (see figure, top of next page).

3. Describe the mechanism of injury in a tibial plateau fracture.
Strong forces directed medially or laterally at the knee joint, combined with axial loading, cause the majority of proximal tibial plateau fractures. Automobile accidents account for 40–60% of all tibial plateau fractures. Other mechanisms include falls from heights, slipping and twisting,

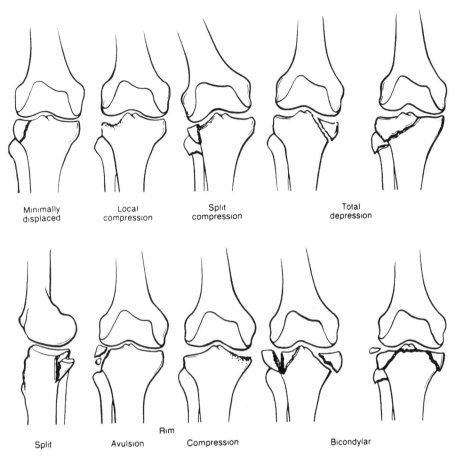

| Minimally displaced | Local compression | Split compression | Total depression |

| Split | Avulsion | Rim Compression | Bicondylar |

Hohl's revised classification of tibial plateau fractures: minimally displaced (22%), local compression (28%), split compression (18%), total depression (13%), split (3%), rim avulsion or compression (5%), and bicondylar (11%). (From Wiss DA: Supracondylar and intercondylar fractures of the femur. In Rockwood CA, Green DP, Bucholz RW (eds): Rockwood and Green's Fractures in Adults, 3rd ed. Philadelphia, J.B. Lippincott, 1991, pp 1778–1797, with permission.)

sport injuries, and motorcycle and bicycle accidents. About 15–14% of fractures include a ligamentous rupture, commonly of the medial or lateral collateral ligaments. Meniscal lesions occur in approximately 20% of all tibial plateau fractures. Some tibial plateau fractures are quite minor and are caused by falls or minor missteps among the elderly.

4. Describe the symptoms of the patient with a tibial plateau fracture.

Most patients have had high-energy trauma and complain of severe pain and swelling of the knee. Instability may be noted when the patient attempts to bear weight. The patient also may complain of tense hemarthrosis.

5. Describe the radiographic findings in a patient with a tibial plateau fracture.

Anteroposterior and lateral radiographs of the knee usually reveal the fracture. If a fracture is suspected but not seen, oblique views or a tunnel view may be taken. Tomograms in the anteroposterior and lateral planes show evidence of plateau fractures Computed tomography (CT) produces excellent images from which to assess depressions and displacements.

6. What are the findings of knee aspiration in patients with a tibial plateau fracture?

Some patients may have a tense hemarthrosis. Aspiration reveals blood in the joint but also may reveal fat. If fat is present in the aspirate, a fracture is surely present.

7. What complications are seen in patients with fractures of the tibial plateau?

Some patients with tibial plateau fractures have a fractured dislocation of the knee. The popliteal artery is usually injured in a knee dislocation. Prompt attention to the arterial pulses and angiography are needed for assessment of the popliteal artery.

8. Describe the indications for conservative treatment in a patient with a tibial plateau fracture.

The major indication is a minimally displaced fracture that shows depression or displacement of < 4 mm. Minimally displaced fractures may involve one or both plateaus. Instability is the most important factor to consider in choosing the treatment for minimally displaced fractures. If the knee is stable to abduction and adduction stress testing, the fracture is considered stable. Stable fractures may be treated with a knee immobilizer, partial weightbearing, or cast bracing. Conservative treatments are maintained until the fracture is united and weightbearing begins.

9. Describe the treatment for tibial plateau fractures with local compression.

Most tibial plateau fractures with > 8 mm of depression should be treated operatively, with restoration of the depressed articular surfaces. Either screw fixation or plate fixation is used. Autogenous bone grafting may be used to support the elevated surface.

10. Describe the treatment for a split-depression tibial plateau fracture.

Bicondylar fractures are generally high-energy fractures associated with a high incidence of vascular and nerve injuries. Soft-tissue damage is likely in the pre- or postoperative period. Bicondylar tibial plateau fractures have the poorest prognosis for functional improvement. Treatment may consist of nonoperative skeletal traction followed by percutaneous pinning and/or cast bracing. Open reduction is used when significant improvement in fracture position is likely and rigid internal fixation is possible.

11. Describe the treatment for a bicondylar tibial plateau fracture.

Bicondylar fractures are generally high-energy fractures associated with a high incidence of vascular and nerve injuries. Soft-tissue damage is likely in the pre- or postoperative period. Bicondylar tibial plateau fractures have the poorest prognosis for functional improvement. Treatment may consist of nonoperative skeletal traction followed by percutaneous pinning and/or cast bracing. Open reduction is used when significant improvement in fracture position is likely and rigid internal fixation is possible.

12. What complications may occur from tibial plateau fracture and its treatment?

Complications include skin loss, compartment syndrome, wound infection, popliteal artery laceration, peroneal nerve palsy, nonunion, malunion, and degenerative arthritis.

13. Describe the etiology of patellar fracture.

The majority of patellar fractures occur in patients between 20 and 50 years of age. The incidence is nearly twice as high in men as in women. They usually result from a direct blow to the knee sustained in a fall or a motor vehicle or pedestrian accident. Fractures also may occur from indirect forces, as in the act of stumbling or partially falling.

14. Describe the classification of patellar fractures.

Transverse fractures in the central or lower third of the patella are the most common type. Vertical fractures may occur but are generally associated with a more comminuted fracture that began as a transverse fracture. Patellar fractures may be displaced or undisplaced.

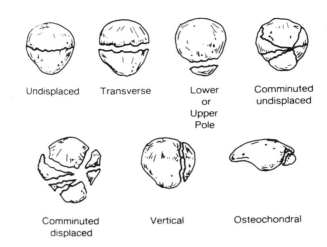

Undisplaced   Transverse   Lower   Comminuted
                               or   undisplaced
                               Upper
                               Pole

Comminuted   Vertical   Osteochondral
displaced

Classification of patellar fractures. (From Wiss DA, Watson JT, Johnson EE: Fractures of the knee. In Rockwood CA Jr, Green DP, Bucholz RW, Heckman JD (eds): Rockwood and Green's Fractures in Adults, 4th ed. Philadelphia, Lippincott-Raven, 1996, with permission.)

15. What treatments are available for patellar fractures?
1. Nonoperative treatment with casting or immobilization
2. Operative treatment with open reduction and internal fixation
3. Partial patellectomy
4. Total patellectomy

16. Describe the indications for nonoperative treatment.
Patients who are able to extend the knee fully have intact retinaculum. Such fractures are usually displaced or have 2–3 mm of acceptable separation. A long leg cast is recommended for 3–4 weeks, followed by quadriceps exercises, straight leg raising, and range-of motion exercises. Partial weightbearing is easily tolerated.

17. Describe the indications for open reduction and internal fixation.
Open reduction and internal fixation are used to reconstruct the patella in patients with displacement and loss of extension. Generally the retinaculum medially and laterally to the patella is torn along with the fracture. The extensor mechanism is no longer in continuity and must be repaired. Operative treatment includes the use of K-wire and tension band or screws.

18. Describe the indication for partial patellectomy.
Partial patellectomy and repair of the extensor mechanism are indicated when there is a small remaining fragment of the patella or quadriceps tendon—usually in an avulsion fracture of the patellar ligament. The lower pole is excised, and the patella tendon is sutured into the remaining patella.

19. What is the indication for total patellectomy?
Total patellectomy is recommended for highly comminuted fractures that have no possibility of repair or reconstruction.

20. Describe the complications from patellar fractures and their treatment.
An occasional patient has an extensor lag. Quadriceps wasting may occur. Fracture fragment separation and loss of fixation occur in as many as 7% of patients. Nonunion may occur postoperatively. Other common problems include patellofemoral pain or osteoarthritic symptoms as a long-term consequence of patellar fracture.

21. What are fractures in the distal one-third of the femur called?
Supracondylar fractures.

22. Describe the classification for supracondylar fractures of the femur.
No classification for supracondylar fractures of the femur is universally accepted, but the AO classification is commonly used. Type A fractures involve the distal shaft, with varying degrees of comminution. Type B fractures are condylar fractures. Type C fractures are T and Y condylar fractures with varying degrees of comminution.

AO/ASIF classification of supracondylar femur fractures. (From Wiss DA: Supracondylar and intracondylar fractures of the femur. In Rockwood CA, Green DP, Bucholz RW (eds): Rockwood and Green's Fractures in Adults, 3rd ed. Philadelphia, J.B. Lippincott, 1991, pp 1778–1797, with permission.)

23. What is the mechanism of injury in supracondylar fractures?

The mechanism of injury is axial loading with varus, valgus, or rotational forces. Supra-condylar fractures are typically seen after high-energy trauma related to motor vehicle or motor-cycle accidents or falls from a height. In the elderly, a slip or fall on a flexed knee frequently leads to comminuted fractures through compromised osteoporotic bone.

24. Describe the initial management for supracondylar fractures.

Patients with supracondylar fractures should be treated with closed skeletal traction with a tibial traction pin. Immediate debridement is necessary for open injuries. Traction is then main-tained if nonoperative treatment is elected. If operative treatment is elected, distraction of the fragments may enhance fracture mobility at the time of surgical intervention .

25. What immediate complications are associated with supracondylar fractures of the femur?

A vascular injury is found in 2–3% of patients. Vessel injury may result directly from lacera-tion or contusion by the fracture fragments or indirectly from stretching that leads to intimal damage. Clinical examination of the leg for signs of ischemia and evaluation of pulses and motor and sensory function are mandatory. If the integrity of the vessels is in doubt, it is wise to proceed with an arteriogram to rule out vascular injury.

26. What are the indications for nonoperative therapy in supracondylar fractures?

1. Nondisplaced or incomplete fractures
2. Impacted stable fractures in elderly osteoporotic patients
3. Significant underlying medical diseases, such as cardiovascular, pulmonary, or neuro-logic problems
4. Severe osteoporosis
5. Severely contaminated open fractures
6. Infected fractures
7. Fractures without joint involvement

27. What are the goals of nonsurgical treatment?

The goals of nonsurgical treatment include a stable, healed fracture with near-normal range of motion of the knee and hip. No more than 7° of malalignment in the mediolateral plane should be accepted. Anterior or posterior angulation should not exceed 7–10°. Limb shortening of 1–1.5 cm is generally well tolerated.

28. Describe the surgical management of supracondylar fractures.

Minimally comminuted fractures involving the medial or lateral condyle are best treated with open reduction, restoration of the articular surface, and internal fixation with AO screws. Severely comminuted fractures should be treated with near-anatomic restoration of the joint using K-wires and screws, followed by a medial and lateral dynamic compression plate. When comminution or defects in the cortex are present, supplemental cortical cancellous bone grafting is necessary. Alternatives are the condylar blade plate, buttress plate, intramedullary nails, and flexible intramedullary nails. External fixation is frequently used in open fractures with signifi-cant soft-tissue wounds or vascular injury.

29. List the long-term complications of supracondylar fractures.

Malunion	Infection	Deep venous thrombosis
Nonunion	Implant breakage	Vascular injury
Loss of knee motion		

BIBLIOGRAPHY

1. Connolly JF, Dehne E, LaFollette B: Closed reduction and early cast-brace ambulation in the treatment of femoral fractures: Results in one hundred and forty-three fractures. J Bone Joint Surg 55A:1581–1599, 1973.

2. Connolly JF, King P: Closed reduction and early cast-brace ambulation in the treatment of femoral fractures: I. an in vivo quantitative analysis of immobilization in skeletal traction and a cast-brace. J Bone
   Joint Surg 55A:1559–1580, 1973.
3. Duwelius P, Connelly J: Closed reduction of tibial plateau fractures: A comparison of functional and
   roentgenographic end results. Clin Orthop 230:116–126, 1988.
4. Mize RD: Supracondylar and articular fractures in the distal femur. In Chapman M (ed): Operative
   Orthopedics. Philadelphia, J.B. Lippincott, 1988, pp 401–412.
5. Muller ME, Allgower M, Willinegger H: Manual of Internal Fixation: Technique Recommended by the
   AO Group. New York, Springer-Verlag, 1979, pp 249–250.
6. Whittle AP: Fractures of lower extremity. In Canale ST (ed): Campbell's Operative Orthopaedics, 9th ed.
   St. Louis, Mosby, 1998, pp 2042–2179.
7. Wiss DA: Supracondylar and intercondylar fractures of the femur. In Rockwood CA, Green DP, Bucholz
   RW (eds): Rockwood and Green's Fractures in Adults, 3rd ed. Philadelphia, J.B. Lippincott, 1991, pp
   1778–1797.

IX. The Lower Leg

82. EXERTIONAL LEG PAIN

David E. Brown, M.D.

1. What is the differential diagnosis of chronic exertional leg pain?
- Medial tibial stress syndrome
- Chronic exertional compartment syndrome
- Stress fracture
- Vascular claudication
- Referred discogenic leg pain
- True shin splints (myositis or tendinitis of the anterior or lateral compartment muscles)

2. What are shin splints?
A shin splint is an inflammatory condition of one or more of the musculotendinous units of the leg. It is most common in the anterior compartment muscles. Repetitive loading of the anterior compartment results in overloading and fatigue, which is often the result of early season conditioning and training errors such as running on hard surfaces, overly rapid increase in training intensity, weak ankle dorsiflexors (anterior compartment), poor shoes, or poor running technique.

3. What is the treatment of common shin splints?
Treatment involves relative rest, icing, antiinflammatory medication, stretching of the antagonist muscle groups, and strengthening of the involved muscle group. Such measures are followed by a gradual return to athletics and activity. Cross-training activities are advised during the initial treatment phase. Immobilization is not recommended. All training errors, biomechanical abnormalities, and improper equipment should be evaluated and corrected.

4. What is medial tibial stress syndrome (MTSS)?
MTSS is an inflammatory condition involving the periosteal attachment of the deep posterior compartment. Pain usually starts after exercise and is relieved by rest. However, symptoms may persist for hours or days after cessation of exercise.

On examination, a localized area of tenderness is found over the posterior medial edge of the distal third of the tibia. Evaluation of the foot may reveal either excessive valgus or varus. The rest of the examination is usually normal. Radiographs are usually normal.

Rest is the primary treatment for MTSS. Cross-training is required, often for an extended period until the stress periostitis resolves. Strength and flexibility of the deep posterior compartment should be emphasized. Abnormal hindfoot and forefoot alignment should be corrected. Recurrences are common.

5. Where is the most common location for stress fractures in the leg?
Stress fractures of the tibia are most common in the proximal third or at the junction of the middle and distal thirds along the posterior medial margin. Fibular stress fractures are most common in the supramalleolar region.

6. Why is a stress fracture of the *anterior* tibia cortex a cause for concern?
An uncommon tibial stress fracture occurs in the anterior tibial cortex, usually in the middle third of the tibia. Because this occurs on the "tension" side of the tibia, it is much more likely to

progress to delayed union or nonunion. Prolonged immobilization and relative rest are required. In some cases, bone grafting of the anterior tibial stress fracture is required to obtain union.

7. Name the various leg compartments and the muscles within each compartment.

The four compartments include the anterior, lateral, superficial posterior, and deep posterior. The anterior compartment consists of the tibialis anterior, extensor digitorum longus, extensor hallucis longus, and peroneus tertius. The lateral compartment includes the peroneus longus and brevis. The superficial posterior has the gastrocsoleus complex, whereas the deep posterior compartment includes the posterior tibialis, flexor hallucis longus, and flexor digitorum longus. Some include the plantaris muscle in the deep posterior compartment.

8. What is *chronic* exertional compartment syndrome?

It is intermittent excessive pressure within an enclosed fascial compartment that occurs only during exercise. Pressures then slowly fall to normal following cessation of exercise, but the pressure falls much more slowly than normal.

9. How does chronic exertional compartment syndrome present?

Athletes typically have pain in the involved compartment that begins at a consistent time in their exercise sessions. Symptoms may then slowly subside after cessation of exercise. They may note numbness in the top of the foot and weakness of ankle dorsiflexion.

10. How is chronic exertional compartment syndrome diagnosed by pressure criteria?

In the presence of appropriate clinical findings, the diagnosis of chronic compartment syndrome exists if: (1) preexercise pressure is $\geq$ 15 mmHg; (2) 1-minute postexercise pressure is $\geq$ 30 mmHg; or (3) 5-minute postexercise pressure is $\geq$ 20 mmHg.

11. What is the incidence of bilaterality in chronic exertional compartment syndrome?

Fifty to 60%.

12. What is the incidence of muscle hernia in patients with chronic exertional compartment syndrome? Which nerve can be compressed by these muscle hernias?

The incidence of muscle hernia is 45%. It usually occurs in the distal third of the lateral compartment where the superficial peroneal nerve exits the compartment and becomes subcutaneous.

13. Which compartment is most commonly involved when a leg muscle hernia is present?

The lateral compartment. On some occasions, the superficial peroneal nerve passes through the anterior compartment, making it susceptible to hernia.

14. What are the treatment options for symptomatic leg muscle fascia hernia?

- Primary repair
- Fascial graft reconstruction
- Fasciotomy

Primary repair has been identified as a causative factor in acute compartment syndrome and is therefore not advised. Fascial graft reconstruction is an acceptable technique, although it is more extensive than fasciotomy. Complete fasciotomy affords relief of symptoms and has not been associated with leg muscle weakness or other significant morbidity, and therefore is the most commonly recommended treatment.

15. When are x-rays positive in the presence of a tibial stress fracture?

At least 14 days must elapse following the onset of symptoms before the characteristic findings of stress fracture are evident. Initially, a single periosteal line may occur along the posterior aspect of the tibia. Later, the subperiosteal region calcifies, resulting in a localized area of sclerosis that is most characteristic of a stress fracture.

16. What is the role of MRI in the evaluation of stress fractures?

MRI is nearly as sensitive as bone scan in detecting stress syndrome. MRI is more accurate in localizing fracture location, does not expose the patient to ionizing radiation, and requires less imaging time. It is preferred over bone scan in the evaluation of femur stress fractures.

17. What is the role of the bone scan in the evaluation of stress fractures?

Technetium bone scan allows for earlier confirmation of a stress fracture. It may become positive within 48 hours of the onset of symptoms. It also is useful in the evaluation of persistent leg pain in which the diagnosis is unclear or if the possibility of multiple stress fractures exists.

18. What is the role of orthotics in the management of MTSS?

One of the primary causes of MTSS is overpronation, which results in excessive motion and tension on the posterior tibialis and soleus muscle attachments. Orthotics may be used to prevent this overpronation. A semirigid orthotic with a medial post that maintains the hindfoot in neutral position is most useful. A recent study in Canada found that hindfoot-forefoot varus may actually be more prevalent. Thus, it appears that any biomechanical foot malalignment may cause MTSS.

19. What is the role of surgery in the treatment of MTSS?

Surgical treatment of MTSS is controversial. Fascial stripping and cauterization of the posterior medial ridge of the tibia have been advocated. However, controlled clinical studies have not been performed. Release of the superficial posterior compartment may be of benefit in resistant cases.

20. Do athletes and military recruits demonstrate different patterns of stress fracture?

Yes. Military recruits most commonly sustain stress fractures of the metatarsals (40%), whereas in athletes, metatarsal stress fractures constitute only 20% of the total number of stress fractures. Of all stress fractures in athletes, 45% affect the tibia and fibula.

BIBLIOGRAPHY

1. Andrish JT, Bergfeld JH, Walheim J: A prospective study on the management of shin splints. J Bone Joint Surg 56A:1697, 1974.
2. AAOS Symposium on the Foot and Leg in Running Sports. St. Louis, Mosby, 1982.
3. Boden BP, Speer KP: Femoral stress fractures. Clin Sports Med 16:307–317, 1997.
4. Detmer DE, Sharpe K, Sufit RL, et al: Chronic compartment syndrome: Diagnosis, management and outcome. Am J Sports Med 13:163, 1985.
5. Fredericson M, Bergman AG, Hoffman KL, et al: Tibial stress reaction in runners. Correlation of clinical symptoms and scintigraphy with a new magnetic resonance imaging grading system. Am J Sports Med 23:472–481, 1995.
6. Holen KJ, Engebretsen L, Grontuendt T, et al: Surgical treatment of medial tibial stress syndrome (shin splint) by fasciotomy of the superficial posterior compartment of the leg. Scand J Med Sci Sports 5:40–43, 1995.
7. Lidor C, Ferris LR, Hall R, et al: Stress fracture of the tibia after arthrodesis of the ankle or the hindfoot. J Bone Joint Surg 79A:558–564, 1997.
8. Mubarak SJ, et al: The medial tibial stress syndrome: A cause of shin splints. Am J Sports Med 10:201, 1992.
9. Pedowitz RA, Hargens AR, Mubarak SJ, et al: Modified criteria for the objective diagnosis of chronic compartment syndrome of the leg. Am J Sports Med 18:35, 1990.
10. Rorabeck CH, Fowler PJ, Nott L: The results of fasciotomy in the management of chronic compartment syndrome. Am J Sports Med 16:224–227, 1988.
11. Siddiqui AR: Bone scans for the early detection of stress fractures. N Engl J Med 298:1033, 1978.
12. Singerman R, White C, Davy DT: Reduction of patellofemoral contact forces following anterior displacement of the tibial tubercle. J Orthop Res 13:279–285, 1995.
13. Sommer HM, Valentine SW: Effect of foot posture on the incidence of medial tibial stress syndrome. Med Sci Sports Exerc 27:800–804, 1995.
14. Styf JR, Korner LM: Chronic anterior-compartment syndrome of the leg: Results of treatment by fasciotomy. J Bone Joint Surg 68A:1338, 1986.

83. ACUTE COMPARTMENT SYNDROME

David E. Brown, M.D.

1. What is acute compartment syndrome?

An acute increase in tissue pressure within the enclosed anatomic space (the muscle compartment that is surrounded by semirigid fascia) results in increased local venous pressure, leading to a decrease in the arteriovenous gradient and thus a decrease in arterial inflow.

2. What are the primary causes of acute compartment syndrome?

Eighty-five percent of cases of acute compartment syndrome are caused by severe trauma associated with fractures or dislocations of the leg. The remainder are generally caused by marked and prolonged increase in exercise intensity, such as a forced prolonged run in a military recruit. A small number are caused by muscle rupture, vascular injury, or prolonged externally applied pressure.

3. What are the symptoms of acute compartment syndrome?

Early symptoms
- Severe pain that increases with passive stretch of the muscles in the compartment
- Tenderness and extreme tightness of the compartment

Late symptoms
- Hypesthesia of nerves traversing the compartment
- Weakness of the muscles in the involved compartment

4. What is a normal intramuscular compartment pressure measurement at rest?

Zero to 10 mmHg.

5. At what pressure does acute compartment syndrome exist?

Any resting pressure above 40 mmHg is indicative of a compartment syndrome. Patients with values between 30 and 40 mmHg may have an impending compartment syndrome and need to be monitored very closely, often with continuous compartment pressure measurements.

6. Name the various leg compartments and the muscles within each compartment.

The four compartments include the anterior, lateral, superficial posterior, and deep posterior. The anterior compartment consists of the tibialis anterior, extensor digitorum longus, extensor hallucis longus, and peroneus tertius. The lateral compartment includes the peroneus longus and brevis. The superficial posterior has the gastrocsoleus complex, whereas the deep posterior compartment includes the posterior tibialis, flexor hallucis longus, and flexor digitorum longus.

7. Which compartment is most commonly involved in an acute compartment syndrome?

The anterior compartment is by far the most commonly involved. The lateral compartment is the next most frequent.

8. How are compartment pressures measured?

Compartment pressures may be measured using a variety of techniques, including needle manometer, wick catheter, slit catheter, and microcapillary infusion. The needle manometer pressure measurements are the easiest to obtain and require the least expensive equipment. An advantage of the wick and slit catheters is that they may be left in place, allowing serial or continuous pressure measurements without the necessity of repeated needle insertion into the leg.

9. Is a compartment syndrome more likely to occur with a closed or open tibia fracture?

A closed tibia fracture. In open tibia fractures, the muscle fascia has frequently been effectively released due to the tissue disruption at the time of injury. However, grade III open fractures *are* associated with increased risk of compartment syndrome, perhaps because of the severity of the injury.

10. What is the risk of compartment syndrome in the presence of popliteal artery injury?

Compartment syndrome does not occur in the presence of popliteal artery occlusion. Rather, it is the *reperfusion* that follows appropriate surgical repair of a popliteal artery injury that places the leg at risk for compartment syndrome. Reperfusion following the repair often leads to marked swelling and increase in intracompartment pressures. Four-compartment release is generally advised following surgical repair of complete popliteal artery injuries.

11. What is the treatment of acute compartment syndrome?

If intracompartment pressures are greater than 40 mmHg and the clinical findings are consistent with compartment syndrome, surgical decompression should be performed immediately. If compartment pressures are between 30 and 40 mmHg, the patient should be monitored closely— if possible, with continuous pressure measurements. All external rigid dressings should be removed. The leg should be positioned at the level of the heart. If this strategy does not promptly relieve symptoms, surgical decompression should be performed.

12. How is surgical decompression performed?

Fasciotomy is generally performed through one of two different methods. The first method, performed through a lateral incision, excises a portion of the proximal fibula. This lateral transfibular approach allows access to all four compartments. However, athletes in contact sports may be symptomatic following partial fibulectomy.

In athletes, it is generally advisable to perform fasciotomy through a technique that uses both a medial and lateral incision. The lateral incision allows access to the anterior and lateral compartments, whereas the medial incision allows access to both posterior compartments.

Regardless of technique, the wounds must be left open. In 5–7 days, delayed primary skin closure and skin grafting are performed. If the compartment syndrome has resulted in muscle ischemia and death, all necrotic muscle must be debrided surgically.

13. Why should the urine be monitored following treatment of acute compartment syndrome?

If muscle ischemia and death has occurred, myoglobinuria may result. The patient should be well hydrated. Renal function must be monitored closely.

14. What clinical problems are most likely to be confused with acute compartment syndrome? How are they differentiated from compartment syndrome?

The most common diagnoses confused with acute compartment syndrome are acute traumatic nerve contusion (neurapraxia), arterial injury, and traumatic hematoma.

Neurapraxia most commonly involves the peroneal nerve. The compartment pressure measurements are normal, and pain is generally not a substantial symptom.

In **arterial injury**, pulses are absent, compartment pressures are normal, and the limb is ischemic. Arterial studies are abnormal.

A large intramuscular **hematoma** may result in significant swelling and tightness of the compartment and occasionally may cause a compartment syndrome. Again, measurement of compartment pressure is essential in ruling out compartment syndrome.

15. What are the complications of compartment pressure release?

1. Neuroma of the superficial peroneal nerve where it exits from the anterior compartment
2. Postoperative infection
3. Unsightly scar

4. Neurologic injury from delayed treatment. Foot drop is most common.

5. If ischemia and death of the muscle has occurred, contractures of the involved compartment will result.

6. Weakness or fatigue of the involved compartments secondary to muscle ischemia and necrosis

7. Pain and weakness of the anterolateral compartments overlying the region of fibulectomy, if performed

16. How much time does a clinician have from the onset of acute compartment syndrome until the occurrence of tissue death and necrosis?

Muscle cell death and subsequent necrosis may occur as early as 4 hours following the onset of compartment syndrome. Muscle tissue rarely remains viable if 8 hours have elapsed prior to restoration of perfusion.

BIBLIOGRAPHY

1. Almdahl SM, Due J Jr, Samdal FA: Compartment syndrome with muscle necrosis following repair of hernia of tibialis anterior. Acta Chir Scand 153(11–12):695, 1987.
2. Azar FM, Pickering RM: Traumatic disorders. In Canale ST (ed): Campbell's Operative Orthopaedics, 9th ed. St. Louis, Mosby, 1998, pp 1405–1416.
3. Blacklidge DK. Kurek JB, Soto AD, et al: Acute exertional compartment syndrome of the medial foot. J Foot Ankle Surg 35:19–22, 1996.
4. Blick SS, Brumback RJ, Poka A, et al: Compartment syndrome in open tibial fractures. J Bone Joint Surg 68A:1348–1353, 1986.
5. Cohen MS, Garfin SR, Hargens AR, Mubarak SJ: Acute compartment syndrome: Effect of dermotomy on fascial decompression in the leg. J Bone Joint Surg 73A:287–290, 1991.
6. Gershuni DH, Mubarak SJ, Yaru NC, Lee YF: Fracture of the tibia complicated by acute compartment syndrome. Clin Orthop 217:221–227, 1987.
7. Gwynne Jones DP, Theis JC: Acute compartment syndrome due to closed muscle rupture. Aust N Z J Surg 67:227–228, 1997.
8. Heppenstall RB, Scott R, Sapega A, et al: A comparative study of the tolerance of skeletal muscle to ischemia: Tourniquet application compared with acute compartment syndrome. J Bone Joint Surg 68A:820–828, 1986.
9. Papalambros EL, Panayiotopoulos YP, Bastounis E, et al: Prophylactic fasciotomy of the legs following acute arterial occlusion procedures. Int Angiol 8:120–124, 1989.
10. Rorabeck CH: The treatment of compartment syndromes of the leg. J Bone Joint Surg 66A:93–97, 1984.
11. Rooser B, Bengtson S, Hagglund G: Acute compartment syndrome from anterior thigh muscle contusion: A report of eight cases. J Orthop Trauma 5:57–59, 1991.

84. ACHILLES TENDON

David E. Brown, M.D.

1. What are the causes of Achilles tendinitis?
- Inflexibility of the tendo Achillis
- Overpronation
- Recent change in shoe wear
- Recent increase in training, especially if it includes hill running

2. What are the signs and symptoms of acute Achilles tendinitis?
- Pain over the distal Achilles tendon
- Swelling
- Painful push-off phase of running or jumping

3. How is acute Achilles tendinitis treated?
1. Relative rest (avoid painful, aggravating activities)
2. Ice and/or contrast treatments
3. Antiinflammatory medication
4. Orthotics/heel lift
5. **Stretching**

If symptoms are severe and recalcitrant to the above measures, a short period of cast immobilization may be necessary.

4. What is the treatment of chronic Achilles tendinitis?
The initial treatment of chronic Achilles tendinitis is the same as for acute injuries. Persistent symptoms, especially in individuals who have a discrete area of thickening in the tendon on physical examination, may be because of a partial tear. The tear may be evaluated by MRI.

5. How should I treat the patient with chronic Achilles tendinitis who is unresponsive to the above conservative management?
If the individual has had symptoms for at least 6 months, has been engaged in a defined physical therapy program, and has symptoms that prevent him or her from participating in athletics or work, surgical treatment may be offered. Preoperative evaluation with MRI is usually involved. The tendon is explored, partial tears of the tendon are surgically debrided, and remaining tissue is repaired as necessary. A thickening of the peritenon should be incised or excised. Satisfactory results are obtained in two-thirds of patients. Proximal tears (> 3 cm above the calcaneus) do better than distal tears.

6. Why isn't cortisone injected into the Achilles tendon when it is either acutely or chronically inflamed?
Injection of the Achilles tendon or its sheath has been implicated as the cause of subsequent Achilles tendon rupture. Corticosteroids markedly decrease the metabolic rate of chondrocytes and fibrocytes, thereby weakening the structural integrity of tendon and articular cartilage.

7. Who is most at risk for sustaining an Achilles tendon tear?
Tears are most commonly seen in males between the ages of 30 and 50 years who are generally recreational athletes or nonathletes engaged in white-collar occupations. During participation in a jumping sport, a sudden forceful contraction of the Achilles causes a rupture. At least 50% of patients who sustain complete tears have had preexisting symptoms of chronic tendinitis.

8. Describe the physical findings in an acute complete Achilles tendon rupture.
A palpable defect in the tendon is present as the proximal tendon retracts following rupture. The gap is usually 2–3 cm long. Within 24–48 hours, marked swelling and ecchymosis usually occur. The patient is able to weakly plantarflex the foot. The Thompson test is positive.

9. What is the Thompson test?
With the patient supine and the affected foot over the end of the table, squeeze the calf and observe for ankle motion. A positive Thompson test occurs when *no* plantar flexion of the ankle occurs when the calf is squeezed. The test is positive in acute complete Achilles tendon tears. In a gastrocnemius muscle tear, no defect in the tendon is present, and the foot plantarflexes as the calf is squeezed during the Thompson test.

10. What is important about the vascular supply to the Achilles tendon?
An area of relative hypovascularity is found 2–5 cm proximal to the Achilles tendon insertion, which is where most Achilles tendon ruptures occur.

11. How are tears of the Achilles tendon treated?

Surgical repair is generally indicated. Sedentary individuals may choose to have the Achilles tear immobilized in an equinus cast for 4–6 weeks, followed by a short-leg walking cast for another 4–6 weeks.

Repair of the Achilles tendon rupture results in improvement in maximum ankle plantar flexion strength, particularly in the aggressive athlete. The risk of re-rupture is much less (2% re-rupture rate in the surgically treated group compared with 8% re-rupture rate in the nonoperative group). However, surgical treatment carries the risk of anesthetic complication, skin and soft tissue breakdown, and neuroma of the sural nerve.

12. How should the patient be rehabilitated after repair of an Achilles tendon rupture?

Rehabilitation is controversial. The conservative approach places the repaired tendon in a cast for up to 3 months. Initially the cast is in an equinus cast so that theoretically the tension is taken off the repair site. The more aggressive approach places the leg in a splint for as little as 1–3 weeks after surgery, followed by a dorsiflexion stop splint, which allows the patient to plantarflex the foot from the neutral position but prevents dorsiflexion past neutral, thereby eliminating excessive tension on the repair site. Animal studies have indicated that early mild tension coupled with motion at tendon repair sites enhances healing by hastening the alignment of collagen fibrils at the repair site. Controlled clinical studies that compare these two methods of rehabilitation have not been performed.

13. How much strain is there on the Achilles tendon repair during weightbearing/walking?

Minimal. Animal studies demonstrate that the strain is not statistically greater than ambulation in a non–weight-bearing cast.

14. Does the plantaris muscle really rupture?

Years ago it was thought that patients with a sudden pop and pain in the medial calf had sustained a rupture of the plantaris muscle, commonly called "tennis leg." However, the plantaris muscle has never been shown to be torn in this setting. On the contrary, plantaris muscle is noted to be present and not ruptured in individuals who have sustained an acute Achilles tendon rupture and is frequently used as a tissue donor source to reinforce the Achilles repair. The injury sustained in this clinical situation is more likely a partial disruption of the medial head of the gastrocnemius muscle belly.

15. What is the treatment of a partial tear of the medial head of the gastrocnemius muscle?

- Heel lift and calf sleeve
- Avoidance of running, jumping, and push-off activities for approximately 4–6 weeks
- Ice massage
- Gentle stretching as tolerated

BIBLIOGRAPHY

1. Incavo SJ, Alvarez RG, Trevino SG: Occurrence of the plantaris tendon in patients sustaining subcutaneous rupture of the Achilles tendon. Foot Ankle 8:110, 1987.
2. James SL, Bates BT, Osterning LR: Injuries to runners. Am J Sports Med 6:40, 1978.
3. Morberg P, Jerre R, Sward L, et al: Long-term results after surgical management of partial Achilles tendon ruptures. Scand J Med Sci Sports 7:299–303, 1997.
4. Motta P, Errichiello C, Pontini I: Achilles tendon rupture. A new technique for easy surgical repair and immediate movement of the ankle and foot. Am J Sports Med 25:172–176, 1997.
5. Nelen G, Martens M, Burssens A: Surgical treatment of chronic Achilles tendinitis. Am J Sports Med 17:754, 1989.
6. Nistor L: Surgical and non-surgical treatment of Achilles tendon ruptures. J Bone Joint Surg 63A:394, 1981.
7. Pritchett JW: C-reactive protein levels determine the severity of soft-tissue injuries. Am J Orthop 25:759–761, 1996.
8. Richardson EG: Disorders of tendons and fascia. In Canale ST (ed): Campbell's Operative Orthopaedics, 9th ed. St. Louis, Mosby, 1998, pp 1889–1925.

9. Roberts JM, Goldstrom GL, Brown TD, et al: Comparison of unrepaired, primarily repaired, and poly-galactin mesh-reinforced Achilles tendon lacerations in rabbits. Clin Orthop 181:244, 1993.
10. Rupp S, Tempelhof S, Fritsch E: Ultrasound of the Achilles tendon after surgical repair: Morphology and function. Br J Radiol 68:454–458, 1995.
11. Shields CL, Redix L, Brewster CE: Acute tears of the medial head of the gastrocnemius. Foot Ankle 5:186, 1985.
12. Thompson TC, Doherty JH: Spontaneous rupture of the tendon of the Achilles: A new clinical diagnostic test. J Trauma 2:126, 1962.
13. Watson TW, Jurist UA, Yang UH, Shen UL: The strength of Achilles tendon repair: An in vitro study of the biomechanical behavior in human cadaver tendons. Foot Ankle Int 16:191–195, 1995.

85. TIBIAL FRACTURES

Matthew A. Mormino, M.D.

1. Describe the appropriate evaluation of a patient with a tibial fracture.

The evaluation of all trauma victims should follow advanced trauma life support (ATLS) protocol. The extremity should be inspected for deformity, tenderness, and crepitus. A baseline neurologic exam should document the status of motor function and sensory response to pinprick and light touch. A vascular exam should include palpation and Doppler evaluation of the dorsalis pedis and posterior tibial pulses. If pulses are absent, the extremity should be gently realigned and the exam repeated. The presence of soft-tissue injuries should be noted. Compartment syndrome may appear early after a tibia fracture and should be looked for. An anteroposterior and lateral x-ray that includes the knee and ankle should be obtained.

2. What are the signs and symptoms of acute compartment syndrome in the leg?

Pain out of proportion to the injury is the hallmark finding. Pain with passive stretch of the toes and ankle and palpably tense compartments are the other important findings. Pulselessness, pallor, paresthesias, and paralysis are findings associated with established or late compartment syndrome. In an awake patient this clinical diagnosis should be treated emergently. Compartment pressure measurements may be relied on to confirm a diagnosis of acute compartment syndrome only in obtunded or anesthetized patients (epidural and spinal anesthesia also may mask the symptoms).

3. How is acute compartment syndrome treated?

Emergent release of all four compartments of the leg (anterior, lateral, superficial posterior, deep posterior) should be performed in all cases of acute compartment syndrome via a lateral incision or medial and lateral incisions.

4. Describe Gustilo's open fracture classification.

Type I: < 1-cm wound, low-energy fracture
Type II: 1–10-cm wound, higher energy fracture
Type III: > 10-cm wound, high-energy fracture
Type IIIA: Moderate periosteal stripping, wound closure not requiring soft tissue flap
Type IIIB: Marked periosteal stripping, wound closure requires soft tissue flap
Type IIIC: Any open fracture with a vascular injury that requires repair

This classification system is the source of endless arguments among orthopaedists; do not feel bad if you cannot accurately classify a fracture. Chances are, neither can your attending.

5. How should an open tibial fracture be treated in the emergency room?

Evaluate and treat all life-threatening injuries according to ATLS protocol. Document the soft-tissue injury and neurovascular exam. Remove gross debris, apply a sterile dressing, and splint the extremity. Probing, irrigating, and culturing of the wound should be done in the operating room as part of a formal irrigation and debridement. Start appropriate antibiotics.

6. Which antibiotics are appropriate for an open fracture?

A first-generation cephalosporin (Ancef) should be given for all open fractures. Add an aminoglycoside (gentamicin) for type III injuries, and add penicillin for barnyard or heavily contaminated wounds. Tetanus status should be assessed and updated or treated appropriately.

7. What are the indications for casting a tibial fracture?

Closed reduction and casting is an option only in closed low-energy fractures in young patients. After an acceptable reduction, the fracture is placed in a long leg cast for 6–8 weeks and then replaced with a short-leg cast or fracture brace until the fracture heals. Healing rates of 90% may be expected. However, recent studies suggest that long-term knee and ankle function is improved in patients treated with operative stabilization.

8. What is an acceptable reduction?

Less than 1 cm shortening, $< 5°$ angulation in any plane, $< 10°$ of malrotation, and $> 50\%$ cortical apposition.

9. What are the indications for operative fixation?

Failure to achieve an adequate reduction, multiple trauma, ipsilateral femoral fracture, bilateral tibial fractures, fractures with compartment syndrome, fractures with vascular injury, and pathologic fractures.

10. When is external fixation recommended?

External fixation is considered the gold standard for treatment of type III open tibial fractures. Recent studies that show similar infection rates and union rates with lower rates of malalignment challenge this practice.

11. When is intramedullary nailing recommended?

Failed closed treatment and unstable fractures are the main indications for intramedullary (IM) nailing. Some authors recommend IM nailing for all open fractures.

12. What are the main differences between reamed and unreamed tibial nailing?

Reamed nailing involves machining the medullary canal to allow intimate endosteal cortical contact and passage of a large diameter nail. The use of a smaller diameter nail without reaming is indicated primarily for open fractures. The main advantage of unreamed tibial nailing is that the medullary blood supply reconstitutes faster (however, it is disrupted by the passage of the nail). The primary disadvantage is that the smaller diameter nail has a less intimate fit and is thus a less stable construct.

13. What is the infection rate for open tibial fractures?

Type I and II: 1–2%; Type IIIA: 3–5%; Type IIIB and C: 40–50%.

14. How are infections managed?

Irrigation and debridement of all necrotic tissue is mandatory. Removal of hardware is indicated if the fracture is healed or if the hardware is loose. The hardware is retained if the fracture is not healed and the hardware is stable. Antibiotics are used to suppress the infection until the fracture is healed and the hardware is removed.

15. What are the soft tissue coverage options for open tibial fractures?

Exposed bone should be covered in 5 days with muscle or fasciocutaneous flaps. In proximal third fractures, use a gastrocnemius flap; in middle third fractures use a soleus flap (however, the soleus is often damaged by the trauma); and in distal third fractures use a free muscle flap.

16. Describe a tibial plateau fracture.

Fractures involving the articular surface of the proximal tibia are termed tibial plateau fractures. They are usually the result of an axial loading mechanism and may involve one or both condyles and often have both split and depressed fractures. Knee ligament injury occurs in 10–20% of such fractures.

17. What are the operative indications for tibial plateau fractures?

This is controversial. Fracture type, patient age, and the patient's functional demands all influence treatment choices. In general, articular stepoff of > 3 mm, depression of > 5 mm, varus or valgus laxity > 10°, and fractures involving the medial plateau are operative indications.

18. What is a Segond fracture?

A Segond fracture is an avulsion fracture of the medial tibial plateau and usually signifies an anterior cruciate ligament injury.

19. What is a tibial pilon fracture?

Fractures that involve the articular surface of the tibia are termed pilon fractures. They usually result from an axial load impacting the talus into the distal tibia. Comminution and massive soft tissue injury reflect the high-energy trauma resulting in such injuries. Surgery is aimed at restoration of the joint surface and preservation of the tenuous soft tissue envelope.

BIBLIOGRAPHY

1. Gustilo RB, Anderson JT: Prevention of infection in the treatment of one thousand and twenty-five open fractures of long bones. J Bone Joint Surg 58A:453–458, 1976.
2. Hansen ST Jr, Swiontkowski MF (eds): Orthopaedic Trauma Protocols. New York, Raven Press, 1993.
3. Mast JW, et al: Fractures of the tibial pilon. Clin Orthop 230:68–82, 1988.
4. Rockwood CA Jr, Green DP, Bucholz RW, Heckman JD (eds): Rockwood and Green's Fractures in Adults, vols. 1 and 2, 4th ed. Philadelphia, J.B. Lippincott, 1996.
5. Schemitsch EH, et al: Comparison of the effects of reamed and unreamed locked intramedullary nailing on blood flow in the callus and strength of union following fracture of the sheep tibia. J Orthop Res 13:382–389, 1995.
6. Whittle AP: Fractures of lower extremity. In Canale ST (ed): Campbell's Operative Orthopaedics, 9th ed. St. Louis, Mosby, 1998, pp 2067–2111.

X. Foot and Ankle

86. ANKLE SPRAINS

Craig R. Mahoney, M.D.

1. In a patient with acute ankle pain, what are the important historical points that need to be covered?

- Mechanism of injury—position the foot was in both before and after the traumatic event
- Location of pain—medial or lateral, proximal or distal
- Weight-bearing ability
- Patient age
- Time of injury
- History of prior injury

2. What are the important physical findings?

Swelling, ecchymoses, tenderness, neurovascular status, range of motion, crepitus, stability, and deformity are all important to note.

3. Which radiographic views are necessary during the initial work-up?

Ankle radiographs include an anteroposterior (AP), lateral, and mortise view. If a foot injury is suspected, an AP, lateral, and oblique view of the foot should each be obtained as well.

4. If no fractures exist, what are the three most likely diagnoses?

An inversion/eversion sprain or a muscular or tendinous injury is most likely. The inversion sprain is most common, constituting approximately 85% of all ankle sprains.

5. Describe the findings consistent with an inversion sprain.

The most obvious finding is the mechanism of rolling over the foot onto the lateral ankle. A previous history of similar sprains is also common. On physical exam anterolateral tenderness and swelling with a positive anterior drawer test should be present (see question 6). Pain is typically not severe enough to inhibit weightbearing, and no bony crepitus should be present.

6. How is the anterior drawer test administered, and what constitutes a positive anterior drawer test?

The test is performed by stabilizing the distal tibia with one hand and grasping the posterior heel with the other. Then, an anterior force is applied to the posterior heel in an effort to displace the talus anteriorly. A large shift anteriorly, or even a palpable clunk in severe cases, indicates a positive anterior drawer test. The uninjured ankle should be examined for comparison.

7. Which lateral ligament is most commonly injured?

The lateral ligament most commonly injured is the anterior talofibular ligament, which is the primary stabilizer of the ankle in plantar flexion. The calcaneofibular ligament is a secondary stabilizer and resists inversion of the talus and calcaneus. The calcaneofibular ligament is usually disrupted in association with a tear of the anterior talofibular ligament. The posterior talofibular ligament is rarely sprained.

8. Describe the findings consistent with an eversion sprain.

An eversion sprain occurs when the foot is caught in a pronated, everted position with concomitant internal rotation of the upper body. Swelling and tenderness is present medially and possibly higher up the leg, indicating a syndesmosis injury. Such patients have pain with an eversion stress to their ankles but have a negative anterior drawer test.

9. Which structure is primarily injured in an eversion sprain?
   The deltoid ligament is primarily injured in an eversion sprain. It originates from the inferior portion of the medial malleolus and attaches to the medial talar neck and body. It functions to stabilize the ankle during eversion and prevents subluxation of the talus.

10. How do you classify ankle sprains?
   Grade I   Negative anterior drawer and talar tilt test
   Grade II   Positive anterior drawer/negative talar tilt test
   Grade III Positive anterior drawer and talar tilt test

11. What is the talar tilt test?
   The talar tilt test examines the integrity of the calcaneofibular ligament and the anterior talofibular ligament. It is performed by grasping the foot and heel while attempting to invert the talus on the tibia.

12. What is a normal talar tilt test?
   Normal individuals rarely have a talar tilt test $> 5°$. A marked difference when compared with the opposite uninjured ankle usually represents insufficiency of the anterior talofibular and calcaneofibular ligaments. Clinically, this is hard to interpret. Stress x-rays are often helpful.

13. When are talar tilt stress x-rays positive?
   When compared with the contralateral normal extremity, a difference of $10°$ is considered a positive test.

14. What is the initial treatment for a mild (grade I) ankle sprain?
   Rest, ice, compression, and elevation (RICE). Protected weight-bearing with early mobilization and range-of-motion and isometric exercises are also involved. If the patient is improving, after 2–3 weeks advance to ankle group muscle strengthening, proprioceptive training, and functional activities with protective bracing.

15. What is the treatment for more severe ankle sprains (grade II or III) and for patients with mild sprains that do not improve?
   Patients with severe sprains or sprains recalcitrant to initial home rehabilitation benefit from a supervised rehabilitation program that progressively advances weightbearing in a protected manner using isometrics or closed kinetic chain exercises. Such patients also often benefit from proprioceptive training. More severe sprains may require compressive bracing for up to 6 months during sports.

16. What structures make up the syndesmotic ligaments and what is their function?
   Four ligaments form the syndesmotic ligament complex: (1) the anterior tibiofibular ligament, (2) the posterior tibiofibular ligament, (3) the transverse tibiofibular ligament, and (4) the interosseous ligament. The four ligaments maintain the integrity between the distal tibia and the fibula and resist the axial, rotational, and translational forces that would otherwise separate the two bones.

17. In a patient with a suspected eversion ankle sprain (see question 8), how is a syndesmosis injury diagnosed? How is it treated?
   Patients have extreme tenderness over the syndesmosis, a positive squeeze test, pain with external rotation of the ankle, and pain with weightbearing. Treatment should be supervised, consisting of RICE, toe-touch weight-bearing until pain-free, gradual mobilization and range-of-motion exercises, and progressive strengthening exercises, and proprioceptive training.

18. Describe the squeeze test.
   The squeeze test is performed by squeezing the distal fibular and tibia together. A positive test is indicated by tenderness over the syndesmosis and is consistent with an injury to this area.

19. What is the treatment for tibiofibular diastasis (complete syndesmosis tear)?

In this injury, the ligaments holding the tibia and fibula have ruptured completely. The mortise needs to be held together with a syndesmosis screw. The distance between the tibia and fibula will be fixed and stable after screw fixation.

20. What are the findings in a patient with a muscle or tendon injury to the ankle?

The patient has swelling or bruising over the injured muscle or tendon. A palpable defect in the injured area may be found along with tenderness. The specific function of the injured muscle should be tested to determine its integrity. No crepitus or significant bony tenderness should be present.

21. What are the three tendon injuries in the ankle that always need to be excluded before diagnosing an ankle sprain?

Achilles tendon rupture

Tibialis posterior tendon dysfunction or rupture

Peroneal tendon instability or rupture

22. What are the hallmark findings in Achilles tendon rupture?

Patients have a history of a sudden, severe pop. They have pain and swelling over the Achilles tendon or calf and may have a palpable defect in their tendon in addition to weak plantar flexion strength and a positive Thompson test.

23. How is the Thompson test conducted?

The patient is placed prone with the affected knee bent at 90°. The calf is squeezed and the foot is examined for plantar flexion. No plantar flexion with squeezing indicates a division in the Achilles tendon complex and and a positive Thompson test.

24. What are the hallmark findings in posterior tibial tendon dysfunction or rupture?

A pre-existing or increased flat foot (pes planus) deformity, swelling or tenderness medially and posterior to the medial malleolus, abduction deformity of the midfoot, decreased heel inversion on heel rise test, or inability to do heel rise.

25. What are the hallmark findings in peroneal tendon instability or rupture?

A history of an external rotation or eversion injury, pain in the lateral ankle and posterior to the lateral malleolus, tenderness along the muscle/tendon unit and, occasionally, dislocatable tendons with resisted eversion/plantar flexion.

26. Despite the correct treatment, what percentage of patients who suffer a grade III ankle sprain will have persistent pain or instability that limits their activities?

Approximately 20–40% of such patients are reported to have residual pain necessitating an alteration in their activities. Often the pain can be localized to the anterior or anterolateral ankle.

27. What is the differential diagnosis for a patient who presents with persistent pain after an ankle sprain?

The possible diagnoses include incomplete rehabilitation, intraarticular injuries, chronic instability, sprain across an adjacent joint, impingement, a meniscoid lesion, sinus tarsi syndrome, and stress fractures.

28. When does impingement occur? How is it treated?

Impingement occurs when the anterior capsule of the ankle is repeatedly traumatized during dorsi and plantar flexion. The trauma may eventually lead to calcifications that form off the anterior edge of the distal tibia. It may be treated nonoperatively with ice and antiinflammatory medications. If the process is recalcitrant to the initial therapy, the spur that forms can be resected arthroscopically.

29. What is sinus tarsi syndrome?

Pain and tenderness over the opening of the sinus tarsi characterize sinus tarsi syndrome. It is accompanied by a sensation of instability that in most cases occurs after trauma. Injecting anesthetic and steroid into the sinus tarsi usually relieves pain; however, some chronic cases may require tissue excision or even subtalar arthrodesis.

30. What is a meniscoid lesion?

A meniscoid lesion is a localized fibrotic synovitis in the lateral compartment of the ankle caused by repetitive sprains. Treatment consists of arthroscopic excision of scar tissue.

31. In the acute setting, when is surgery indicated for an ankle sprain?

Never. Studies have shown no advantage in surgical repair for ankle sprains when compared with nonoperative treatment.

32. What are the indications for surgical repair of a chronic ankle sprain?

Failure of nonoperative treatment with residual mechanical symptoms of instability, episodes of giving way, and chronic pain are the most commonly reported indications for surgical repair of a chronic ankle sprain. Isolated mechanical instability by itself in the absence of giving-way episodes is not an appropriate reason. Less than 1% of patients with ankle sprains will require surgery.

33. What are the different operations that may manage chronic ankle instability?

Approximately 50 procedures are designed to stabilize the chronically sprained ankle and may be classified into two groups: (1) anatomic reconstructions and (2) nonanatomic reconstructions.

34. Describe an anatomic ankle reconstruction.

An anatomic ankle reconstruction repairs the injured ligament secondarily with or without augmentation. Examples of this are the Brostrom repair and the Gould modification of the Brostrom repair. Brostrom originally found it possible to repair chronic ankle ligament injuries by direct suture. Later techniques involving shortening of the ligaments and directly reimplanting them into bone have been highly successful. Gould later reinforced the anterior talofibular ligament with the extensor retinaculum and reinforced the calcaneofibular ligament with the lateral talocalcaneal ligament.

35. Describe a nonanatomic ankle reconstruction.

A nonanatomic reconstruction substitutes another structure or material to take the place of a damaged ligament. An example of this is the Chrisman-Snook modification of the Elmslie procedure, which uses half of the peroneus brevis tendon to reconstruct both the anterior talofibular ligament and the calcaneofibular ligament.

Left, Brostrom repair. The anterior talofibular and calcaneofibular ligaments are reimplanted into bone, achieving an anatomic reconstruction. *Right,* Crisman-Snook repair. One-half of the peroneus brevis tendon is used to reconstruct both the anterior talofibular ligament and the calcaneofibular ligament.

BIBLIOGRAPHY

1. Adamson C, Cymet T: Ankle sprains: Evaluation, treatment, rehabilitation. Md Med J 46(10):530–537, 1997.
2. Brown DE: Ankle and leg injuries. In Mellion MB, Walsh M, Shelton GL (eds): The Team Physician's Handbook, 2nd ed. Philadelphia, Hanley & Belfus, 1997, pp 579–592.
3. Larkin J, Brage M: Ankle, hindfoot, and midfoot injuries. In Reider B: Sports Medicine: The School Aged Athlete. Philadelphia, W.B. Saunders, 1991, p 366.
4. McBryde A: Disorders of ankle and foot. In Grana WA, Kalenak A (eds): Clinical Sports Medicine. Philadelphia, W.B. Saunders, 1991, p 466.
5. Povacz P, Salzberg FU, Wels KM, et al: A randomized, prospective study of operative and non-operative treatment of injuries of the fibular collateral ligaments of the ankle. J Bone Joint Surg 80A:345–351, 1998.
6. Renstrom PA: Persistently painful sprained ankle. J Am Acad Orthop Surg 2:270–280, 1994.
7. Wexler RK: The injured ankle. Am Fam Physician 57(3):474–480, 1998.

87. FOOT AND ANKLE TRAUMA

Scott T. McMullen, M.D.

1. What is a Jones fracture?

It is a fracture of the proximal fifth metatarsal diaphysis approximately 1.5 cm from the tip of the tuberosity. It has a potential for nonunion and must be distinguished from the oblique avulsion fracture of the tuberosity of the fifth metatarsal, which tends to heal without complication.

2. What is a march fracture?

A march fracture is a stress fracture of a metatarsal. It carries this name because of its frequent occurrence in military personnel.

3. What are the main principles in dealing with fractures and dislocations of the ankle?

1. Reduction of the injury should be performed as soon as possible.
2. The reduction must be maintained during the healing period with either external immobilization such as a cast or internal fixation devices.
3. All joint surfaces must be reduced anatomically to help diminish the risk of post-traumatic arthritis.

4. What is the ankle syndesmosis?

It is the relationship or articulation between the distal tibia and fibula, and is maintained by the interosseous membrane, the anterior/inferior tibiofibular ligament, the posterior inferior tibiofibular ligament, the posterior talofibular ligament, and the inferior transverse ligament.

5. What complications may occur following ankle fractures or dislocations?

Posttraumatic arthritis	Nonunion
Reflex sympathetic dystrophy (RSD)	Malunion
Neurovascular injury	Infection (particularly if the fracture was open or operated on)

6. What is a worrisome complication of fractures of the talar neck?

Avascular necrosis (AVN) of the talar body.

7. What is the radiographic appearance of AVN of the talus?

Increased density of the avascular body is seen compared with the surrounding bone, which is vascular and undergoing disuse resorption. Hawkin's sign is the presence of subchondral osteopenia and excludes the diagnosis of AVN. Bone scanning or magnetic resonance imaging also may be helpful in the diagnosis of AVN.

8. Which x-ray views are necessary when evaluating an injured ankle?
Anteroposterior, lateral, and mortise views. The mortise view is taken with the leg internally rotated approximately 15–20°, which aligns the beam perpendicular to the intermalleolar line.

9. What is a pylon fracture?
A pylon fracture is a distal tibial metaphyseal fracture with extension into the joint surface, usually with extensive comminution.

10. When evaluating a person with a calcaneus fracture, you must consider injuries to what other areas?
It is important not to overlook potential spinal injuries. A typical mechanism in both fractures is axial loading. Other associated fractures include femoral neck fractures and tibial plateau fractures.

11. Name two complications of calcaneal fractures.
1. Posttraumatic arthritis involving the subtalar joint and possibly the calcaneal cuboid joint
2. Impingement of the peroneal tendons laterally secondary to calcaneal widening

12. Can a compartment syndrome develop in the foot?
Yes. One must consider surgical decompression if this is diagnosed.

13. What are the compartments of the foot?
The four osteofascial compartments of the foot are:
1. The medial compartment consists of the abductor hallucis and flexor hallucis brevis.
2. The lateral compartment contains the abductor digiti minimi, flexor digitorum brevis, and opponens digiti minimi.
3. The central compartment contains the flexor digitorum brevis, the lumbricals, the quadrates plantae, and the adductor hallucis.
4. The interosseous compartment contains the interosseous muscles.

14. What are the common mechanisms of ankle fractures?

Adduction	External rotation
Abduction	Vertical loading

15. How are ankle fractures classified?
The two most common are the Lauge-Hansen and the Danis-Weber AO classification systems.

16. What is the Lauge-Hansen classification?
The Lauge-Hansen classification is based on the suspected mechanism of injury. In each category, the injury begins in a specific anatomic location and progresses sequentially about the ankle, creating the injury patterns described.
Supination adduction (SA)
I. Transverse avulsion type fracture of the fibula below the level of the tibial plafond
II. Vertical fracture of the medial malleolus
Supination external rotation (SER)
I. Disruption of anterior tibiofibular ligament
II. Spiral oblique fracture of the distal fibula originating near the level of the tibial plafond
III. Disruption of the posterior tibiofibular ligament or fracture of posterior malleolus
IV. Oblique fracture of medial malleolus or rupture of deltoid ligament

Pronation adduction (PA)

I. Transverse fracture of medial malleolus or rupture of deltoid ligament

II. Rupture of syndesmotic ligaments

III. Short horizontal or oblique fracture of the fibula above the level of the ankle joint

Pronation external rotation (PER)

I. Transverse fracture of the medial malleolus or disruption of the deltoid ligament

II. Disruption of anterior tibiofibular ligament

III. Oblique fracture of the fibula approximately 4–5 cm above the level of the tibial plafond

IV. Rupture of the posterior tibiofibular ligament or avulsion fracture of the posterior lateral tibia

Pronation dorsiflexion (PD)

I. Fracture of medial malleolus

II. Fracture of anterior margin of tibia

III. Supramalleolar fracture of fibula

IV. Transverse fracture of posterior tibial surface

17. **What is the Danis-Weber AO classification system?**

It is based on the level of the fibula fracture.

Type A, fibular fracture below syndesmosis

1. Isolated fracture
2. With associated fracture of medial malleolus
3. With associated posterior medial tibia fracture

Type B, fibular fracture at level of syndesmosis

1. Isolated
2. With associated medial malleolus or deltoid ligament injury
3. With associated medial lesion and fracture of posterior lateral tibia

Type C, fibular fracture above syndemosis

1. Isolated fibular fracture
2. Comminuted fibular fracture
3. Proximal fracture of the fibula

18. **What is an injury to the tarsal metatarsal joint area called?**

This joint is known as Lisfranc's joint. Injuries may include disruption of the ligaments supporting the joints and associated fractures. For subtle injuries, displacement may be seen only on a weight-bearing oblique view of this region. Anatomic reduction is mandatory.

19. **How are talus fractures classified?**

The Hawkins classification system is used:

Type I: Nondisplaced vertical fracture of the talar neck

Type II: Displaced fracture of the talar neck with subluxation or dislocation of the subtalar joint with the ankle joint remaining intact

Type III: Displaced fracture of the talar neck with dislocation of the body of the talus from both the subtalar and ankle joints

The risk of AVN increases as the amount of displacement increases.

20. **What is unique about the blood supply to the talus?**

Approximately 60% of the talus is covered by articular surface. Thus, only limited areas are available for vascular perforation. Most of the vascularity of the body of the talus is supplied in retrograde fashion. Displaced fractures of the neck pose the risk of AVN.

21. **On the mortise view, the distance between the medial malleolus and medial border of the talus is known as the medial clear space. What is its typical distance?**

Normally, this space is symmetric with the superior clear space between the talus and distal tibia. A space > 4 mm is considered abnormal, indicating lateral talar shift and a need for either closed or open reduction.

BIBLIOGRAPHY

1. Hawkins LG: Fractures of the neck of the talus. J Bone Joint Surg 52A:991–1002, 1970.
2. Jones R: Fracture of the base of the fifth metatarsal by indirect violence. Ann Surg 35:697–700, 1902.
3. Lauge–Hansen N: Fractures of the ankle combined experimental-surgical and experimental-roentgeno-logic investigations. Arch Surg 60:967–985, 1950.
4. Manoly A II: Compartment syndromes of the foot: Current concepts. Foot Ankle 10:340–344, 1990.
5. Myerson MS: Experimental decompression of fascial compartments of the foot with a basis for fas-ciotomy in acute compartment syndrome. Foot Ankle 8:308–314, 1988.
6. Rockwood CA Jr, Greene DP, Bucholz RW, Heckman JD (eds): Fractures in Adults, vols. 1 and 2, 4th ed. Philadelphia, Lippincott-Raven, 1996.
7. Whittle AP: Fractures of lower extremity. In Canale ST (ed): Campbell's Operative Orthopaedics, 9th ed. St. Louis, Mosby, 1998, pp 2043–2066.

88. FOREFOOT SYNDROMES

Scott T. McMullen, M.D.

HALLUX VALGUS

1. What is a bunion?

The term bunion is used to describe a deformity of the great toe metatarsophalangeal (MTP) joint in which there is a medial prominence and lateral deviation of the great toe. Bunion is derived from the Latin word *bunio*, which means turnip. Bunion deformity is more correctly called hallux valgus.

2. What is hallux valgus?

Hallux valgus is static subluxation of the great toe MTP joint with lateral deviation of the great toe. Occasionally it is associated with medial deviation of the first metatarsal.

3. Are narrow shoes the only cause of the hallux valgus deformity?

No. Shoewear may play a large role in its development, particularly in feet that are symptomatic. The deformity does occur, however, in societies and cultures where shoewear is limited.

4. What are possible factors affecting the development of hallux valgus?
- Heredity
- Flat feet (pes planus)
- Metatarsus primus varus
- Hypermobile first metatarsal cuneiform joints
- Abnormal length of first metatarsal
- Joint hyperlaxity

5. What is the normal first MTP joint angle (HV angle)?

The normal first MTP joint angle is $\leq 15°$.

6. What is the normal intermetatarsal angle (IMA = the angle between the first and second metatarsals)?

The normal intermetatarsal angle is $\leq 9°$.

7. Can a painful hallux valgus deformity be treated without operative intervention?

Yes. Shoewear modification to increase the width of the toe box, which relieves direct pressure, may be helpful. Pads or splints also may help to relieve symptoms.

8. What is hallux interphalangeus?

It is lateral deviation of the great toe secondary to deformity within the proximal phalanx or at the interphalangeal (IP) joint. It may be seen with a hallux valgus deformity.

9. What is the primary goal of surgery in the hallux valgus deformity?

The primary goal is to restore the normal anatomic relation of the great toe MTP joint.

10. List the surgical options for hallux valgus deformity.

1. Medial eminence resection (simple bunionectomy)
2. Distal soft tissue correction at the MTP joint
3. Distal soft tissue correction with osteotomy of the proximal metatarsal
4. Osteotomy of the distal aspect of the first metatarsal (Chevron osteotomy)
5. Resection of a portion of the proximal phalanx (Keller procedure)
6. Fusion of the metatarsal phalangeal joint
7. Fusion of the metatarsocuneiform joint and distal soft tissue procedure (Lapidus)

11. What are the main indications for performing various hallux valgus surgeries?

Isolated distal soft-tissue procedures can be used only if a congruent joint, normal IMA, and HV angle < 30° are present.

Chevron osteotomy has similar indications, but also may be used with an incongruent joint. It can correct an IMA < 15°.

Proximal osteotomy with distal soft-tissue realignment can correct any IMA and hallux valgus angle, and thus is especially useful when the IMA is > 15° and/or the HV angle is > 30°.

The main indications for fusion of the MTP joint include degenerative disease, hallux valgus deformity following neurologic injury, and rheumatoid arthritis. It also is a salvage procedure for a failed hallux surgery. The Keller resection arthroplasty may be beneficial in an older, low-demand patient. The Lapidus procedure is indicated if significant hypermobility of the first metatarsocuneiform joint is present.

12. What are common complications associated with metatarsal osteotomy?

- Nonunion
- Dorsiflexion at the osteotomy
- Plantar flexion at the osteotomy
- Shortening of the metatarsal
- Avascular necrosis of the metatarsal head (with distal osteotomy)

13. What results can be expected from hallux valgus surgery?

If careful preoperative planning is performed and indications for operative procedures are followed closely, one can expect 90% of patients to have good results.

14. Is pes planus related to the development of juvenile hallux valgus?

Pes planus has been believed to be related to development of juvenile hallux valgus; however, a recent study found no relationship between pes planus and juvenile hallux valgus.

15. What deformity can result if too much of the MTP head of the medial great toe is removed?

Instability develops and the MTP joint may deviate into a varus position. Correction of this deformity is treated with a transfer of the extensor hallucis longus tendon.

16. Is the hallux valgus deformity seen only in adults?

No. The deformity may develop during the teen or preteen years and is known as a juvenile hallux valgus.

17. In addition to the valgus deformity at the MTP joint, what other abnormalities may be present?

There may be pronation of the great toe and lateral displacement of the sesamoids from under the head of the first metatarsal.

18. What is hallux rigidus?

Hallux rigidus is a degenerative process that occurs with the MTP joint of the great toe. Typically, bony proliferation is present on the dorsal aspect of the metatarsal head, which limits dorsiflexion. Surgical treatment (cheilectomy) consists of generous resection of dorsal osteophytes.

LESSER TOE DEFORMITIES

19. What is a hammer toe?

A hammer toe is a deformity in which flexion of the proximal interphalangeal (PIP) and distal interphalangeal (DIP) joints exists, creating a prominence over the dorsal aspect of the PIP joint. Subluxation or dislocation of the MTP joint dorsally also may occur.

20. What is a claw toe?

A claw toe is hyperextension at the MTP joint, flexion of the PIP joint, and either flexion or extension at the DIP joint.

21. What is a mallet toe?

A mallet toe is hyperflexion at the DIP joint. Typically it is a fixed deformity.

22. What are claw toes often associated with?

They are often associated with neurologic dysfunction with weakness or loss of the intrinsic muscles of the foot. This may be secondary to central nervous system disorders such as stroke or traumatic head injury, peripheral nerve injuries, or peripheral neuropathy such as Charcot-Marie-Tooth syndrome.

23. What is a flexible flexed toe?

Essentially, it is a flexible hammer toe deformity. If the deformity is truly flexible, pushing up on the metatarsal head will straighten the toes.

24. What is a bunionette?

This prominent, painful area on the lateral aspect of the fifth metatarsal head is also referred to as a tailor's bunion.

25. What are the treatment options for hammer toe deformity?

1. Relief of local irritation by increasing the height of the shoe toe box and direct padding.
2. Transfer the flexor digitorum longus to the extensor mechanism (effective only in the flexible flexed toe variety)
3. PIP fusion

26. What if a hammer toe deformity of the second toe is found next to a hallux valgus deformity?

Generally, one would need to correct the great toe alignment prior to correcting the second toe. Correcting only the second toe results in a high risk of recurrence of the deformity.

27. What is metatarsalgia?

Metatarsalgia is pain in the region of the MTP joints. Palpation in the involved metatarsal heads typically elicits extreme point tenderness.

28. What are the characteristic deformities seen in the forefoot of the rheumatoid patient?

Subluxation and dislocation of the metatarsal phalangeal joints in the dorsal direction are common. One also may see hallux valgus deformity and flexion deformities in the IP joints of the lesser toes. Such deformities are a result of the chronic synovitis and destruction of the normal supporting structures of these joints.

29. What painful joint process in the forefoot area may contribute to deformity at the MTP joint level?

MTP joint synovitis. This has been reported both as a traumatic and a nontraumatic entity. The nontraumatic entity may lead to attenuation of the capsule ligamentous structures and resultant instability and deformity at the MTP joint.

30. What symptoms and findings are associated with MTP joint synovitis?

Metatarsal phalangeal joint synovitis. Pain may be sharp in nature. There may be a sense of fullness in the forefoot area, and its symptoms often mimic interdigital neuritis, an important diagnosis from which to distinguish it. Palpation elicits tenderness over the MTP joint, and subluxation stress testing causes pain. There may be evidence of instability.

BIBLIOGRAPHY

1. Kilmartin TE, Wallace WA: The significance of pes planus in juvenile hallux valgus. Foot Ankle 13:53–56, 1992.
2. Jahss MH: Disorders of the Foot and Ankle: Medical and Surgical Management, 2nd ed. Philadelphia, W.B. Saunders, 1991.
3. Johnson KA: Surgery of the Foot and Ankle. New York, Raven Press, 1989.
4. Lapidus PW: Operative correction of metatarsus varus primus in hallux valgus. Surg Gynecol Obstet 58:183, 1934.
5. Mann RA, Coughlin MJ (eds): Surgery of the Foot and Ankle, 6th ed. St. Louis, Mosby, 1993.
6. McBride ED: Hallux valgus, bunion deformity: Its treatment in mild, moderate, and severe stages. J Int Coll Surg 21:99, 1954.
7. Mizel MS, Michelson JD: Nonsurgical treatment of monarticular, nontraumatic synovitis of the second metatarsophalangeal joint. Foot Ankle Int 18:424–426, 1997.
8. Rossie WR, Ferreira JC: Chevron osteotomy for hallux valgus. Foot Ankle 13:378–381, 1992.
9. Thordarson DB, Leventen EO: Hallux valgus correction with proximal metatarsal osteotomy: Two-year follow-up. Foot Ankle 13:321–326, 1992.
10. Trepman E, Yeo SJ: Nonoperative treatment of metatarsophalangeal joint synovitis. Foot Ankle Int 16:771–777, 1995.

89. ANKLE ARTHROSCOPY

David E. Brown, M.D.

1. When was the first ankle arthroscopy performed?

It was performed in 1939 in Japan by Dr. K. Takagi.

2. What are the chief indications for ankle arthroscopy?

1. Loose bodies
2. Osteochondritis dissecans/osteochondral fractures
3. Osseous impingement/osteophytes
4. Lateral soft tissue impingement lesions/chronic synovitis
5. To facilitate ankle arthrodesis
6. Unexplained pain, swelling, or mechanical symptoms

3. What are the contraindications for ankle arthroscopy?

1. Abnormal neurovascular status
2. Severe swelling or edema
3. Severe arthrofibrosis or degenerative arthritis with restricted joint volume that cannot be overcome with mechanical joint distraction

4. What are the complications of ankle arthroscopy?

1. Nerve injury (usually neurapraxia), most commonly involving the superficial peroneal nerve, which is at risk from the anterolateral portal. The sural nerve is at risk from the posterolateral portal, whereas the saphenous nerve is at risk from the anteromedial portal.

2. Vascular injury. The dorsalis pedis is at risk from the anterocentral portal. Posterior tibial artery injury may occur from the posteromedial portal.

3. Infection

4. Thrombophlebitis

5. Iatrogenic joint scuffing usually related to inadequate distraction or improper portal placement

5. Describe the common portals used in ankle arthroscopy.

Anteromedial—just medial to the anterior tibialis tendon at the level of the joint line.

Anterolateral—immediately lateral to the peroneus tertius tendon at the level of the joint line.

Anterocentral—through or immediately medial to the common extensor tendons at the level of the joint line.

Accessory Anterolateral—1 cm distal and 0.5 cm medial to the anterolateral portal (usually used only for small inflow cannula)

Posterolateral—lateral to the Achilles tendon at the level of the posterior joint space. This should enter the joint just medial to the transverse tibia-fibula ligament. Placement may be obtained through the use of a switching stick from the anterolateral portal.

Posteromedial—immediately medial to the Achilles tendon at the level of the posterior joint line. (This is an uncommon high-risk portal.)

6. Is distraction necessary for ankle arthroscopy? What types of distraction are available?

Mechanical joint distraction is often necessary to achieve satisfactory joint visualization and allow safe instrumentation within the joint. Operative techniques limited to the anterior aspect of the joint generally do not require distraction. Distraction may be achieved *noninvasively* with the use of a clove/hitch device that wraps around the foot and ankle. A weight is then attached to this device to provide distraction. Alternatively **invasive** distraction, using tibial and calcaneal pins with a mechanical distraction device, may be used.

7. Which arthroscopes should be used for ankle arthroscopy?

A standard 4-mm, 30-degree arthroscope is typically used. Especially when mechanical distraction is used, the standard 4.0-mm scope provides good illumination and the widest field of view. Occasionally a 2.7-mm or 1.9-mm scope is needed in a tight joint with posterior pathology. A variety of mini-probes, graspers, curettes, rongeurs, power shavers, and burs are available.

8. Describe and discuss anterolateral soft tissue impingement lesions.

The anterolateral impingement lesions generally are a localized area of fibrosis or synovitis that occurs after an ankle injury. Symptoms include persistent anterolateral ankle pain, swelling, and catching. If these symptoms do not respond to a prolonged period of conservative treatment including rest, immobilization, and antiinflammatory medication, then arthroscopic surgical resection of the impingement lesion may be required.

9. Are ankle joint spurs amenable to arthroscopic resection?

Anterior tibiotalar impingement spurs are amenable to arthroscopic diagnosis and resection. Commonly, associated loose bodies or degenerative lesions also are amenable to arthroscopic care.

Scranton and McDermott compared open resection with arthroscopic resection. All but the most severe spurs are amenable to arthroscopic resection. Those managed arthroscopically recovered in half the time of those treated by arthrotomy and resection.

10. What is the etiology and treatment of osteochondral lesions of the talus?

Osteochondral lesions of the talus may occur from trauma or idiopathic osteonecrosis. Many terms have been used to describe these lesions, including osteochrondritis dissecans, transchondral talar dome fracture, osteochondral fracture, and talar dome fracture. Treatment includes cast immobilization, resection, drilling, internal fixation, osteochondral mosaicplasty, and bone grafting. Nearly all lesions are amenable to arthroscopic treatment.

11. Describe the Berndt and Hardy classification of osteochondral lesions of the talus.

Type I: Compression fracture
Type II: partially detached osteochondral fragment
Type III: Completely detached fragment but nondisplaced
Type IV: Completely detached fragment, displaced

BIBLIOGRAPHY

1. Alexander AH, Lichtman DM: Surgical treatment of transchondral talar-dome fractures (osteochondritis dissecans): Long-term follow-up. J Bone Joint Surg 62A:646–652, 1980.
2. Berndt AL, Harty M: Transchondral fractures (osteochondritis dissecans) of the talus. J Bone Joint Surg 41A:988–1020, 1959.
3. Ferkel RD, Guhl J, Van Buecken K, et al: Complications in ankle arthroscopy: Analysis of the first 518 cases. Orthop Trans 16:726–727, 1992–1993.
4. Ferkel RD, Karzel RP, Del Pizzo, et al: Arthroscopic treatment of anterolateral impingement of the ankle. Am J Sports Med 19:440–446, 1991.
5. Ferkel RD, Scranton PE: Current Concepts Review: Arthroscopy of the Ankle and Foot. J Bone Joint Surg 75A:1233–1241, 1993.
6. Hangody L, Kish G, Karpati Z, et al: Treatment of osteochondritis dissecans of the talus: Use of mosaicplasty technique—A preliminary report. Foot Ankle Int 18:628–634, 1997.
7. McGinty JB: Operative Arthroscopy, 2nd ed. New York, Lippincott-Raven, 1996.
8. Phillips BB: Arthroscopy of lower extremity. In Canale ST (ed): Campbell's Operative Orthopaedics, 9th ed. St. Louis, Mosby, 1998, pp 1542–1550.
9. Scranton PE, McDermott JE: Anterior tibiotalar spurs: A comparison of open versus arthroscopic debridement. Foot Ankle 13:125–129, 1992.

90. RHEUMATOID FOOT DISEASE

Jeffrey A. Senall, M.D., and Todd A. Kile, M.D.

The incidence of rheumatoid arthritis (RA) in the general population is 2 to 3 per 1,000, 90% of whom eventually develop foot involvement. The ravages of RA, when left unchecked, deprive patients of the ability to ambulate effectively.

1. RA begins in the feet in what percentage of cases?

Seventeen percent. Pedal involvement with RA tends to be progressive and bilateral. Cash found that 21% of patients had involvement of the feet within the first year of disease. This rose to 53% after 3 years. In patients with longstanding RA, approximately 90% had involvement of the feet.

2. Which region of the foot is most often involved?

The forefoot is affected in up to 89% of RA patients with a predilection for the synovium of the metatarsophalangeal (MTP) joints.

3. What other areas are typically involved?

The midfoot and hindfoot are more commonly affected than the forefoot (up to 67% of adults). The sites most often involved are the talonavicular joint (39%), the subtalar joint (29%), and the calcaneocuboid joint (25%).

4. What is the most common deformity associated with rheumatoid foot disease?

Hallux valgus develops in 70–80% of patients. Hammer toes are also common, occurring in 50–80% of patients.

5. List some of the nonarticular manifestations of RA and their effects on foot function.

Extraosseous involvement often is present before other evidence of systemic disease.

1. Inflammation of soft tissues leads to attenuation of ligaments and tendons, which leads to flatfoot deformity (46% of patients). Posterior tibialis and peroneal tendons are most commonly involved. Rupture is caused by eroded bone surfaces, tendon degradation, or previous corticosteroid injection.

2. Rheumatoid nodules (immune complex-mediated vasculitis) occur in 20–30% of patients, and may develop over extensor surfaces of joints or areas of bony prominence. They usually herald a more malignant form of arthritis.

3. Vasculitis (inflammatory destruction of blood vessels by immune-complex deposition) results in digital infarcts, cutaneous ulcers, and diffuse rashes about the foot and ankle (rashes are rare in seronegative patients, and should alert clinicians to other systemic effects).

4. Neurologic involvement (evident in 46% of patients) due to nerve compression or neuropathy may be present.

6. Is hindfoot varus or valgus more common in RA?

In patients who continue weightbearing, **hindfoot valgus** is more common. The combined loss of subtalar cartilage and bone, ligamentous laxity, and posterior tibial tendon dysfunction or rupture contribute to this deformity. **Hindfoot varus** is more common in patients with severe knee flexion contractures who have experienced long periods of recumbency and in patients with juvenile rheumatoid arthritis.

7. Give a differential diagnosis for pain and swelling in the foot.

1. Fracture
2. Infection
3. Tumor
4. Sarcoidosis
5. Hemophilia
6. RA
7. Spondyloarthropathies (Reiter's) are commonly found at the insertion of the Achilles tendon or the origin of the plantar fascia
8. Psoriatic arthritis should be considered when the interphalangeal joints are affected more than other joints or if ankylosis is present.

8. Why do calluses develop beneath the metatarsal head?

The combination of dorsal dislocation of the MTP joints, causing downward pressure on the metatarsal heads, and distal retraction or atrophy of the plantar fat pad results in painful metatarsalgia and eventually callosity.

9. What is the most specific radiographic finding in RA?

Periarticular osteoporosis. Other common findings include soft-tissue swelling, loss of joint space, and juxtaarticular erosions at the insertion of the ligaments. Late findings include subluxation and dislocation.

10. Radiographs of which part of the body are more likely to provide information than radiographs of any other region?

Standing radiographs of the feet. One study of 200 patients found radiographic changes in 19% of feet and 9% of hands during the first 6 months of disease. In another study of 105 patients with definite or classic RA, 26% had foot changes without hand changes. No patients had positive hand films with negative foot films.

11. What are the nonoperative options for management of the rheumatoid foot?

Consultation with rheumatologic specialists to optimize pharmacotherapy is key. Acute phases are relieved with rest, splinting, and periods of brief immobilization, followed later by directed mobilization to preserve joint motion. Judicious use of injectable glucocorticoids is sometimes helpful. As progression is inevitable, physical therapy becomes more important to maintain range of motion and strength. Hot soaks and contrast baths may be beneficial.

12. Why do shoewear modifications make a difference in the patient with a rheumatoid foot?

By controlling instability and relieving pressure, many of the more disabling hindfoot and forefoot deformities may be delayed or alleviated, thereby allowing the patient to continue effective ambulation.

13. Of all operations done for RA, what percentage involve the foot and ankle?

Twenty-five to 35% of all operations done for RA involve the foot and ankle.

14. Does surgical treatment cure the rheumatoid foot?

No. With continued weightbearing and progression of the disease, all treatment, operative and nonoperative, should be considered palliative.

15. Preoperative evaluation of the rheumatoid patient should include radiographic assessment of the foot and what other area?

The cervical spine also should undergo radiographic assessment for C1–C2 instability.

16. Name the three surgical options for severe RA in the ankle.

1. Synovectomy may be beneficial in patients with significant ankle symptoms unresponsive to conservative therapy early in the course of the disease. Indications include patients with persistent synovitis for 4–6 months who are unresponsive to immobilization and intraarticular steroid injection with articular cartilage of 3–4 mm in width remaining on a standing ankle mortise radiograph.

2. Arthrodesis may be the procedure of choice for the rheumatoid patient with high functional demands and joint involvement limited primarily to the ankle.

3. Total ankle arthroplasty should be reserved for patients with low functional demands and involvement primarily of the ankle without deformity or instability in other joints. Bone density must be sufficient to support the arthroplasty components.

17. When hindfoot fusion becomes necessary, should a triple arthrodesis of the talocalcaneal, talonavicular, and calcaneocuboid joints be performed routinely to provide stability?

No. Only the affected joints should be fused.

18. When is an isolated talonavicular joint arthrodesis indicated?

When it is painful, the only joint destroyed, and when the hindfoot is still flexible or in neutral. This procedure has been shown to prevent later hindfoot deformity.

19. What is the only indication for surgical intervention in the rheumatoid forefoot?

Pain. Deformity or difficulties with fashionable shoewear in the absence of pain are not sufficient reasons for surgery.

20. What is the procedure of choice for painful hallux valgus in the rheumatoid forefoot?

Arthrodesis of the MTP joint. Resection arthroplasty (Keller procedure) is usually reserved for the elderly patient with fragile connective tissues and the need for immediate weightbearing.

21. What is the most important aspect of surgical treatment for the lesser toe deformities in the rheumatoid foot?

Adequate bone resection.

CONTROVERSY

22. In a patient who presents with both ankle and subtalar disease, which joint should be fused?

Occasionally, ankle pain may be referred from other sites (e.g., subtalar joint, peroneal or posterior tibial tendons). Thus it is imperative that the origin of the pain be identified, usually by careful physical examination, selective diagnostic injections, and imaging studies. If indeed both the subtalar and ankle joints are involved, both should be included in the arthrodesis. Some authors advocate a "pantalar" (tibiotalar, talonavicular, and talocalcaneal) arthrodesis. A relatively recent and innovative method stabilizes the arthrodesis with an intramedullary nail inserted retrograde through the calcaneus and talus and into the tibia to achieve rigid internal fixation. Early results are encouraging.

BIBLIOGRAPHY*

* Please see Bibliography of Chapter 92.

91. THE DIABETIC FOOT

Timothy C. Fitzgibbons, M.D.

1. Why all the fuss about the foot in diabetes? Certainly the other involved organ systems are more important?

There is no question that the various system failures associated with diabetes are more life-threatening; no problem, however, is more emotional, or, in one sense, more disabling than development of a diabetic foot ulcer.

2. Why not amputate the foot and ankle once they become infected?

The obvious answer, of course, is the patient's emotional attachment to his or her extremity. Some patients resist amputation at almost any cost. Of more importance, however, are the costs involved. The cost of a below-the-knee amputation, in terms of prosthetic fitting and loss of productiveness, has been shown on average to be more expensive than limb salvage. Certainly there is a point at which limb salvage is not feasible, but each patient has to be assessed individually.

3. What are the two most common complications of diabetes that affect the foot?

The two most common complications of diabetes that affect the foot are peripheral neuropathy and peripheral vascular disease.

4. What is peripheral neuropathy in diabetics?

Peripheral neuropathy in diabetics may have many different patterns, but the primary problem is the progressive loss of protective sensation in the foot and ankle.

5. What does the term neuropathic mean?

Neuropathic refers to a process that occurs as a result of peripheral neuropathy.

6. What is the incidence of peripheral neuropathy affecting the foot in diabetics?

Some signs of neuropathy occur in 10–15% of diabetics; 8–14% of patients have neuropathy at the time of diagnosis. Studies have shown a 20–50% incidence of neuropathy in patients who have had diabetes at least 25 years.

7. What is neuropathic ulceration?

Neuropathic ulceration is an erosion of the skin and subcutaneous tissue that occurs in diabetic patients because they lack protective sensation. Whereas the normal individual with a foreign object or pressure point in the shoe has discomfort and takes the shoe off, the diabetic is unable to feel the pressure and continues walking to the point that erosion occurs through the skin and subcutaneous tissue, leading to ulceration.

8. Why are diabetic ulcerations difficult to heal?

The combination of the inability to protect the foot, the high incidence of peripheral vascular disease, and the patient's inability or lack of desire to comply with treatment recommendations makes ulceration an especially difficult problem.

9. What is the incidence of peripheral vascular disease in diabetic patients?

The literature supports an increased incidence of peripheral vascular disease in diabetic patients. In one study of patients who had diabetes for less than 1 year, 22% had some vascular calcification on plain radiographs.

10. What is the concept of "small vessel disease"? How does it affect treatment recommendations?

Diabetes tends to cause occlusion and dysfunction at the capillary and arteriole level. The common teaching is that diabetics are not candidates for peripheral revascularization because the disease affects the smallest vessels. All diabetics, however, should be evaluated for possible revascularization of larger vessels to improve general perfusion to the extremity, which aids in healing of ulcers. Newer techniques of small vessel revascularization are being perfected and may be even more helpful.

11. What is the recommended treatment for diabetic foot problems?

The most important treatment recommendation for diabetic foot problems is prevention. Once diabetic ulceration occurs, it is extremely hard to heal, and the patient is committed to long-term treatment, non–weight-bearing status, and sometimes multiple surgeries.

12. How does one prevent diabetic ulcers?

The first stage of treatment is always the same. The patient must be taught to understand the disease, including the subtle progressive neuropathic changes and the risks of ulcerations. This can be extremely difficult, especially in a young diabetic male. Once the patient accepts and understands the disease, instruction in the do's and don'ts of foot care (see table below) and fitting the patient with special shoes with inlays can begin.

Instructions for Diabetic Patients: Do's and Don'ts

Do's
- Use your eyes to check for problems when feeling is lost in the feet. If your vision is impaired, have your family help you.
- Check your feet every day for blisters, cuts, scratches, and nail problems. Use a mirror to see the bottom of your feet.
- Check your shoes every day for foreign objects and rough spots that could cause sores.
- Wash your feet every day. If you have dry skin, use a small amount of lotion containing lanolin on the surfaces of your feet. Keep the skin dry between the toes.
- Make sure your shoes and socks are not tight on your feet. Shoes should have extra room in the toe box and a soft upper material that can "breathe." Rotate your shoes, and do not wear new shoes more than a few hours at a time. If you have fitting problems, ask about accommodative or prescription shoes.
- Make sure your physician checks your feet at every visit. Tell the shoe salesperson that you are a diabetic.

Table continued on following page.

Instructions for Diabetic Patients: Do's and Don'ts (Continued)

Dont's
• Don't walk barefoot. You could injure your foot on sharp objects or rough surfaces without knowing it.
• Don't use heat on your feet, which may cause a burn. Don't soak in hot water. Don't use a heating pad. Wear socks to keep your feet warm at night.
• Don't use chemicals or sharp instruments to trim calluses. Small cuts and blisters will become infected.
• Don't cut into the corners when trimming nails. Cut nails straight across. Use cotton to pack skin away from nails.
• Don't use tobacco. It impairs circulation in the foot.

13. What are "diabetic shoes"?

The most common diabetic shoe used today is the extra-depth shoe with a custom-molded plastizote inlay. The extra depth allows decompression of the bottom of the foot, removes pressure from all bony prominences, and also allows room for the inlay.

14. How do you treat a diabetic ulcer?

All patients with diabetic ulcers should be evaluated in the same fashion. Radiographs must be obtained to rule out infection. A peripheral vascular examination must be done to quantify the amount of perfusion to the foot. Referral to a vascular surgeon with vascular studies should be considered for all patients to determine whether perfusion can be increased. All ulcers must be debrided of any necrotic or infected tissue. Proper antibiotics should be used when necessary. If plantar ulcers are present, the patient must be off-loaded.

15. What is "off-loading"?

Off-loading is the process by which the patient is prevented from putting pressure on the bony prominence that caused the ulcer. Off-loading can be done with crutches or a walker and sometimes is facilitated by special temporary shoes.

16. Describe the proper technique of wound care.

Most authorities believe that wound dressings should be moist. Various types of alternating saline and antibiotic solutions can be used. It is best to avoid the use of cytotoxic agents, such as hydrogen peroxide and Betadine, because they kill cells that aid in healing as well as bacteria.

17. What about growth factor and its use in diabetic ulcers?

Platelet derived growth factors, which are proteins normally produced by the host to heal wounds, may be absent in the wounds of patients with diabetes. The evidence continues to mount that such growth factors are important in wound healing. The most common source of growth factor is from the platelets of the patient's own blood. The theory is that the patients cannot get such growth factor proteins to their ulcers because of circulation problems; therefore, by extracting it from their platelets and applying it to the wounds directly they may benefit. The process is complicated and expensive but appears effective. It is important, however, that patients' ulcers are properly debrided, free of infection, and that any possible revascularization to ensure growth factor's effectiveness has been performed. Recently, growth factor solutions that are not processed from patients' own blood have been introduced. Use of such prescription growth factors is encouraging.

18. What is the Charcot foot?

The Charcot foot is a syndrome peculiar to diabetes. Patients present with swelling, inflammation, warmth, and deformity that are inconsistent with their history. The usual differential diagnosis is fracture, cellulitis, or deep vein thrombosis. Destructive changes on radiographs are out of proportion to historical trauma. This inflammatory process is peculiar to patients with neuropathic disease and is not completely understood. Initial treatment is rest and immobilization. The consensus in the literature is against surgery in the Charcot foot, except under conditions in which nonsurgical treatment has failed. Wound-healing and bone-healing problems are common.

For that reason, after initial rest and immobilization, treatment consists of custom-molded shoes to fit the deformed foot.

19. What are the surgical options for the diabetic foot ulcer?
The goal of all surgery in diabetic foot ulcers is to close the wound and maintain as much function as possible. Standard treatments have included extensive debridement of the ulcer with off-loading and eventual granulation by secondary intention; primary amputations of toes or portions of the foot are indicated in certain patients. Recently, a two-stage approach with eventual secondary closure has been described and has been quite successful.

BIBLIOGRAPHY

1. Gould JS: The Foot Book. Baltimore, Williams & Wilkins, 1988.
2. Jahss MH (ed): Disorders of the Foot and Ankle: Medical and Surgical Management, 2nd ed. Philadelphia, W.B. Saunders, 1997.
3. Kumagai SG, Mahoney CR, Fitzgibbons TC, McMullen ST: Treatment of diabetic (neuropathic) foot ulcers with two-stage debridement and closure. Foot Ankle Int 19:160–165, 1998.
4. Levin ME, O'Neal LW, Bowker JH (eds): The Diabetic Foot, 5th ed. St. Louis, Mosby, 1992.
5. Mann RA, Coughlin MJ (eds): Surgery of the Foot and Ankle, 6th ed. St. Louis, Mosby, 1993.

92. ARTHRITIS AND ARTHROPLASTY OF THE FOOT AND ANKLE

Jeffrey A. Senall, M.D., and Todd A. Kile, M.D.

1. What radiologic views are needed for proper evaluation of a patient with a foot or ankle disorder?
• Standing, anteroposterior (AP), lateral, and mortise radiographs of the ankle.
• Standing, AP, lateral, and oblique radiographs of the foot.

2. What serologic tests are useful in patients suspected of having an inflammatory arthritis?
Complete blood cell count (CBC), blood chemistry, rheumatoid factor (RF), antinuclear antibody (ANA), erythrocyte sedimentation rate (ESR), and the histocompatibility antigen HLA-B27.

3. List the major categories of arthritides that affect primarily the foot and ankle.
1. Crystal-induced arthritis
2. Seronegative spondyloarthropathies
3. Degenerative joint disease or osteoarthritis
4. Seropositive or rheumatoid arthritis (RA)

4. What type of crystal causes arthritis in gout?
Arthritis in gout is caused by the needle-like sodium urate crystals, which are strongly negatively birefringent under polarized light.

5. Where does gout present in the foot and ankle?
Of initial gouty attacks, 50–75% involve the metatarsophalangeal (MTP) joint of the great toe, clinically termed acute podagra. Of all gout patients, 90% experience one or more attacks in their toes. Involvement of the ankle and medial midpart of the foot is also common.

6. **In what other mammal does gout occur?**

None. Humans are the only mammal that lacks the enzyme uricase, which is needed to oxidize uric acid to the more soluble allantoin. Thus, purine metabolism in humans produces the relatively insoluble uric acid, which must be cleared by the kidney.

7. **How is acute gouty arthritis diagnosed?**

The classic history consists of abrupt onset of excruciating pain with erythema and swelling, usually at night, over the first MTP joint. The attack may be precipitated by minor trauma, binge drinking, or consumption of purine-rich foods. Most commonly it occurs without provocation. It also may occur without hyperuricemia. Diagnosis is confirmed by aspirating synovial fluid and demonstrating the presence of uric acid crystals within the polymorphonuclear leukocytes.

8. **What is the proper medical management for acute gouty arthritis?**

Symptomatic treatment consisting of elevation and rest of the foot and nonsteroidal antiinflammatory drugs (NSAIDs) at maximum doses (e.g., 75 mg indomethacin followed by 50 mg orally 4 times/day with food) usually provides the most rapid relief. Intravenous colchicine is reserved for patients who cannot tolerate NSAIDs or steroids.

9. **What radiologic feature distinguishes gouty arthritis?**

Destructive bony lesions remote from the articular surface and periarticular destruction (ratbite lesions) are often seen in chronic disease.

10. **What is pseudogout?**

Pseudogout is the most frequently recognized form of calcium pyrophosphate deposition disease (CPPD). Deposits of the weakly positively birefringment, polygonal calcium pyrophosphate dihydrate crystals in synovial joints can mimic acute gout. The knee is the most commonly affected joint, but the ankle, talonavicular, subtalar, and first MTP joints also may be affected.

11. **What is chondrocalcinosis?**

The term chondrocalcinosis should be used as a radiographic or pathologic description for calcium pyrophosphate noted in articular cartilage or menisci and should not be confused with an actual clinical diagnosis. Chondrocalcinosis also may be noted on radiographs of patients with advanced degenerative joint disease.

12. **Name the serologic spondyloarthropathies that affect the foot and ankle.**
   • Ankylosing spondylitis
   • Reiter's syndrome (most common)
   • Psoriatic arthritis
   • Arthropathy of inflammatory bowel disease

13. **What are the radiologic differences between the spondyloarthropathies and the inflammatory arthropathies?**
   • Intraarticular ankylosis
   • Calcification within the adventitia
   • Lack of osteopenia

14. **List some clinical features of the spondyloarthropathies and the inflammatory arthropathies.**
   • Inflammation of the site of ligamentous or tendinous insertions (enthesopathy)
   • Axial skeleton involvement, such as sacroiliitis or spondylitis
   • Sites of extraarticular inflammatory disease such as skin, mucous membranes, genitourinary tract, and gut

- Increase prevalence of HLA-B27 haplotype in Caucasian patients
- Associated with peripheral arthritis
- Asymmetric involvement of distal joints (commonly the MTP joint), and inflammation of soft tissues of entire toe (sausage digits)
- Often present with heel pain (Achilles tendinitis, calcaneal bursitis, plantar fasciitis)

15. What are the most common causes of arthrosis of the ankle?

Previous trauma or malalignment secondary to lower extremity trauma or other causes are most common. Examples include: Pilon fractures, trimalleolar fractures with large posterior fragment, tibial fracture malunions (especially varus or extension), calcaneal fracture malunions, posterior tibial tendon rupture (hindfoot valgus), and subtalar coalitions or fusions.

16. List some conservative treatment options for patients with ankle arthrosis.

Change in activities, NSAIDs, cane, ankle braces, intraarticular injections, shoes with rocker bottom soles or solid ankle cushion heel (SACH), physical therapy, custom ankle-foot orthotics, and casting.

17. What are surgical treatment options for patients with ankle arthrosis?

Debridement (either open or arthroscopic), ligament reconstruction for lateral ankle instability as a cause of mild arthrosis, joint distraction arthroplasty (controversial), corrective tibial osteotomy for malalignment of the distal tibia, ankle reconstruction for fracture malunion, or arthrodesis.

18. What can be done to repair isolated ankle arthrosis (impingement)?

Anterior cheilectomy or removal of the osteophytes from the anterior aspect of the distal tibia and talus via a standard arthrotomy or arthroscopically.

19. What is the standard treatment for advanced arthrosis and failed medical and other nonsurgical treatment?

Ankle arthrodesis.

20. What is the optimum position of ankle arthrodesis?

- Neutral dorsiflexion–plantar flexion
- Hindfoot valgus 5–10°
- Neutral mediolateral displacement
- Posterior translation of the talus ≤ 1 cm (to decrease the anterior lever arm of the foot and decrease overloading of the midfoot joints)

21. How much tibiopedal motion is retained after ankle arthrodesis?

Approximately 30–40% of normal motion is retained through Chopart's (talonavicular) and Lisfranc's (tarsometatarsal and calcaneocuboid) joints.

22. Describe the various methods for achieving ankle arthrodesis.

The most important aspect of arthrodesis is rigid fixation. The numerous variations used include internal compression screws, external fixation devices, internal fixation with plates, and screws or staples and percutaneous pins. The trend is toward internal fixation with large cancellous screws (6.5 or 7.0 mm), which has high success rates. At least two screws are necessary for adequate fixation. Supplemental fibular onlay grafting has been shown to add stability. Joint debridement prior to fixation may be done using open methods or arthroscopically in selected patients.

23. What are the advantages of arthroscopic ankle arthrodesis?

- Minimal bone resection preserves anatomy and overall appearance and size of the foot and ankle.

• Patients are more likely to be able to wear normal shoes
• A statistically shorter time to fusion

24. Who is *not* a suitable candidate for arthroscopic arthrodesis?
Patients with significant malalignment or poor bone quality are not candidates for arthroscopic arthrodesis.

25. Why is total ankle arthroplasty not as common as total knee or total hip arthroplasty?
The increased force per unit area across the ankle joint, coupled with higher shear stresses, poor bone stock (particularly in the talus), and a tenuous blood supply, produce significantly higher rates of complications compared with total knee arthroplasty. Sepsis, loosening, and fractures are common complications.

26. Who is a good candidate for total ankle arthroplasty?
A patient with RA with a painful ankle having little or no deformity and adequate bone stock.

27. List the contraindications of total ankle arthroplasty.

Patient	Ankle
Youth (< 60 years old)	Hindfoot malalignment
Osteoarthrosis (primary or post-traumatic)	Avascular necrosis of the talus
Peripheral neuropathy	Painful arthrodesis
Corticosteroid use	Pseudoarthrosis
Vascular insufficiency	Distorted anatomy
Paralysis of muscles around the ankle	Sepsis
	Poor bone stock
	Neuropathic arthropathy

28. What variables are associated with a higher rate of failure of a total ankle arthroplasty?
• Previous operative procedure on the ipsilateral foot or ankle
• ≤ 57 years of age

29. How does a total ankle arthroplasty fail?
The most common mode of failure is loosening and subsidence of the talar component.

30. What is the treatment for failed total ankle arthroplasty?
Treatment combines repeated arthrodesis of the ankle with interposition of an intercalary bone graft to minimize shortening.

31. Define triple arthrodesis.
Arthrodesis of the talonavicular, calcaneocuboid, and subtalar joints.

32. What are the indications?
• Significant arthrosis in 2 or 3 hindfoot joints
• Rigid hindfoot valgus deformity
• Certain neuromuscular foot deformities

33. Which of the three hindfoot joints has the highest incidence of nonunion following a triple arthrodesis?
The talonavicular joint.

34. What are the common causes of subtalar joint arthrosis?
Intraarticular calcaneus or talus fractures and subtalar instability are common causes of subtalar joint arthrosis.

35. List the symptoms of patients with subtalar joint arthrosis.

Symptoms include lateral ankle and hindfoot pain, pain with weightbearing, difficulty ambulating on uneven terrain, painful and restricted hindfoot motion, and tenderness over the sinus tarsi.

36. Define hallux rigidus.

Hallus rigidus is a painful degenerative affliction of the first MTP joint associated with painful dorsiflexion, increased bony bulk about the joint, and loss of dorsiflexion. Radiographic features include joint space narrowing and a large dorsal osteophyte.

37. What is the treatment of hallux rigidus?

Cheilectomy—removal of the dorsal 20–30% of the first metatarsal head—relieves the dorsal impingement and increases MTP dorsiflexion in adults with pain and large dorsal osteophytes. It has the advantage of being a simple procedure with low morbidity. Cheilectomy is indicated in a patient with painful hallux rigidus and > 50% of the articular cartilage remaining.

38. What is a Moberg procedure and when is it indicated?

A Moberg procedure (dorsiflexion osteotomy of the proximal phalanx) is indicated in a younger patient with limited dorsiflexion of the hallux metatarsophalangeal joint and no dorsal prominence.

39. What are the indications for first MTP joint arthrodesis?

• A painful or damaged joint
• Unstable joint
• Degenerative arthrosis, especially with hallux valgus or failed cheilectomy
• Rheumatoid arthritis (often combined with resection of metatarsal heads 2–5)
• Salvage for total joint arthroplasty, hallux valgus surgery, or other MTP joint operations

40. What are the contraindications for a first MTP joint arthrodesis?

Acute infection and patients who find a stiff joint undesirable.

41. What is the desired position for a first MTP joint arthrodesis?

Ten to 20° valgus of the MTP joint and 10–15° dorsiflexion of the MTP joint, which provides neutral alignment of the hallux with the toe just touching the ground when standing with the ankle dorsiflexed to 90°.

42. What are the indications for resection arthroplasty (Keller procedure)?

A Keller resection arthroplasty (resection of the base of the proximal phalanx) is indicated only in elderly, low-demand patients with painful hallux rigidus, plantar ulceration, or painful hallux valgus, patients with failed silicone arthroplasty, septic arthritis, or in patients where an arthrodesis is not indicated.

43. Why is a Keller arthroplasty not recommended?

A Keller arthroplasty is not recommended because of its complications, which include: recurrence of deformity (hallux valgus), cock-up toe deformity, shortening of the first ray, loss of flexion power of the hallux, transfer metatarsalgia, and stress fractures of the lateral metatarsals.

44. When was the first MPT joint replacement performed and by whom?

The first procedure was performed in 1952 by Al Swanson. The implant—a metal head with an intermedullary stem—failed because of resorption and bone loss about the stem.

45. What is the most widely used and studied implant for metatarsophalangeal joint arthroplasty?

Silicone elastomer (Silastic) implants.

46. What are the indications for MTP joint arthroplasty?
- Osteoarthritis of the first MTP joint with or without hallux valgus
- Failure of other procedures resulting in damage to the joint or bone loss
- Expectations that can be reasonably met and an understanding of possible long-term problems
- A cooperative patient
- The surgery must be within the surgeon's ability

47. List the complications of MTP joint arthroplasty.
1. Infection
2. Breakage of the implant
3. Implant particulation and medullary lysis
4. Cortical osteophyte proliferation
5. Synovitis
6. Possible lymphadenopathy
7. Recurrence of hallux valgus
8. Stress fractures of lateral metatarsals due to transfer
9. Hallux extensus deformity (cock-up toe)

48. What can be done for failed MTP joint arthroplasty?
- Removal of the device (resection arthroplasty)
- Replacement of the device if broken
- Arthrodesis of the MTP joint with or without interpositional bone graft

CONTROVERSIES

49. Is total ankle arthroplasty ever appropriate?
A recent report of the Mayo Clinic's experience with cemented polyethylene total ankle arthroplasty showed disappointing results, with loosening and subsidence of the talar component as a mode of failure. Many patients required implant removal and arthrodesis of the ankle. Additionally, difficulties with arthrodesis due to bone loss are encountered during revision surgery. Results such as these have led many to abandon this procedure. A biologically fixed, minimally constrained ankle prosthesis incorporating the creation of a synostosis between the distal tibia and fibula has recently been developed and reviewed with favorable results. Only time will tell if this will tilt the scales back in favor of total ankle arthroplasty or broaden its indications.

50. Is metatarsophalangeal joint arthroplasty safe?
The effects that implantable silicone devices have on the body have been seen, and the media has made many Americans and lawyers aware of complications associated with their use. Cases of silicone synovitis and lymphadenopathy have been reported using such devices in the foot. Until independent clinical studies (studies not associated with the manufacturer) supporting silicone devices are done, caution should be exercised in using them. Many authors do not recommend using silicone implants.

BIBLIOGRAPHY

1. Campbell DC, Papagelopoulos PJ: Reconstruction of the great toe: Implant and nonimplant options. In Morrey BF (ed): Reconstructive Surgery of the Joints. New York, Churchill Livingstone, 1996, pp 1811–1830.
2. Claridge RJ, Hart MB, Jones RA, Johnson KA: Replacement arthroplasties of the ankle and foot. In Jahss MH (ed): Disorders of the Foot and Ankle, 2nd ed. Philadelphia, W.B. Saunders, 1991, pp 2647–2687.
3. Clayton ML, Winter WG (eds): The Rheumatoid Foot. Clin Orthop 340:7–94, 1997.
4. Hansen ST: The ankle and foot. In Kelley WN, Ruddy S, Harris ED, Sledge CB (eds): Textbook of Rheumatology, 5th ed. Philadelphia, W.B. Saunders, 1997, pp 1759–1772.

5. Kitaoka H, Newman SR: Arthritis and deformities of the hindfoot and ankle. In Lutter LD, Mizel MS, Pfeffer GB (eds): Orthopaedic Knowledge Update: Foot and Ankle. Rosemont, IL, American Academy of Orthopaedic Surgeons, 1994, pp 283–294.
6. Kitaoka H, Johnson KA: Ankle replacement arthroplasty. In Morrey BF (ed): Reconstructive Surgery of the Joints. New York, Churchill Livingstone, 1996, pp 1757–1769.
7. Lachiewicz PF: Rehumatoid arthritis of the ankle: The role of total ankle arthroplasty. Semin Arthroplasty 6(3):187–192, 1995.
8. Mizel MS, Sobel M: Disorders of the Foot and Ankle. In Miller MD (ed): Review of Orthopaedics, 2nd ed. Philadelphia, W.B. Saunders, 1996, pp 223–243.
9. Saltzman CL, Johnson KA: The ankle and foot. In Kelley WN, Harris ED Jr, Ruddy S, Sledge CB (eds): Textbook of Rheumatology, 4th ed. Philadelphia, W.B. Saunders, 1993, pp 1855–1872.
10. Solomon G: Inflammatory arthritis. In Jahss MH (ed): Disorders of the Foot and Ankle: Medical and Surgical Management, 2nd ed. Philadelphia, W.B. Saunders, 1991, pp 1681–1702.
11. Strauss E, Missirian J (eds): Arthritis, foot and ankle. Clin Orthop Research 349:9–138, 1998.
12. Thompson FM, Mann RA: Arthritides. In Mann RA, Coughlin MJ (eds): Surgery of the Foot and Ankle, 6th ed. St. Louis, Mosby, 1993, pp 615–713.
13. Toolan BC, Hansen ST: Surgery of the rheumatoid foot and ankle. Curr Opin Rheumatol 10:116–119, 1998.
14. Wapner K, Hecht PF: Arthritis in the midfoot and forefoot. In Lutter LD, Mizel MS, Pfeffer GB (eds): Orthopaedic Knowledge Update: Foot and Ankle. Rosemont, IL, American Academy of Orthopaedic Surgeons, 1994, pp 295–305.

93. LESIONS OF NERVES IN THE FOOT

John A. Schneider, M.D.

1. Name the five major nerves entering the foot at the level of the ankle.

Medially, the **posterior tibial nerve** divides into the medial and lateral plantar nerve branches. Anteromedially, the **saphenous nerve** parallels the saphenous vein. The **deep peroneal nerve** courses with the anterior tibial artery deep to and between the extensor hallucis longus and the extensor digitorum longus tendons. Anterolaterally, the **superficial peroneal nerve** branches into the medial and intermediate cutaneous nerves. The **sural nerve** runs to the Achilles tendon with the short saphenous vein.

2. List the common causes of foot pain.

Interdigital neuroma	Peripheral vascular disease
Lumbar spine disorders	Diabetic neuropathy
Plantar fasciitis	Tenosynovitis
Plantar fibromatosis	Tarsal coalition
Peripheral neuritis	Reflex sympathetic dystrophy
Tarsal tunnel syndrome	

3. What is Morton's neuroma (interdigital neuritis)?

Morton's neuroma is a perineural thickening of the common digital nerve of the second or third interspace of the foot. It is most commonly seen in women (female-to-male ratio 4:1). The etiology is uncertain; possibilities include anatomic factors, direct trauma, and extrinsic pressure.

4. Describe the symptoms of Morton's neuroma.

Morton's neuroma usually presents as pain on the plantar aspect of the foot between the metatarsal heads, which is often associated with burning or tingling of the involved toes. Pain increases with activity and with the wearing of shoes with a narrow toe box. Typically the pain is resolved with removal of the shoe and massage of the foot.

5. What diagnostic and/or radiographic tests are helpful in diagnosing Morton's neuroma?

The diagnosis of a Morton's neuroma is based on history and physical examination. In one-third of patients the nerve and its neuroma can be palpated. It is important to differentiate metatarsal phalangeal joint tenderness from interdigital tenderness. Typically, pain is elicited with palpation of the neuroma in the interdigital space or by compression of the metatarsal heads. Rarely, radiographic studies are required for the diagnosis.

6. What is the nonsurgical management of Morton's neuroma?

Nonsurgical treatment should always be tried first because approximately 20% of patients will have complete resolution of symptoms. The goals should be to alleviate pressure on the nerve by decreasing tension on the intermetatarsal ligament and to reduce compression of the forefoot, which may be accomplished through the use of shoes with a wide toe box, firm sole, and a more rigid arch support. Metatarsal pads also may help to relieve pressure on the nerve. Antiinflammatory medication rarely offers any benefit. Local corticosteroid injection may be helpful in relieving symptoms, but repeated injections are contraindicated.

7. Do all patients improve after excision of a Morton's neuroma?

No. In a recent large review, 20% of patients considered the operation to be either a failure or only marginally beneficial. Therefore, it is important to inform the patient that surgical excision does not always provide relief.

8. What is the tarsal tunnel? What structures lie within it?

The tarsal tunnel is a fibro-osseous tunnel formed by the flexor retinaculum or laciniate ligament, the medial wall of the calcaneus and talus, and the medial malleolus. The tunnel contains the **t**ibialis posterior tendon, flexor **d**igitorum longus tendon, posterior tibial **a**rtery and **v**ein, tibial **n**erve and flexor **h**allucis longus tendon, respectively from anterior to posterior. The mnemonic **T**om, **D**ick **A**nd **V**ery **N**ervous **H**arry may be helpful in remembering the order of the structures.

- **T** = tibialis posterior
- **D** = flexor digitorum longus
- **A** = posterior tibial artery
- **V** = posterior tibial vein
- **N** = tibial nerve
- **H** = flexor hallucis longus

9. Define tarsal tunnel syndrome.

Tarsal tunnel syndrome is analogous to carpal tunnel syndrome and involves compression of the posterior tibial nerve or its branches (the calcaneal branch, lateral plantar nerve, and medial plantar nerve). It was first described in 1962 by Keck. The cause of the syndrome can be identified in only 50% of cases. Etiologies include fracture callus, ganglion of the tendon sheath, lipoma, exostosis, engorged venous plexus, and excessive pronation of the hind foot.

10. What are the most common symptoms of tarsal tunnel syndrome?

Patients with tarsal tunnel syndrome complain of plantar numbness, diffuse plantar burning, and tingling pain that increases with activity and decreases with rest. Occasionally, the pain radiates along a branch of the posterior tibial nerve or proximally along the posterior tibial nerve.

11. How is tarsal tunnel syndrome diagnosed?

Three criteria have been proposed by Mann:

1. Characteristic pain (see question 8).
2. Positive Tinel's sign over the tarsal tunnel.
3. Positive electromyelogram (EMG) documenting entrapment of the posterior tibial nerve or one of its branches.

12. How is tarsal tunnel syndrome treated?

Conservative treatment consisting of nonsteroidal antiinflammatory medications (NSAIDs) and local corticosteroid injection may provide relief of symptoms. Orthotics may help to reduce tension on the nerves by limiting pronation in the patient with a hindfoot deformity. When conservative modalities fail, surgical treatment consisting of tarsal tunnel release is indicated.

13. What is reflex sympathetic dystrophy?

Reflex sympathetic dystrophy (RSD) presents with symptoms of burning pain, swelling, and vasomotor dysfunction. The cause is poorly understood, although RSD is thought to represent an abnormal autonomic response to trauma. The severity of the syndrome ranges from minor causalgia after injury to a major mixed nerve. Major causalgia results in marked vasomotor changes indicated by cool, moist skin; edema of the foot and ankle; and severe dystrophic changes, including demineralization of the bones of the foot.

14. How is RSD treated?

The mainstay of treatment for RSD involves early clinical recognition and vigorous physical therapy. If the condition is severe, lumbar sympathetic blocks are both diagnostic and therapeutic. If sympathetic blocks have been successful and symptoms continue to recur, sympathectomy may be considered.

15. What is the most common cause of peripheral nerve injury about the foot?

The most common cause of peripheral nerve injury about the foot is surgical incision. The sural nerve and superficial peroneal nerves over the dorsum of the foot are most frequently affected.

16. What other nerve entrapment syndromes have been described?

Several other less common nerve entrapment syndromes have been described. **Sural nerve entrapment** presents as pain and/or numbness over the lateral aspect of the foot. Pain and numbness over the anterolateral lower leg extending across the ankle joint to the dorsum of the foot is seen in **superficial peroneal nerve entrapment**. The area of pathology typically exists where the **superficial peroneal nerve** exits through a short, fibrous tunnel through the deep fascia of the lateral compartment. In **anterior tarsal tunnel syndrome**, the deep peroneal nerve may be entrapped by the inferior or superior extensor retinaculum or the extensor digitorum brevis. Trauma is the most common precipitating factor. Symptoms include neuritic pain over the dorsum of the foot.

BIBLIOGRAPHY

1. Baxter DE: Functional Nerve Disorder in the Athlete's Foot, Ankle and Leg. Rosemont, IL, American Academy of Orthopaedic Surgeons. Instructional Course Lectures 42:185–194, 1993.
2. Baskin JL: Nerve entrapment syndromes of the foot and ankle. J Am Acad Orthop Surg 5:261–269, 1997.
3. Mann RA: Diseases of the nerves of the foot. In Mann RA, Coughlin MJ (eds): Surgery of the Foot and Ankle, 6th ed., St. Louis, Mosby, 1993.
4. Mann RA, Reynolds JD: Interdigital neuroma: A critical clinical analysis. Foot Ankle 3:238, 1983.
5. Weinfeld SB, Myerson MS: Interdigital neuritis: Diagnosis and treatment. J Am Acad Orthop Surg 4:328–335, 1996.

94. TENDINITIS AND FASCIITIS OF THE FOOT AND ANKLE

Brian E. Brigman, M.D.

1. Which tendons cross the ankle joint? What do they do?
Achilles tendon (gastrocnemius and soleus) and plantaris tendon: ankle plantar flexors.
Flexor hallucis longus (FHL): flexes the great toe and plantarflexes the foot.
Flexor digitorum longus (FDL): flexes the lesser toes and plantarflexes the foot.
Tibialis anterior: dorsiflexes the ankle and inverts the foot.
Extensor hallucis longus (EHL): extends the great toe and dorsiflexes the ankle.
Extensor digitorum longus (EDL): extends the lesser toes and dorsiflexes the ankle.
Tibialis posterior: plantarflexes and inverts the foot.
Peroneus brevis, peroneus longus, and peroneus tertius: evert and plantarflex the foot.

2. How is the vascular supply of the above tendons different from that in the the hand? How does this affect them?
The large, extrinsic tendons of the foot have a segmental blood supply. Vessels at the musculotendinous junction and insertion supply each end of the tendon. In areas of low friction, mesotendinous vessels supply the tendon. These tendons rely relatively more on perfusion than diffusion, which may account for increased intratendinous degeneration seen in the foot compared to the hand.

3. What is posterior tibial tendon dysfunction (PTTD)?
PTTD is a spectrum of degenerative change of the posterior tibial tendon that often occurs at the site of relative hypovascularity just distal to the medial malleolus. Obesity, diabetes, hypertension, seronegative spondyloarthropathies, steroid exposure, and previous trauma may be predisposing factors.

4. List the stages of PTTD.
Stage I: Medial ankle pain and swelling with mild posterior tibial tendon weakness
Stage II: Posterior tibial tendon disruption with a flexible flatfoot deformity
Stage III: Posterior tibial tendon disruption with a rigid flatfoot deformity

5. What is the "too many toes" sign?
In advanced cases of PTTD, the flatfooted patient will stand with hindfoot valgus and forefoot abduction. When viewed from behind, the foot appears to have too many toes.

Too many toes sign.

6. What else is notable on physical exam of a patient with PTTD?

Weakness of inversion may be noted. The patient may have difficulty with single heel raise (heel remains in valgus; arch is unchanged).

7. What is the treatment for PTTD?

Stage I: Antiinflammatory medications and a trial of immobilization
Stage II: Controversial—orthotics vs. surgical reconstruction (synovectomy, tendon transfer)
Stage III: Hindfoot arthrodesis, if symptoms warrant

8. Where does the peroneus longus tendon insert?

The peroneus longus turns anteriorly around the tip of the lateral malleolus (where it is superficial to the peroneus brevis), under the trochlear process of the calcaneus, and medially about the lateral aspect of the cuboid to reach the base of the first metatarsal, where it inserts.

9. What are the symptoms of peroneal subluxation?

A snapping sensation combined with pain and swelling behind the lateral malleolus.

10. How can peroneal subluxation be reproduced on physical exam?

It may be reproduced by resisting dorsiflexion in a plantarflexed, everted foot.

11. Describe the treatment options for subluxing peroneal tendons.

In the acute setting, immobilization for 3–6 weeks is usually sufficient. Surgical correction of chronic subluxing peroneal tendons may be recommended. Procedures include repair, reattachment or reconstruction of the peroneal retinaculum, rerouting the peroneal tendons, or deepening the peroneal groove.

12. Which peroneal tendon is prone to develop longitudinal tears?

Peroneus brevis.

13. How do peroneal tears present?

Pain and swelling behind the lateral malleolus may be present, typically after an inversion injury to the ankle.

14. What is the treatment for a peroneus brevis tear?

Nonsurgical treatment, including NSAIDs, stretching, a lateral heel wedge, or short-term cast immobilization usually will suffice. If necessary, surgical debridement of the tendon or tenodesis to the peroneus longus may be considered.

15. Define dancer's tendinitis.

Stenosing tenosynovitis, or tendinitis, of the flexor hallucis longus (FHL) may be a result of direct blunt trauma or previous laceration or repetitive impact or excessive plantarflexion, as in the ballet dancer's *en pointe* position.

16. Where does stenosing tenosynovitis of the FHL usually occur?

It usually occurs in one of three sites: within the sheath behind the medial malleolus, at the start of the fibroosseous tunnel between the medial and lateral talar tubercles, or between the hallux sesamoids.

17. Describe the symptoms of FHL tendinitis.

The symptoms are pain, swelling, and crepitance posterior to the medial malleolus, exacerbated with active or passive motion of the hallux interphalangeal joint.

18. What is the treatment for FHL tendinitis?

Conservative treatment, including NSAIDs, stretching exercises, training modifications or short-term immobilization, usually is sufficient.

19. Where and when does plantar fasciitis usually hurt?

Most patients describe pain and tenderness near the medial aspect of the calcaneal tuberosity at the insertion site of the plantar aponeurosis. The pain is typically most severe with the first few steps in the morning, then subsides, only to return after prolonged activity.

20. What nerve entrapment syndromes may mimic plantar fasciitis?

Tarsal tunnel syndrome (entrapment of the tibial nerve beneath the flexor retinaculum) or entrapment of branches of the tibial nerve (the lateral plantar nerve specifically) can cause heel pain similar to plantar fasciitis.

21. What is the significance of an associated heel spur?

Up to 50% of patients with plantar fasciitis have an associated spur. The spur actually lies in the origin of the flexor digitorum brevis on the tuberosity. The pain is usually not directly associated with the spur and spur removal usually is not necessary.

22. What is the treatment for plantar fasciitis?

Nonoperative management, including orthotics, NSAIDs, and stretching, will improve symptoms in the vast majority of patients. Local steroid injections also may be considered. Recalcitrant cases may benefit from plantar fascia release.

23. What is lederhosen syndrome?

Plantar fibromatosis is a proliferative fibroplasia of the plantar aponeurosis similar to Dupuytren's contracture. Patients present with nodularity of the aponeurosis, frequently in the medial, non–weight-bearing region.

24. What is the treatment for plantar fibromatosis?

Nonoperative treatment, including modification of footwear, is the first line of treatment. For large, painful lesions, surgical resection of the lesion should include wide margins. Recurrence rates are high.

BIBLIOGRAPHY

1. Almekinders LC: Tendinitis and other chronic tendinopathies. J Am Acad Orthop Surg 6:157–164, 1998.
2. Canale ST (ed): Campbell's Operative Orthopaedics, 9th ed. St. Louis, Mosby, 1998.
3. Netter FH: Atlas of Human Anatomy. Summit, NJ, Ciba-Geigy, 1989.
4. Saltzman C, Bonar S: Tendon problems of the foot and ankle. In Lutter LD, Mizel MS, Pfeffer GB (eds): Orthopaedic Knowledge Update: Foot and Ankle. Rosemont, IL, American Academy of Orthopaedic Surgeons, 1994, pp 269–283.

95. THE CHILD'S FOOT

Paul W. Esposito, M.D., FAAP

1. How is a congenital vertical talus (CVT) identified clinically at birth?

CVT is a rigid deformity that is more accurately defined as a convex pes valgus. It also has been described as a Persian slipper foot. CVT is characterized by a rigid equinus contracture of the hindfoot with an everted or valgus heel, marked dorsiflexion, and abduction of the mid and forefoot, creating a "rockerbottom" foot. This deformity is almost always associated with other congenital neuromuscular abnormalities, such as myelomeningocele, arthrogryposis multiplex congenita, or other syndromes.

2. How is CVT differentiated from a postural or positional deformity such as calcaneovalgus?

The calcaneovalgus foot has an extremely supple heel in a calcaneus posture (i.e., the exact opposite of an equinus contracture). Although the forefoot may be dorsiflexed to the point that it abuts the anterior tibial crest, it easily stretches downward into forefoot equinus. The lack of rigidity clearly differentiates calcaneovalgus from CVT.

3. Is it possible to document radiographically that a deformity is a CVT as opposed to a more benign deformity?

Lateral radiographs obtained in a neutral weight-bearing and plantarflexed position are the key in CVT. These x-rays usually demonstrate the inability of the talus to rotate upward into a more horizontal position with plantarflexion (one of the primary problems in CVT is that the navicular joint is in a flexed, dislocated position on the neck of the talus). Thus, in the neutral weight-bearing position, the talus is vertical and the calcaneus is in equinus, producing an increased talocalcaneal angle. In flexible or oblique talus foot, plantarflexion returns the talocalcaneal angle to normal (approximately 35°). Other findings include concavity on the dorsal aspect of the neck of the talus in the older toddler and subluxation or dislocation of the calcaneocuboid joint.

4. Besides the rigid equinus and dislocation of the talonavicular joint, what other pathologic findings are present in CVT?

The extensor tendons and the tibialis anterior are contracted to varying degrees. Anterior subluxation of the peroneals and posterior tibialis may be present, which in effect makes them dorsiflexors of the foot. Contractures of the dorsal talonavicular, calcaneocuboid, posterior capsule, and calcaneofibular ligaments also may be present.

5. What is the initial treatment of CVT?

The initial treatment is casting to bring the forefoot out of dorsiflexion. Almost all patients eventually require an extensive operative release if their associated health problems allow.

These operative procedures may be done as one global procedure or in two different surgical stages.

CLUBFOOT

6. What is the inheritance pattern for idiopathic clubfoot?

A paper by Dietz strongly implicates a single major gene defect rather than a multifactorial inheritance pattern. Many patients, however, have no family history of clubfoot.

7. What is the incidence of idiopathic clubfoot?

Approximately 1 in 1,000, with a male-to-female ratio of approximately 2:1.

8. What other conditions may be associated with clubfoot?

- Myelodysplasia
- Sacral agenesis
- Arthrogryposis multiplex congenital
- Amniotic band syndrome (congenital constriction bands)

9. Are clubfeet in patients with myelomeningocele treated differently than isolated club feet?

The rigid, teratologic clubfeet seen in association with myelomeningocoele, rarely, if ever respond to conservative treatment. The operative treatment of the severe form is more aggressive, requiring excision of all the tendons of the foot to leave the foot flail but balanced. Residual, unopposed muscle function always will lead to recurrent deformity. This type of rigid clubfoot is most commonly seen in patients with a high lumbar or thoracic meningocele.

10. What are the clinical and pathologic findings in clubfoot?

The hindfoot is in equinus and varus. The talus also is in equinus and is medially rotated, with a short, deformed head and neck. The navicular is markedly displaced medially and may be palpated as it abuts against the medial malleolus. The cuboid also may be medially displaced. The midfoot and forefoot are adducted and plantarflexed with contractures of the plantar fascia, abductor hallices, and short plantarflexors. The gastrocsoleus and posterior tibialis muscles, as well as the ligaments and joint capsules of the ankle, subtalar joint, and midfoot, are shortened.

11. What is the initial treatment of clubfoot?

Almost all surgeons agree that casting or strapping should begin as soon after birth as possible. Serial casting allows rapid resolution of postural deformities that may mimic clubfoot. A true clubfoot may worsen with time despite casting.

12. What are the principles of casting for clubfoot?

1. The forefoot cavus component is corrected by molding the forefoot.
2. The forefoot adductus and dislocation of the navicular on the talus are corrected.
3. The hindfoot varus is treated by externally rotating the anterior aspect of the calcaneus by placing a valgus mold on the heel.
4. If correction is proceeding satisfactorily, the equinus is corrected.
5. No forceful dorsiflexion is ever applied.

13. Is casting always effective?

The success rate with casting alone varies from center to center, based on the skill of the orthopedist and the severity of the clubfoot. Most surgeons use casting as long as improvement is occurring. By 3–4 months of age, it is evident that almost all true clubfeet require some surgical release, varying from percutaneous lengthening of the Achilles tendon to a complete plantalar release. Persistent manipulation in resistant feet may lead to a rockerbottom foot.

14. Is there any way to document whether casting alone is correcting the clubfoot?

A dorsiflexion lateral radiograph with a normal talocalcaneal angle indicates correction of the clubfoot. The first metatarsal should always line up with the talus and the cuboid should line up with the calcaneus on both the AP and lateral x-rays.

15. What are some of the most common persistent static deformities after a primary clubfoot release?

Persistent forefoot adduction and supination are believed to result from inadequate release of the calcaneocuboid joint and plantar fascia. Intraoperative radiographs may help in recognition and prevention of this problem. A more extensive medial release, including the navicular medial cuneiform joint, may be required.

16. What causes residual dynamic adductovarus deformity in a child with a completely corrected clubfoot on static examination?

Peroneal weakness with relative overactivity of the anterior tibialis in midswing phase may cause dynamic adductovarus. If no fixed deformity such as hindfoot varus is present, a split anterior tibial tendon transfer may remedy the problem. Transfer of the entire anterior tibialis (Garceau procedure) has been done in the past but involves the risk of an overcorrected (abducted) forefoot.

17. What deformity may result from the loss of function in the peroneus longus tendon after surgery for clubfoot?

Dorsal bunion may occur because the peroneus longus functions as a depressor of the first metatarsal head.

18. What deformity results from overzealous release of a clubfoot?

Soft tissue overcorrection may cause a severe flat foot. Occasionally, the calcaneus may dislocate laterally from the talus.

MISCELLANEOUS CONDITIONS

19. How does a metatarsus adductus differ from a clubfoot?

In metatarsus adductus, which may be familial or positional, only the forefoot is involved. The hindfoot is in a neutral or even mildly valgus posture.

20. What radiographic classification is used for metatarsus adductus?

Berg's classification is as follows:
Simple—isolated forefoot adductus
Complex—forefoot adductus and lateral translation midfoot
Skewfoot—forefoot adductus and hindfoot valgus
Complex skewfoot—adductus, hindfoot valgus, and lateral translation midfoot

21. Should children with metatarsus adductus be treated at birth?

Rarely is a metatarsus adductus rigid enough to require treatment at birth. Approximately 85% of cases resolve with manipulation and/or without treatment. Some controversy exists as to the time of treatment, but if the child has a stiff residual adductus that does not respond to stretching or if a crease in the mid arch is present, treatment with serial casting, special shoes, or orthoses may be effective at age 3–4 months. After 1–2 years of age, capsulotomies may be performed coupled with a fractional lengthening of the abductor hallucis. After the age of approximately 5 years, osteotomies may be necessary.

22. What functional problems do children with residual metatarsus adductus have?

Impingement pressure on the first metatarsal head and the base of the fifth metatarsal occurs. The impingement is caused by shoes; thus, in cultures in which shoes are not worn, it is not a functional problem.

23. What kind of shoes should be recommended for normal toddlers with flat feet (asymptomatic flexible pes planus)?

Shoes have been shown to have no effect on the development of arches. The normal developmental pattern is gradual improvement in the arch until about 5–6 years of age, regardless of shoe wear. Shoe wedges or orthotics also have been shown to be ineffective in changing torsional alignment.

24. What are the requirements of a good shoe for normal children?

Shoes should be quadrangular in shape, flexible, flat with no heel elevation, porous to prevent skin maceration, and moderately attractive. They should be lightweight, extended above the ankle in young children (to prevent the shoe from falling off), and acceptable in appearance. Expense has little to do with the quality of the shoe.

25. Are there any indications for treatment of pes planovalgus?

Yes. Pes planovalgus should be treated if pain in the arch or the shin is present. Children with painful arches should be evaluated for underlying neurologic disease, Kohler's disease, os naviculare, or tarsal coalition. Custom-molded medially posted orthotics may be helpful. It is extremely rare for any child with flexible flat foot to require surgery.

26. Is toe walking (intermittent equinus) normal in toddlers?

Intermittent toe walking is common in normal children. However, close neurologic examination, an in-depth history, and serial follow-up examinations should be done, especially if other signs of developmental delay are evident. Toe walking may be one of the first signs of subtle spastic diplegic cerebral palsy. Unilateral toe walking may be seen in mild spastic hemiplegia, spinal cord anomalies, or tumors of the central nervous system. Idiopathic toe walking is therefore a diagnosis of exclusion, and a positive family history is frequently present.

27. What is cleft foot?

This extremely rare deformity is also known as lobster claw foot, split foot, and ectrodactyly. A varying degree of absence of the middle portion of the foot is present, including metatarsals and phalanges. Cleft foot is an autosomal dominant disorder with varying penetrance. It is most commonly bilateral, often in association with lobster claw hands. If a large cleft is present in the feet, treatment involves complex plastic surgical flaps as well as bony procedures, depending on the nature of the abnormality.

28. What are the osteochondroses? Which bones in the child's foot are involved?

Kohler's disease involves the navicular joint and presents as arch pain in a relatively young child. It is diagnosed by radiographs that show sclerosis or fragmentation of the navicular joint. Generally it is self-limited without long-term deformity or symptoms, but may necessitate a period of casting and/or orthotics. Frieberg's disease involves the second metatarsal head and causes pain in the forefoot. It usually presents in late adolescence.

29. What is the most common cause of heel pain in the preadolescent or early adolescent?

In the past, such heel pain was known as Sever's disease (i.e., osteochondrosis of the calcaneal apophysis). However, x-rays of the asymptomatic side frequently show more fragmentation and involvement than on the radiographs of the affected side. The heel pain is now believed to be secondary to inflexibility of the Achilles tendon and plantar fascia in a rapidly growing child. It responds to stretching, heel pads, and occasional casting. Other causes of heel pain may include stress fractures, bone cysts, tumors, and osteomyelitis of the calcaneus.

30. What is the likely pathology in an adolescent child with a symptomatic flat foot and a painful bump on the medial arch?

An os naviculare (accessory navicular) may cause a progressive and painful flat foot. The insertion of the posterior tibialis is superior to its normal insertion and thus does not elevate the arch adequately. This may be treated with a simple excision of the ossicle if the child does not respond to orthotic and or cast treatment.

31. What is a common cause of a stiff, painful flat foot in an adolescent?

A common cause is tarsal coalition, which frequently presents as recurrent sprains and pain in the medial subtalar joint or sinus tarsi. The most common sites of a coalition (fibrous or bony bridge) are in the middle facet of the talocalcaneal joint and the calcaneonavicular joint. Physical examination reveals varying degrees of stiffness. Oblique radiographs demonstrate the calcaneonavicular bridge, but commuted tomography (CT) is the best method to diagnose a talocalcaneal coalition. The Harris axial view of the subtalar joint may demonstrate medial talocalcaneal coalition if the medial facet is obliquely oriented and irregular or fused, but it is not as reproducible and reliable as CT. Coalitions can be excised if conservative treatment fails with results dependent on the size of the coalition and the extent of secondary changes in the involved joints.

BIBLIOGRAPHY

1. Ankle and Foot: Pediatric aspects. Orthopaedic Knowledge Update 2. Rosemont, IL, American College of Orthopaedic Surgeons, 1990, pp 603–612.
2. Asirvatham R, Stevens PPM: Idiopathic forefoot-adduction deformity: Medial capsulotomy and abductor hallucis lengthening for resistant and severe deformities. J Pediatr Orthop 17:496–500, 1997.
3. Berg EE: A reappraisal of metatarsus adductus and skewfoot. J Bone Joint Surg 68:1185–1196, 1986.

4. Berman A, Gartland JJ: Metatarsal osteotomy for the correction of adduction of the fore part of the foot in children. J Bone Joint Surg 53A:498–506, 1971.

5. Comfort TK, Johnson LO: Resection for symptomatic talocalcaneal coalition. J Pediatr Orthop 18:283–288, 1998.

6. Cummings RJ, Lovell WW: Current concepts review: Operative treatment of congenital idiopathic club foot. J Bone Joint Surg 79A:2208–1112, 1988.

7. Heyman CH, Herndon CH, Strong JM: Mobilization of the tarsometatarsal and intermetatarsal joints for the correction of resistant adduction of the fore part of the foot in congenital club foot or congenital metatarsus varus. J Bone Joint Surg 40A:200–302, 1958.

8. Jacobsen ST, Crawford AH: Congenital vertical talus. J Pediatr Orthop 3:306–310, 1983.

9. Johnston CE II, Roach JW: Dorsal bunion following clubfoot surgery. Pediatr Orthop 8:1036–1040, 1985.

10. Kodros SA, Dias LS: Single stage surgical correction of congenital vertical talus. J Pediatr Orthop 19:42–48, 1999.

11. Kumar SJ, Cowell HR, Ramsey PL: Foot problems in children. American Academy Orthopaedic Surgeons: Instructional Course Lectures, pp 235–251, 1982.

12. Neto J, Dias LS, Gabrieli AP: Congenital talipes equinovarus in spina bifida: Treatment and results. J Pediatr Orthop 16:782–785,1996.

13. Olney BW, Asher MA: Excision of symptomatic coalition of the middle facet of talocalcaneal joint. J Bone Joint Surg 69A:539–544, 1987.

14. Ponseti, IV, Becker JR: Congenital metatarsus adductus: The results of treatment. J Bone Joint Surg 78A:448–453, 1992.

15. Ponseti IV, Becker JR: Congenital metatarsus adductus: The results of treatment. J Bone Joint Surg 48A:702–711, 1966.

16. Rebbeck TR, Dietz FR: The genetics of idiopathic clubfoot. Paper No. 19, p 34. Am J Hum Genet 53:1051–1063, 1993.

17. Staheli LT: Rotational problems in children. J Bone Joint Surg 75A:939–949, 1993.

18. Staheli LT: Shoes for children: A review. Pediatrics 88:371–375, 1991.

19. Stark JG, Johanson JE, Winter RB: The Heyman-Herndon tarsometatarsal capsulotomy metatarsus adductus: Results in 48 feet. J Pediatr Orthop 7:305–310, 1987.

20. Tarraf YN, Carroll NC: Analysis of the components of residual deformity in clubfeet presenting for reoperation. J Pediatr Orthop 12:207–216, 1992.

21. Wood VE, Peppers TA, Shook J: Cleft-foot closure: A simplified technique and review of the literature. J Pediatr Orthop 17:501–504, 1997.

INDEX

Page numbers in **boldface type** indicate complete chapters.